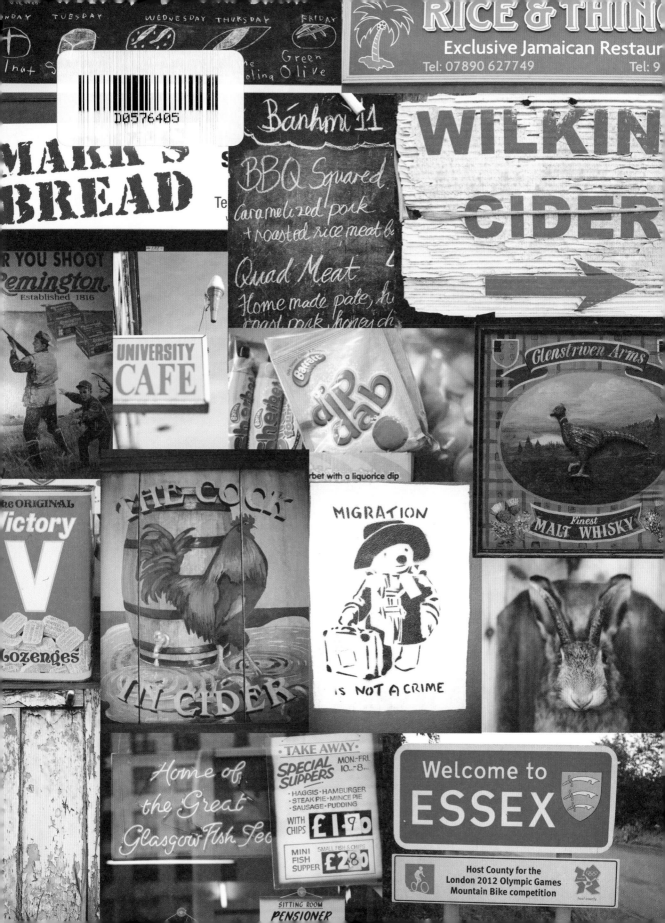

JAMIE'S GREAT BRITAIN

MICHAEL JOSEPH
AN IMPRINT OF
PENGUIN BOOKS

Also by Jamie Oliver

Photography by *'Lord' David Loftus*
Design by *Interstate Associates*

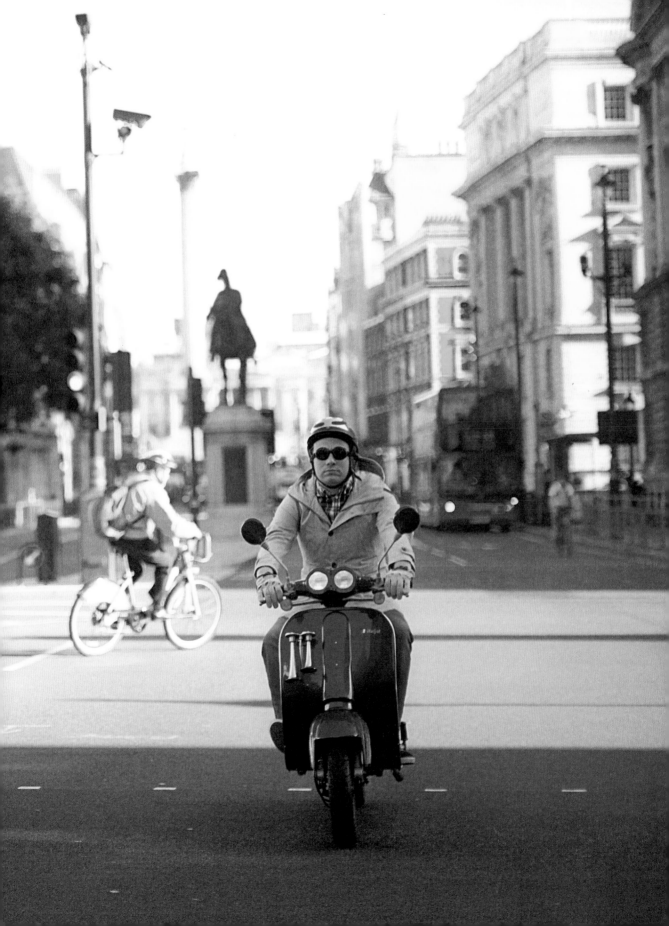

Michael Joseph

Published by the Penguin Group

Penguin Books Ltd
80 Strand
London WC2R ORL, England

Penguin Group (USA) Inc.
375 Hudson Street
New York, New York 10014, USA

Penguin Group (Canada)
90 Eglinton Avenue East, Suite 700
Toronto, Ontario, Canada M4P 2Y3
(a division of Pearson Penguin Canada Inc.)

Penguin Ireland
25 St Stephen's Green
Dublin 2, Ireland
(a division of Penguin Books Ltd)

Penguin Group (Australia)
250 Camberwell Road
Camberwell, Victoria 3124, Australia
(a division of Pearson Australia Group Pty Ltd)

Penguin Books India Pvt Ltd
11 Community Centre,
Panchsheel Park, New Delhi - 110 017, India

Penguin Group (NZ)
67 Apollo Drive
Rosedale, Auckland 0632, New Zealand
(a division of Pearson New Zealand Ltd)

Penguin Books (South Africa) (Pty) Ltd
24 Sturdee Avenue
Rosebank, Johannesburg 2196, South Africa

Penguin Books Ltd, Registered Offices:
80 Strand, London WC2R ORL, England

www.penguin.com
www.jamieoliver.com

First published 2011
3

Copyright © Jamie Oliver, 2011
Photography copyright © David Loftus, 2011
Illustrations copyright © Sroop Sunar, 2011

The moral right of the author has been asserted

Printed in Germany by Mohn media
Colour reproduction by Altaimage Ltd

A CIP catalogue record for this book
is available from the British Library

ISBN: 978-0-718-15681-7

Dedicated to Rose Gray, my old boss

Rose was undoubtedly one of the most influential foodies, chefs and restaurateurs of the past century. Her food, philosophies, natural flair, style, simplicity and unforgiving single-mindedness in pursuit of perfection have defined many of the great things that happen in food today. And although the strings to her bow were many, her greatest achievement was inspiring the hordes of future chefs lucky enough to learn from her and Ruth Rogers at the River Café to go on to incredible things and make their own mark on the country and the world.

I'm merely one of the many chefs blessed to pass through that kitchen in the twenty-plus years she ran it. And I, like all the others, will carry on cooking with a little bit of Rose Gray ranting, in the back my head, that I should try harder, always expect more, and do anything to source and use the best ingredients.

Love, respect and fond memories as always, Rose.
28 January 1939 – 28 February 2010

PS Love to all the family: *David, Hester, Lucy, Ossie, Dante and the rest of Rose's beautiful army xxxx*

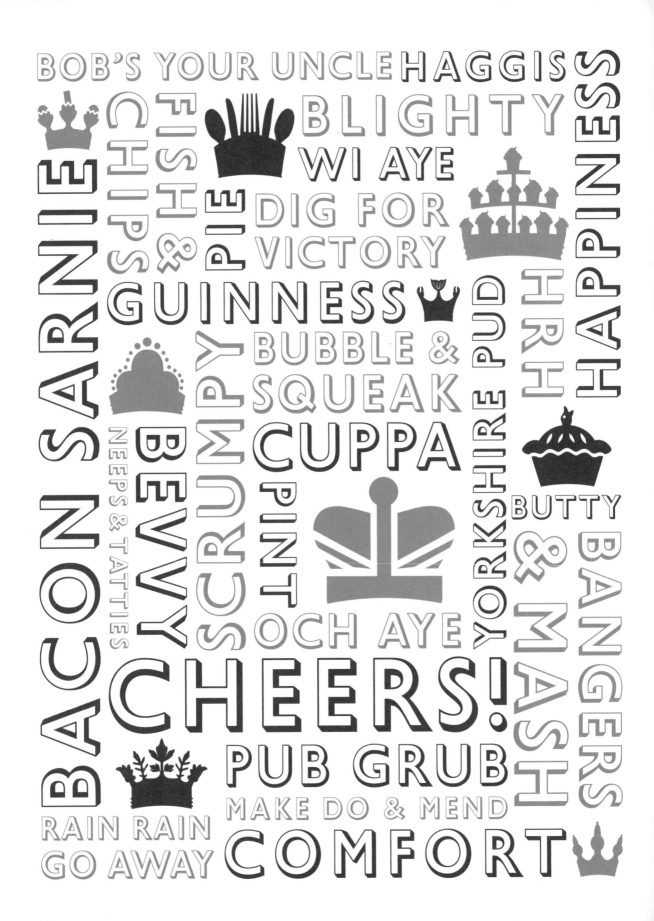

When Britain hosts the Olympic Games in 2012 for the first time since 1948, the world will be looking at what we do and how we do it. Thankfully, it's coming at a really great moment...

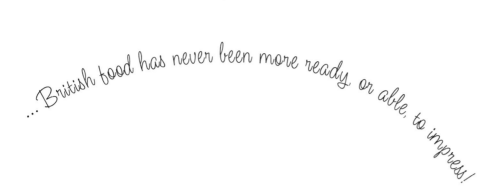

...British food has never been more ready, or able, to impress!

JAMIE'S

AS A TEENAGER GRADUATING FROM WESTMINSTER CATERING COLLEGE, I WAS ENTERING THE WORKFORCE AT THE SAME TIME AS BRITAIN WAS COMING OUT OF SOME PRETTY BLEAK YEARS FOR FOOD. ALTHOUGH HISTORICALLY BRITAIN HAD BEEN FAMOUS FOR SOME SPECTACULARLY RICH FOOD TRADITIONS, A MIGHTY INDUSTRIAL REVOLUTION, TWO WORLD WARS ACCOMPANIED BY YEARS OF FOOD RATIONING AND THE RISE OF PROCESSED FOODS, AMONG OTHER THINGS, SOON PUT AN END TO OUR IMPRESSIVE FOOD CULTURE. WHERE BRITAIN'S FOOD HAD ONCE BEEN RESPECTED AND ADMIRED BY FOREIGN VISITORS, IT WAS INSTEAD KNOWN FOR BEING FAIRLY CONFUSED AND UNINSPIRING. YES, WE STILL HAD

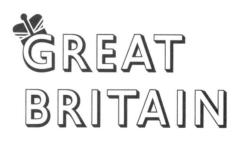

GREAT BRITAIN

INCREDIBLE RESTAURANTS, BUT LARGELY THEY WERE FOR THE RICH; GOOD FOOD HADN'T BEEN DEMOCRATIZED FOR THE WORKING OR MIDDLE CLASSES. BUT THINGS WERE CHANGING…

MANY CHEFS, PRODUCERS AND ARTISANS ALL AROUND BRITAIN BEGAN RETRACING OLD RECIPES, REDISCOVERING SOME OF OUR GREAT INGREDIENTS AND FOCUSING ON SIMPLICITY AND QUALITY. THEY USED THAT KNOWLEDGE TO STEER BRITAIN BACK TOWARDS THE RICH FOOD CULTURE IT HAD ONCE HAD. A BRITISH FOOD RENAISSANCE HAD DEFINITELY BEEN IGNITED, AND IT'S STILL GOING STRONG TODAY. AS I WALKED OUT OF COLLEGE THAT LAST DAY, I WAS DETERMINED TO SEE THE WORLD, EXPLORE AND LEARN AS MUCH AS I COULD. OVER THE YEARS I'VE DONE THAT, AND AS I FINISH WRITING THIS BOOK (LUCKY NUMBER THIRTEEN), **I'M NOT A TEENAGER ANY MORE, I'M A FATHER WITH FOUR KIDS AND A DIFFERENT PERSPECTIVE ON MY OWN COUNTRY, AND IT'S DEFINITELY ONE THAT I'M PROUD TO SHARE WITH YOU HERE.** IT REALLY FEELS LIKE I'VE COME FULL CIRCLE AND IT'S NICE TO FOCUS ON HOME. SO MUCH HAS BEEN ACHIEVED IN OUR FOOD INDUSTRY, AND THIS IS THE PERFECT TIME TO WRITE A BOOK ON BRITISH FOOD. IN 2012, BRITAIN WILL BE HOSTING THE OLYMPICS FOR THE FIRST TIME SINCE 1948, AND THE WORLD WILL BE LOOKING AT WHAT WE DO, AND HOW WE DO IT. THANKFULLY, IT'S COMING AT A REALLY GREAT MOMENT FOR BRITISH FOOD. I'M HAPPY TO SAY WE'VE NEVER BEEN MORE READY OR ABLE TO IMPRESS. YES, THERE'S A UNION JACK ON THE COVER, AND OF COURSE IT'S GOOD TO BE LOYAL AND PATRIOTIC ABOUT YOUR COUNTRY, BUT SOMETIMES IF YOU CLING ON TOO TIGHTLY TO ANY KIND OF PATRIOTISM, YOU

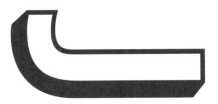

CAN MISS OUT ON THE INCREDIBLE THINGS THAT ARE HAPPENING ON THE PERIPHERY. BECAUSE OF THAT, I TEND TO GO ON INSTINCT. I'LL TASTE ANYTHING, REGARDLESS OF

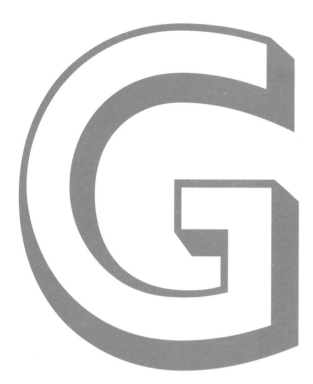

WHETHER IT'S BRITISH, SPANISH, ITALIAN, INDIAN, FRENCH OR YEMENI, AND WAIT FOR MY TONGUE TO TALK TO MY BRAIN. GREAT FOOD IS ABOUT HOW YOU FEEL, NOT WHERE YOU'RE FROM. I HAVEN'T WRITTEN THIS BOOK TO SAY 'WE'RE BETTER'; I'VE WRITTEN IT TO CELEBRATE MY FAVOURITE BRITISH RECIPES, SHARE A FEW OF OUR STORIES, AND REALLY SHOUT ABOUT THE WONDERFUL FOOD WE HAVE HERE. OUR WEATHER MAY BE UNPREDICTABLE, BUT IT GIVES US ORCHARDS OF BEAUTIFUL FRUIT, GREAT SOIL FOR VEGETABLES AND THE MOST WONDERFUL LUSH GRASS THAT FEEDS OUR ANIMALS, GIVING US AMAZING MEAT, MILK AND CHEESES IN RETURN. THERE IS SO MUCH TO CELEBRATE. AS I WROTE THIS BOOK, I FOUND I WAS CONSTANTLY DEBATING WITH MYSELF EXACTLY WHAT THE TERM 'BRITISH FOOD' MEANS. WALK DOWN ANY BRITISH HIGH STREET AND IT'S CLEAR TO SEE THAT OUR FOOD EMBRACES MUCH MORE THAN A HANDFUL OF OLD RECIPES. OUR HISTORY HAS BEEN ONE OF INVASION, EXPLORATION, COLONIZATION AND IMMIGRATION, AND THE EVIDENCE OF THAT IS EVERYWHERE: ON OUR PLATES, IN OUR SUPERMARKETS AND IN OUR CUPBOARDS. SOME OF THE THINGS WE NOW THINK OF AS QUINTESSENTIALLY BRITISH ACTUALLY ARRIVED LONG AGO WITH IMMIGRANTS CARVING OUT NEW LIVES HERE. A GREAT EXAMPLE OF THIS IS FISH AND CHIPS – FIRST INTRODUCED BY LONDON'S JEWISH IMMIGRANTS IN THE 1800s AND NOW THOUGHT OF AS A BRITISH DISH THE WORLD OVER.

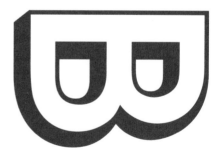

I LIKE TO THINK OF GREAT BRITAIN AS A MAGPIE NATION BECAUSE THROUGHOUT OUR HISTORY WE SEEM TO HAVE COLLECTED BEAUTIFUL FLAVOURS FROM ELSEWHERE AND WORKED THEM INTO OUR OWN CULTURE. TRULY ICONIC BRITISH CONDIMENTS LIKE PICCALILLI, WORCESTERSHIRE AND HP SAUCE ARE ALL HEAVILY INFLUENCED BY INDIAN FLAVOURS; OUR BELOVED MEAT PIE CAN BE TRACED TO INVADING ROMAN SOLDIERS (AND ANCIENT EGYPT BEFORE THAT). IN MY MIND, ONE OF THE MOST EXCITING AND UNIQUE THINGS ABOUT BEING BRITISH IS OUR ABILITY TO BE OPEN-MINDED AND WILLING TO EMBRACE ANYTHING THAT LOOKS AND TASTES GOOD FROM ANY NEW NEIGHBOUR. I SEE THIS WITH BRITISH KIDS ALL THE TIME, WHETHER THEIR ROOTS ARE WEST INDIAN, EUROPEAN, JAMAICAN OR INDIAN – THEY ALL ADMIRE AND RESPECT EACH OTHER'S FOOD AND GO JUST AS MAD FOR JERK CHICKEN OR RICE AND PEAS AS THEY WILL FOR A ROAST DINNER OR BEAUTIFUL CURRY. SO IN THIS BOOK YOU'LL FIND DISHES INSPIRED BY SOME OF OUR IMMIGRANT COMMUNITIES, OLD AND NEW, SANDWICHED BETWEEN RECIPES FROM MY CHILDHOOD, MY PARENTS' CHILDHOOD, EVEN MY NAN'S CHILDHOOD AND BEYOND.

AND TO ME, THAT'S WHAT BRITAIN TODAY IS: A TAPESTRY AND PATCHWORK QUILT THAT EMBRACES THE BEST OF THE OLD TRADITIONS AS WELL AS THE NEWER ADDITIONS TO OUR REPERTOIRE, WHICH ARE JOYFUL, COLOURFUL AND RESOURCEFUL IN THEIR OWN RIGHT.

ONE THING'S FOR SURE, EVERY TIME I WROTE A RECIPE FOR THIS BOOK, I HAD TO RESTRAIN MYSELF FROM STARTING EACH INTRO WITH THE SENTENCE 'THIS DISH WILL MAKE YOU SO HAPPY', BUT I SWEAR, IT'S TRUE. THIS IS BEAUTIFUL COMFORT FOOD AT ITS BEST – UNFUSSY AND UNPRETENTIOUS, BUT FULL OF LIFE. YOU CAN'T FORCE IT, OR PRETEND; IT JUST IS WHAT IT IS. I KNOW THAT IF YOU COOK THE RECIPES FROM HERE YOU WILL BE REWARDED WITH GOOD TIMES, BRILLIANT WEEKENDS AND BIG HAPPY SMILES ALL AROUND THE TABLE … I'M SO EXCITED ABOUT THAT.

This is beautiful comfort food at its best – unfussy and unpretentious, but full of life.

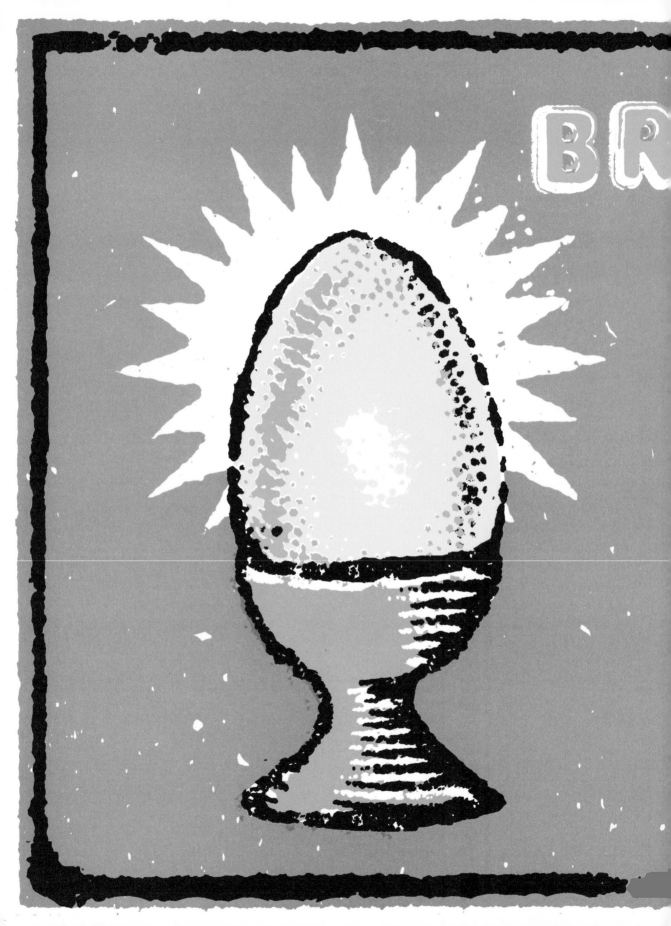

EAKFASTS

Britain is the home of the cooked breakfast, and our 'full English' of eggs, toast, crispy bacon, black pudding, sausages and baked beans (aka 'the full monty') is copied all over the world. Scotland, Wales and Northern Ireland each have their own variations on cooked breakfasts – all equally delicious. If you look back in time it's easy to see how this cooked breakfast tradition came about: people needed a big meaty meal to sustain them until midday – a pretty little pastry and a shot of espresso would never have been enough. Admittedly, over the last fifty years, dodgy cafés that don't really care about the quality of the food they're serving have given breakfast a bad name. But there are still plenty of places doing it well. So whether your style is a few crispy rashers of good bacon inside a soft white bap (or bacon butty as we like to call it), a cooked breakfast, omelette, kedgeree, or any one of the other beautiful things in this chapter, when made with love and quality ingredients these are all a great start to the day.

ONE-PAN BREAKFAST
... THE RETURN OF THE MIDNIGHT PAN-COOKED BREAKFAST

I wrote a similar recipe to this in my second book, and weirdly had more feedback on that than on any other recipe in the book! People still talk about it, and I've even noticed a few restaurants make this now. What can I say? People love a cooked breakfast. I came up with this method years and years ago because I'd often come home late after work (and a drink or two, if I'm honest) with a massive craving for a cooked midnight breakfast. But I wouldn't want to dirty too many pots and pans and get a rollicking from my mum in the morning, so I'd cook all the elements in the one pan. **Admittedly it's not the healthiest thing in the world, so you're probably best to share it with one other lucky person. If you're feeling generous you can make it for even more people – a dozen if you like! Just roast or grill loads of sausages, bacon and black pudding, combine everything in one huge tray once cooked, crack in twelve eggs and whack it back under the grill for brilliant results.** Preheat the grill on your oven to high and put a frying pan (about 26cm in diameter) on a high heat. Add a drizzle of **olive oil**. Cut a **quality pork sausage** lengthways and open it out like a book. This way it cooks nice and quick and gets crispy. Add a 2cm thick slice of **quality black pudding** to the pan with the sausage, and 2 rashers of **quality smoked streaky bacon**. Keep an eye on the pan, but try not to turn anything for 2 minutes so it all gets nicely golden. Flip everything over and do the other side. If the bacon or black pudding start looking perfect, remove them to a plate for a couple of minutes while you quarter a **field mushroom** (or a few **button mushrooms**) and get it going in the pan. You can allow the sausage to get charred or slightly overcooked; it won't hurt. Continue cooking for a few minutes, then drop 3 or 4 halved **cherry tomatoes** into the pan and poke them with a knife to get them sagging. Pour away any fat if necessary, then put the bacon and black pudding back into the pan. Make sure everything is spread out nicely, then make two gaps towards the edges of the pan and crack in 2 large **free-range eggs**. Move the pan around so the egg whites almost surround everything, like a big egg Frisbee touching all the other ingredients. Cook for 1 minute, then pop the pan into the middle of the oven under the hot grill for 2 minutes, or until the eggs are cooked to your liking. Serve in the pan with a stack of hot toast and a bottle of HP sauce.

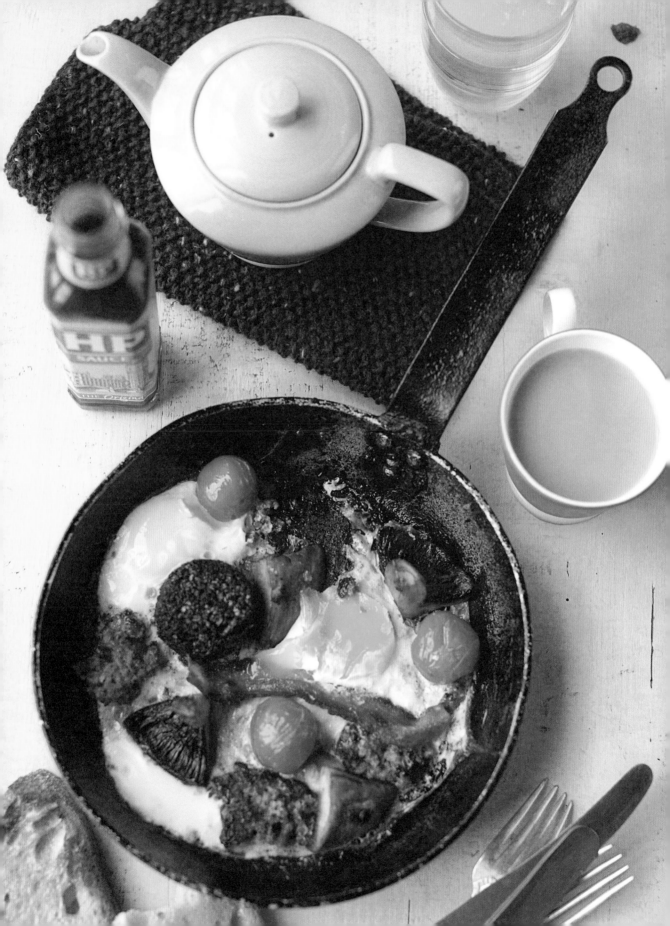

BUBBLE & SQUEAK

Bubble and squeak is a dish created out of leftovers and it's become one of our great British recipes. The first recorded recipes for it were written in the early 1800s, when any roasted shredded meat or vegetables left over from Sunday's dinner would be fried in the pan the next day to create this big and beautiful veggie patty. But it's so damn good you shouldn't have to wait for leftovers to enjoy it, so I'm giving you this recipe as a guide. As long as you use 60% potato, you can make the rest up using whatever you've got to hand - vegetables, crumbled chestnuts, herbs, crispy bacon or leftover meat.

In the cockney cafés they call this 'bubble', and serve it alongside eggs for breakfast. Because it often sits in the pan for ages getting dark and crispy, it tends to take on a fairly dark grey and rather ugly colour, but ironically, those are often the tastiest bubble and squeaks of all.

SERVES 8

- 1kg fluffy potatoes, such as Maris Piper
- 600g mixed vegetables, such as carrots, swede, turnips, parsnips, kale, Brussels sprouts … anything you like!
- olive oil
- 2 knobs of butter
- a few sprigs of fresh herbs, such as rosemary, sage, thyme or whatever you have knocking about in the fridge, leaves picked and chopped
- sea salt and white pepper

Peel and trim all the vegetables, cutting the root veg into 2.5cm dice. Bring a pan of salted water to the boil, add the vegetables and cook for around 10 minutes, or until they are all cooked through. If you're using swede or turnips, put them in about 5 minutes earlier than everything else as they take slightly longer to soften up. If using kale, just blanch this for a few minutes right at the end. Once cooked, drain all the vegetables and leave to steam dry for a few minutes.

Put a medium non-stick frying pan (roughly 26-28cm) over a medium heat and add a lug of olive oil and a couple of knobs of butter. Once nice and hot, add the fresh herbs, then the cooked vegetables. Season well with salt and pepper, then mash everything up in the pan. Pat everything into a flat layer and cook for 3 or 4 minutes, until a lovely golden crust starts forming underneath. Fold those crispy bits back into the mash, then pat and flatten down and repeat the process for about 15 or 20 minutes. Concentrate on building up flavours, character and crispiness.

Halfway through the cooking, flip it over using a fish slice, or like a pancake if you're brave. If it breaks don't worry, just push it back together. Let it crisp up on the underside then nick a bit and taste it. This is the time to correct the seasoning. Once you're happy, serve it with a smear of HP sauce and whatever else you fancy.

PS: What do you do with leftover bubble and squeak? Well, it's a rare occasion that you'll need to worry about that, but you can always push it back into the pan, grate over some cheese and pop it under the grill, or even use it as a topping for a shepherd's pie.

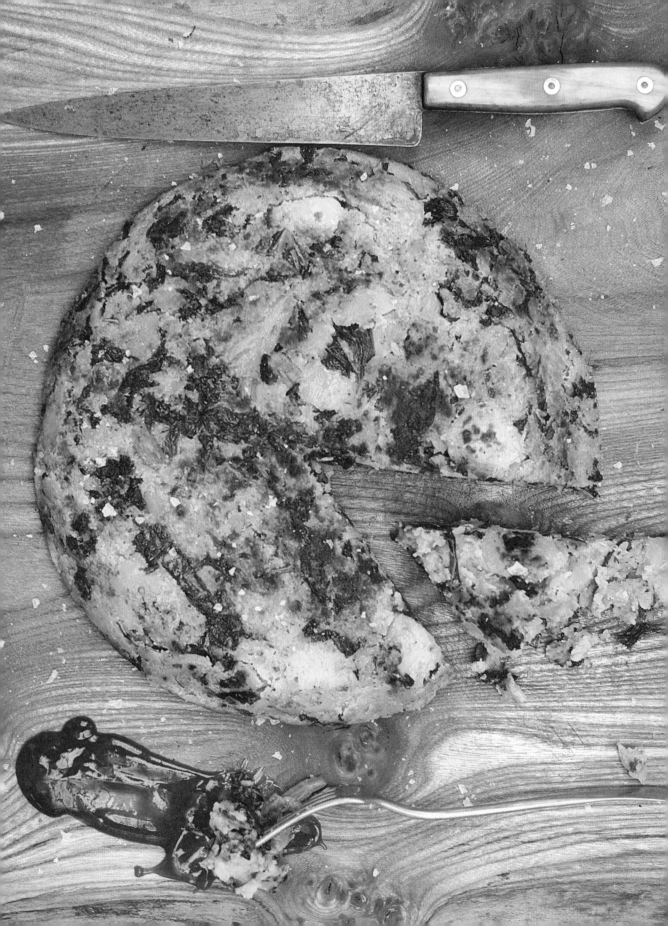

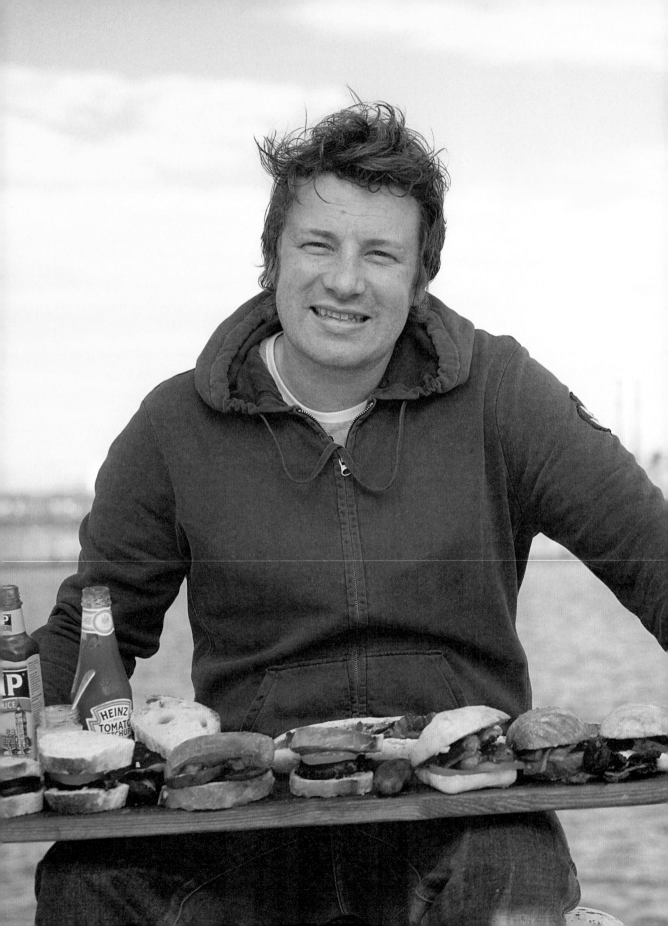

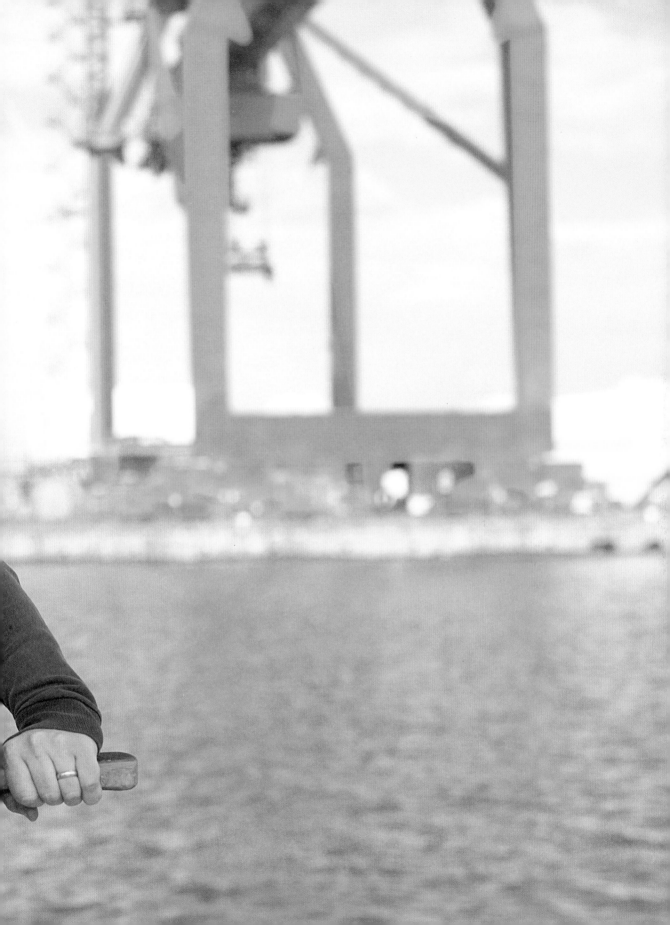

BREAKFAST BUTTY

A breakfast butty is a humble old meal, but once you're really good at making these simple little beauties and have got used to that feeling of ultimate pleasure in the morning, or, to be frank, at any time of day (even late at night after a visit to the pub), you'll become, as many do, a breakfast butty aficionado. First and foremost, why am I having this random conversation with you about something so simple? The truth is, I'd say seven out of ten of the breakfast butties you get are miserable, anaemic, fat-ridden, soggy, filthy little fellas. So, there are certain things you've got to ask for or do to make this story have a happy ending. To start with, you need sauces. I may have travelled the world, but Heinz ketchup and HP sauce remain a must. Choose one or the other, or take advantage of both and blend a little of each with a few drops of Worcestershire sauce and smear it on to the bread. Now, while we're talking about bread, remember that butter, sausages, bacon and sauces all keep pretty happily in the fridge, but if bread is a day old it can lose that beautiful muggy softness that makes grabbing the sarnies such a pleasure, as well as the ability to suck up juices. So, if you are lumbered with stale bread, when you've got your chosen filling almost to crisp, golden perfection, put two slices of bread together and pop them as one into the toaster, to give you two crisp, crunchy outsides. Peel them open to reveal a soft, spongy inside, and act fast because the moisture doesn't last long at all. Thinly butter it, jam it full of filling, smear it with sauce, then slice it up and eat it before it dries up like an old prune. There are lots of trendy breads that can be used, and I even make some, but deep down, a softer, spongier bread holds the breakfast butty closest to its heart. With butter, the general rule is to use it, but not too much. Definitely don't use marg – if you're on a health kick, I'd rather you don't use anything at all and just let the moisture of your filling make a difference. Whether you want chipolatas or Cumberlands, just keep it simple and go for a high-quality, high-meat-content (no less than 70%) sausage. Cook under the grill or roast, and take it to the limit, not black, but golden, perfect and sizzling. The same goes for bacon and black pudding. Take it to the edge, and it'll stick to the bread and give incredible flavour. If you're a sucker for a bit of crunch, you could run a knife down the sausage to increase the surface area and get it much crispier. Bacon is very simple, but back, streaky, whatever you choose, you have to use smoked and it has to be quality. I don't see any point in cheap bacon. Black pudding also makes a marvellous sandwich filler: cut it just over 1cm thick, cook it in the oven or a dry pan until crispy on the outside, and the thickness will allow it to be soft and heavenly on the inside. A simple egg butty can be a beautiful thing. Soft-boiled, peeled and squashed with a fork, poached, fried or scrambled eggs are all good as long as they're cooked to perfection. For the vegetarians out there, or for anyone who's after a slightly lighter sandwich, a drizzle of olive oil and a sprinkle of salt and pepper on a simply roasted or grilled tomato or a lovely flat or Portobello mushroom can be exceptional, especially if you kiss it with a tiny bit of butter towards the end of cooking. Back to the story – you've got your perfect bread (or a nice crusty roll that's soft on the inside, which I forgot to mention), butter (or not), fillings and sauces. And there's really nothing else to say except if it's done quickly and to perfection, it can be an absolutely wonderful mobile treat. Good luck, and spread the word! Next time you go to a café, remember all these points, ask for crispy fillings and be fussy about what they give you.

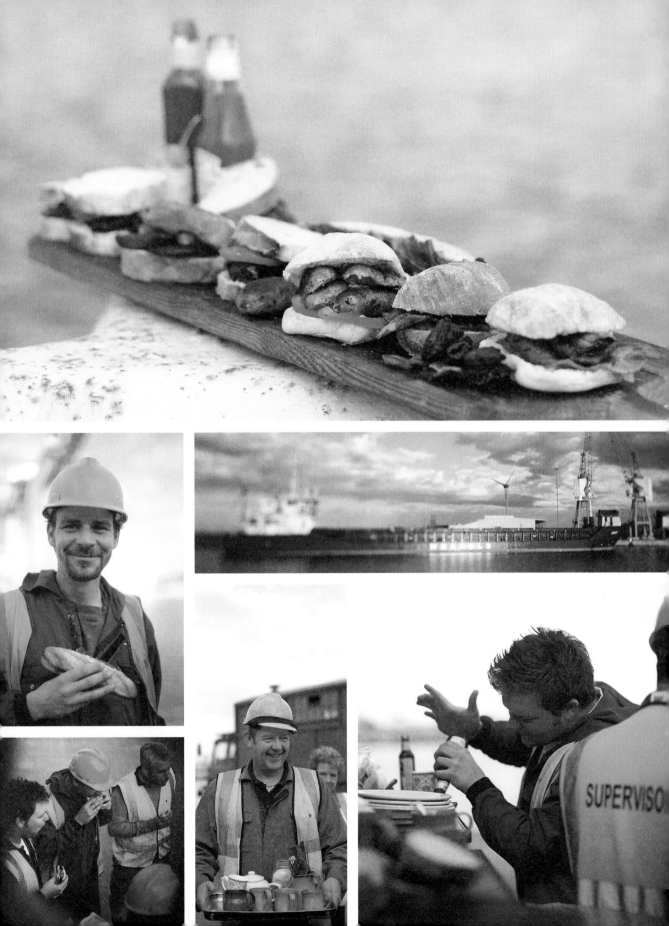

EASIEST HOMEMADE YOGHURT
... BEAUTIFUL SUMMER FRUIT COMPOTES

Why would you make your own yoghurt, you ask? Because it's great fun turning plain old milk into delicious thick live yoghurt, that's why. All you need to make this happen is a few spoonfuls of natural live yoghurt. Some brands can work better than others, so if you don't have any luck with this method change to another brand of live yoghurt and try again. It's so rewarding. I've also given you some simple recipes for lovely fruit compotes. They each go brilliantly with yoghurt, and make the flavours fresh and electric.

SERVES 4 TO 6 AS A COMPOTE WITH YOGHURT

For the yoghurt
- 1 litre semi-skimmed milk
- 4 heaped tablespoons natural live yoghurt

For the compote
- 400g of your chosen fruit
- 2-3 heaped tablespoons golden caster sugar, to taste

Pour all of the milk into a large pan (with a lid) and gently bring to a simmer over a low heat. Turn the heat off and leave the milk to cool until it's the temperature of tepid water (this will take roughly 30 minutes). At this point, whisk in the 4 heaped tablespoons of natural live yoghurt, then pop the lid on the pan and leave it on the kitchen counter overnight to let the live culture work its magic. Once it has set into yoghurt, cover it with clingfilm and put it into the fridge to be used up within the week. Now you know how it's done, you'll never need to buy yoghurt again. Just keep using a few spoonfuls of your old homemade stuff to make your next batch. Amazing!

To make the compote, simply put your chosen fruit into a pan on a medium to high heat (destone cherries or plums first, if using). Add 2 to 3 heaped teaspoons of the sugar and any other ingredients you need to flavour the compote, (see above) then put the lid on and simmer for around 5 minutes, or until the fruit is lightly cooked but still holding its shape. Remove from the heat and leave to cool, then either serve with a dollop or two of your homemade yoghurt, or decant to a bowl, cover with clingfilm and keep in the fridge until needed.

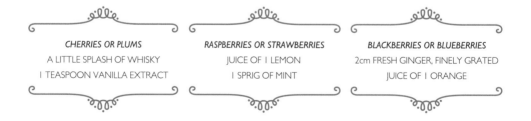

CHERRIES OR PLUMS
A LITTLE SPLASH OF WHISKY
1 TEASPOON VANILLA EXTRACT

RASPBERRIES OR STRAWBERRIES
JUICE OF 1 LEMON
1 SPRIG OF MINT

BLACKBERRIES OR BLUEBERRIES
2cm FRESH GINGER, FINELY GRATED
JUICE OF 1 ORANGE

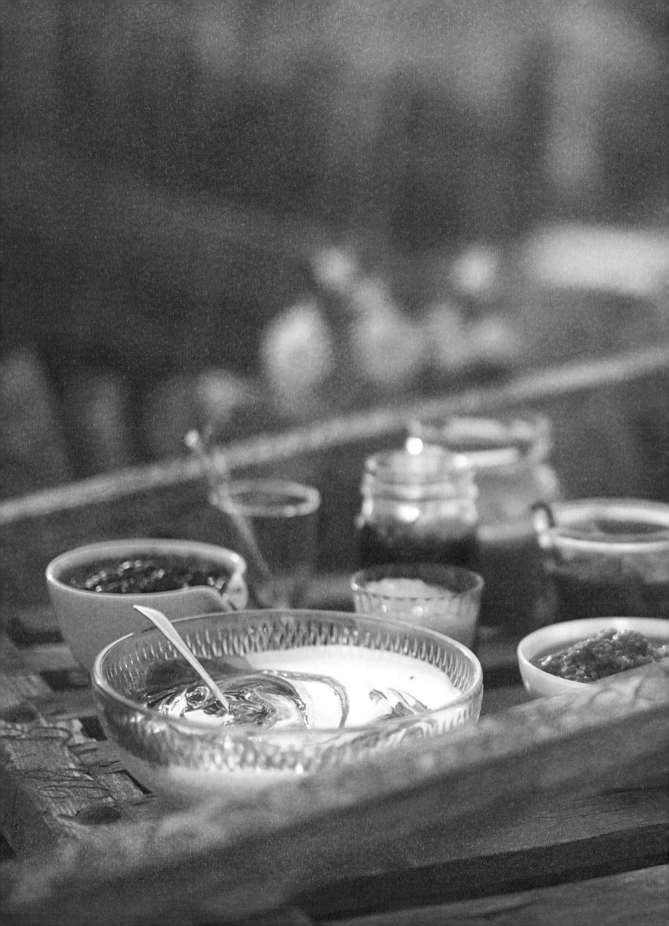

YEMENI PANCAKES

These incredible pancakes will definitely ruffle some feathers on a Sunday morning (in a good way). They're soft and delicious, and all the little holes that pop up on the top are perfect for a smear of butter, honey or any of the traditional things you want to drizzle over a pancake. The texture is phenomenal; I was introduced to this style of pancake by the ladies of the Yemeni community in Cardiff's Tiger Bay. They've been making these pancakes here for over 200 years now, so I say they deserve a place in this book. I've adapted their recipe to make it a bit more accessible for everyday cooking, but without compromising the end result. In their culture, they'd serve these with savoury food and use them to mop up lovely meat stews – but they're equally delicious this way.

MAKES 12 PANCAKES

- 1 x 7g sachet of dried yeast
- 1 teaspoon runny honey
- 2 large free-range eggs
- 400ml milk

- 175g self-raising flour
- 175g cornmeal
  or fine semolina flour
- sea salt

- olive oil
- *optional:* fresh raspberries,
  a knob of butter and runny
  honey, to serve

Dissolve the yeast in a bowl with a couple of good splashes of warm water and the runny honey, then leave in a warm place for around 20 minutes. Beat the eggs in a large bowl and whisk in the milk. Gently whisk in the yeast mixture, then add the flour, semolina and a pinch of salt. Whisk for a minute or so, until the mixture is thick enough to coat the back of a spoon. If it feels too dense and isn't pourable, let it down with a splash more milk. Cover the bowl with a tea towel and set aside for around 1 hour.

When you're ready to start cooking, put a large non-stick frying pan over a medium heat and rub a little olive oil on to it with some kitchen paper. Once hot, pour a ladle of the pancake mixture into the pan and sort of tilt the pan all around so the batter spreads out into a large circle. Loads of little holes should start bubbling and appearing on top; cook for 2 minutes to allow the bubbles to form properly, then turn the heat down to low and pop a lid on the pan. Continue to cook for a further 2 minutes, or until the pancake is golden on the bottom and cooked through. After you've cooked the first one, review the temperature and adjust it so that each pancake comes off the pan soft and floppy. Serve with the holey side facing up, with raspberries, a knob of butter and a drizzle of runny honey.

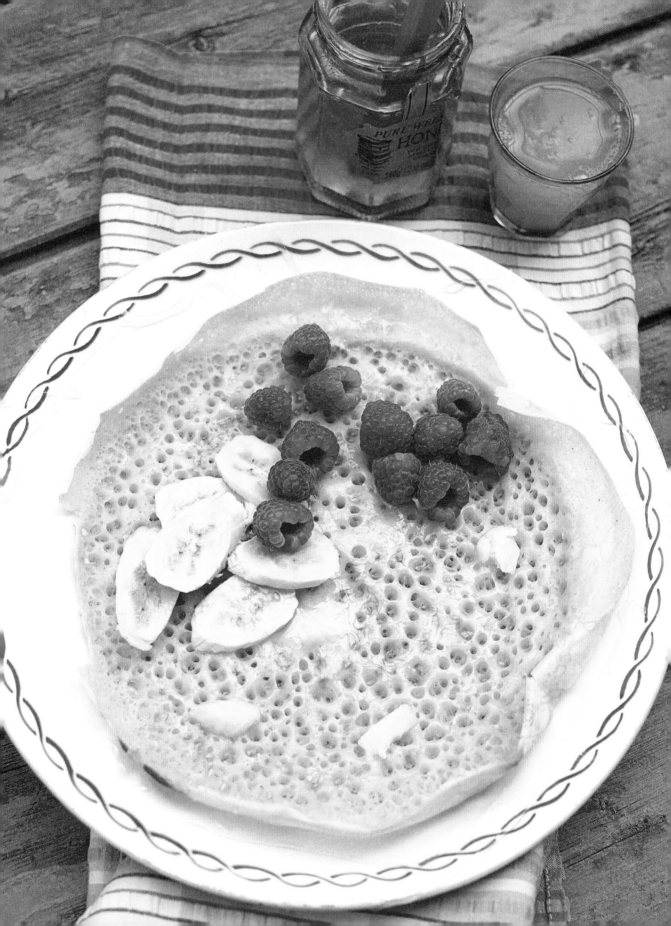

GLASGOW POTATO SCONES
BEST SCRAMBLED EGG • SMOKED SALMON

During a stay in Glasgow I was introduced to these incredible potato scones. I didn't grow up eating these, but they're beautiful and so easy. A bit like bubble without the squeak. This was my first attempt at mastering them and it turned into this lovely breakfast, which I made in a pretty little flat in Glasgow's West End. It's the posh area of town and is full of beautiful shops and neighbourhoods. Well worth a visit.

This dish is the best brunch I can think of, besides maybe kedgeree. I never would have thought of putting this much flour with potatoes, but it works brilliantly. Give them a go with bangers, stews, on their own, or as part of this lovely brunch ... I assure you this is one of the nicest ways to start the day, ever.

SERVES 4

- 500g floury potatoes, such as Maris Piper, skins on
- sea salt and ground pepper
- 100g plain flour
- a small bunch of fresh chives
- 2 knobs of butter
- ½ a level teaspoon baking powder
- olive oil
- 5 large free-range eggs
- 200g really good-quality smoked salmon
- a few pinches of washed watercress, to serve
- extra virgin olive oil
- 1 lemon, cut into wedges, to serve

Cut the potatoes into 2.5cm chunks and cook them in boiling salted water for around 7 minutes, or until tender. Drain them, allow them to cool, then return them to the empty pan and add the flour. Lightly mash everything together but try to avoid stirring it up too much. Finely slice the chives and add them to the potatoes with a knob of butter and the baking powder, then mash a few more times. (If you like, you can grate a little cheese into the mixture at this point – it's delicious.) Season, then use your clean hands to bring the mixture together. Pinch off a little, taste and adjust the seasoning, then divide into 4 balls and dust with flour.

Put a large frying pan (roughly 32cm) on a medium heat and add a drizzle of olive oil. Add the potato balls (you may need to cook them in batches) and pat them down so they're almost flat – 2cm thick is about right. Cook for around 10 minutes, turning them every few minutes until golden on both sides.

Meanwhile, beat the eggs so they are broken and marbled. Season and put aside. When your potato scones are perfectly cooked, divide them between your plates, then take the pan off the heat and add a knob of butter. Once bubbling, pour in the eggs and put back on a low heat. Don't be tempted to stir aggressively, use a rubber spatula to just sweep up the cooked layer of egg from the bottom of the pan every time it forms, so the uncooked egg can get down there and set. This will give you the nicest texture. The key to good scrambled egg is getting the perfect ratio of cooked silky egg and slightly less-cooked curds. To achieve that, you need to remove it from the heat once it looks three-quarters cooked – trust me. It will carry on cooking and by the time you mix it around one more time and serve, it will be gold.

Arrange a piece of smoked salmon on top and add a pinch of watercress. Drizzle over a little extra virgin olive oil and serve with wedges of lemon for squeezing over.

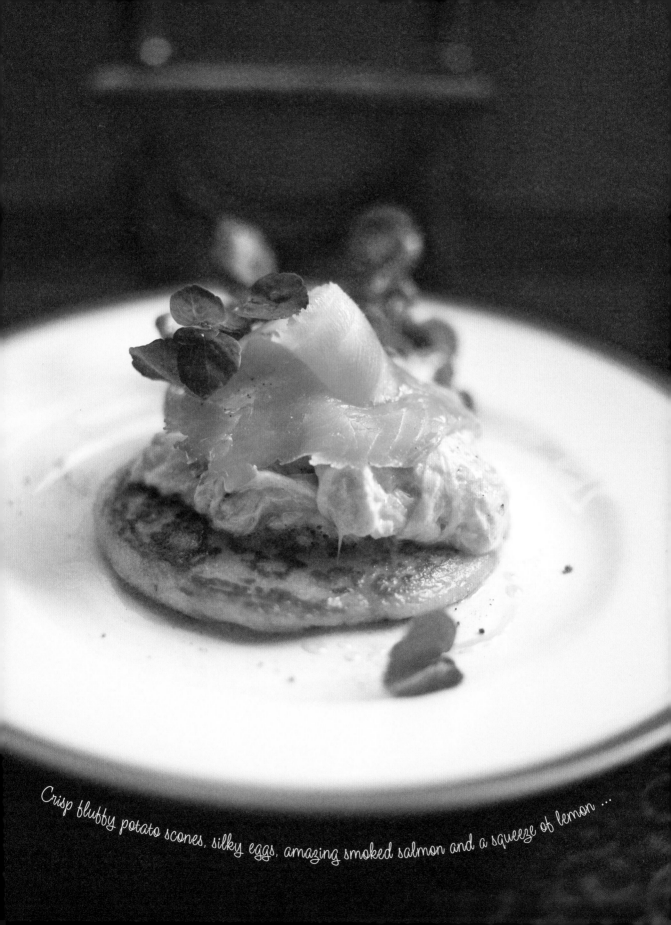

Crisp fluffy potato scones, silky eggs, amazing smoked salmon and a squeeze of lemon ...

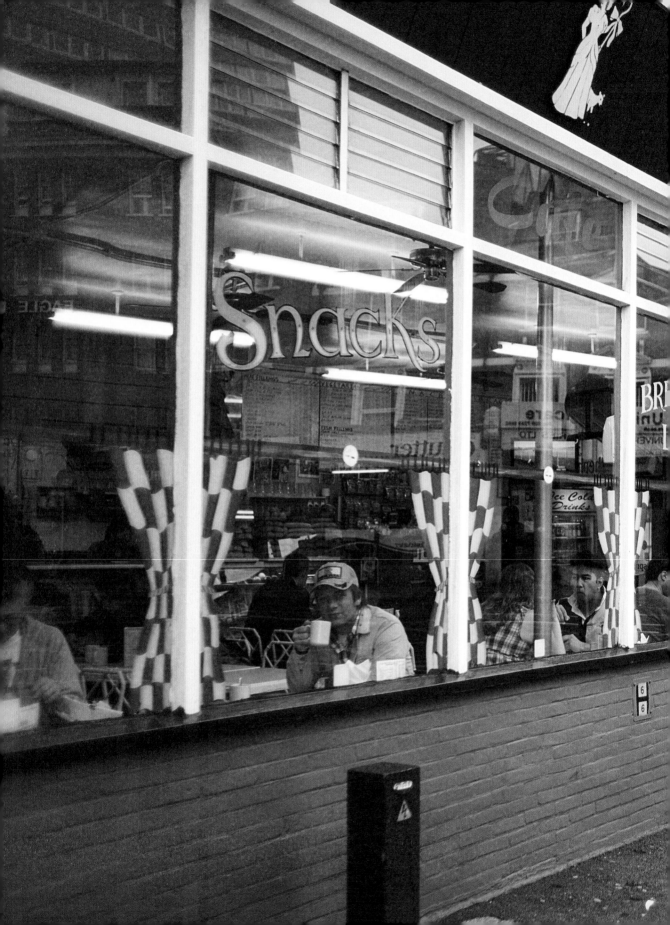

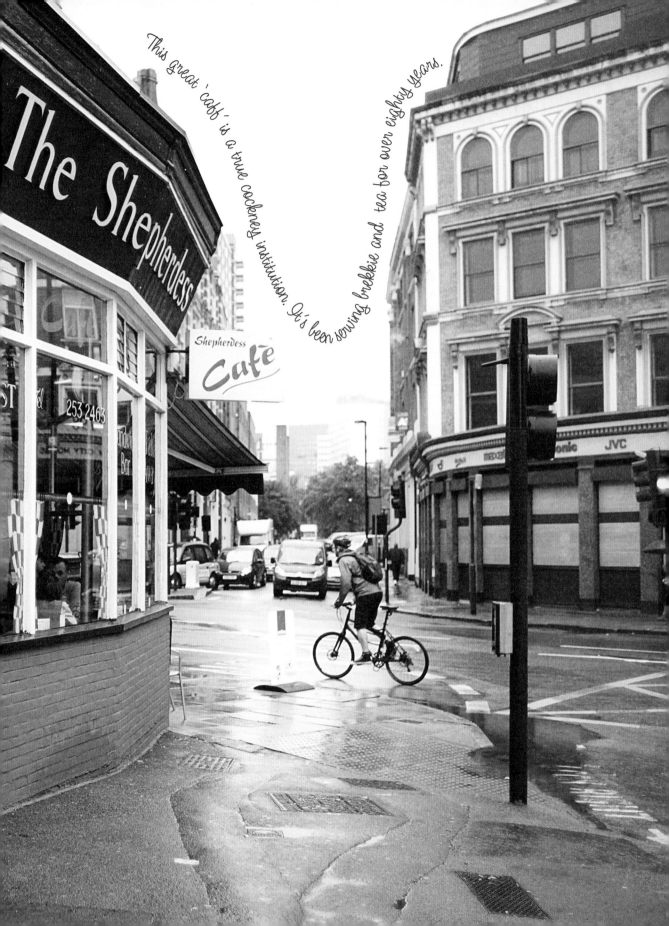

This great 'caff' is a true cockney institution. It's been serving brekkie and tea for over eighty years.

OLD BOY'S OMELETTE

FRIED BREAD CHUNKS • MUSHROOM SLICES

I love the idea of frying little crispy chunks of bread at the same time as the bacon, then simply cooking them right into an omelette. It's a little twist on a classic but well worth trying, and absolutely perfect for a Sunday morning. Serve with HP sauce and ketchup, and your favourite Sunday paper.

SERVES 1

- olive oil
- 1 slice of sourdough bread, crusts removed
- 1 field mushroom, brushed clean
- 1 rasher of quality smoked streaky bacon, cut into 2cm pieces
- 2-3 large free-range eggs
- sea salt and ground pepper
- Cheddar cheese, for grating

Preheat a small frying pan (roughly 20cm) over a medium to high heat and add a drizzle of olive oil. Cut your bread into 2cm cubes and your field mushroom into 1cm slices and add both to the pan with your chopped bacon. Spend a few minutes getting some nice colour happening, and turning things every so often. It's important to look after everything in the pan and keep in mind that things will cook at different speeds. Have a small plate nearby, and if anything starts looking primo – take it out until everything else catches up.

Beat your eggs in a bowl and season. Return anything you've taken out back to the pan, spread it out evenly, then pour in the eggs and move the pan around so they completely cover the base of it. As the eggs begin to set, gently push the set eggs around with a wooden spoon – they'll ruffle up like skirts of beautiful silk. Turn the heat off, and keep moving and folding until the raw egg stops moving around. Quickly grate over a tiny bit of cheese. You want the omelette to look slightly underdone, because when you turn it out it carries on cooking and will be absolutely perfect when you tuck in. Ultimately if it's perfectly cooked in the pan, it will be overcooked when you serve it – it might sound like I'm over-egging the omelette, but overcooked egg is what you get on an aeroplane. Perfect eggs are what you get in your own kitchen: velvety, soft, silky and delicious. Good luck!

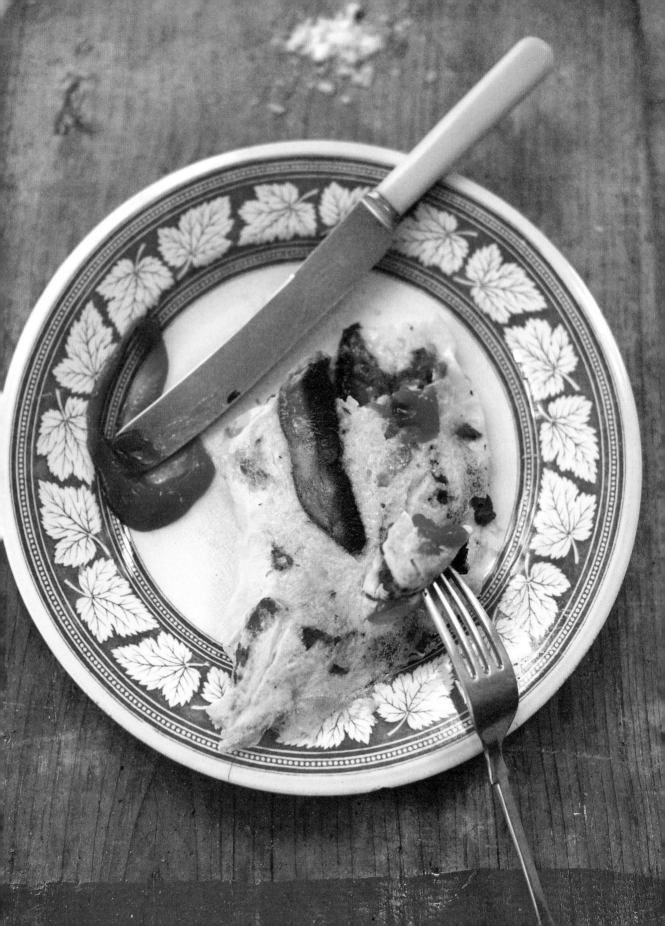

BREAKFAST CRUMPIES

Crumpies are my new delicious invention and are a cross between a crumpet and a Yorkshire pudding. They can be whizzed together quickly, then poured into a Yorkshire pudding mould and banged into the oven to get lovely and crisp on the top and bottom, and knotty, chewy and bubbly inside. They're perfect with butter, or whatever other lovely condiments you've got hanging around the cupboard. My wife loves strawberry jam with hers, Daisy loves Marmite, Poppy loves a drizzle of honey, and personally I like a little scrambled egg with a blob of ketchup or brown sauce (or both) on the plate and, depending on how I feel, a little chilli sauce.

MAKES 12

- vegetable oil
- 500g strong bread flour
- 1 teaspoon caster sugar
- 1 x 7g sachet easy action yeast
- a good pinch of bicarbonate of soda
- 2 teaspoons sea salt

Preheat the oven to 170°C/325°F/gas 3 and grease a 12-hole muffin tin with some vegetable oil. Place all the other ingredients in a bowl and pour in 600ml of tepid water. The water needs to be warm enough to activate the yeast, but not so hot that it kills it.

Whisk everything together until you've got a loose batter that is just combined - this should only take a few seconds. Leave to stand for 10 minutes to let the yeast do its job. When the mixture is a spoonable, sticky consistency, but still quite wet, spoon it into the muffin tin. Fill each hole until it's almost level with the top of the tin and cook for around 35 minutes, or until the crumpies are risen and golden. Remove to a wire rack for a few minutes to cool slightly, then serve while still warm with anything you fancy.

HERE ARE A FEW IDEAS TO GET YOU STARTED:

CREAM CHEESE

JAM AND BANANA

A FEW SLICES OF COOKED HAM

SOME BEAUTIFUL SLICES OF CHEESE

SMOKED SALMON AND A WEDGE OF LEMON

SLICED STRAWBERRIES WITH CREAM OR YOGHURT

SOME SNAPPED UP PIECES OF CRISPY BACON

A SPOONFUL OF QUALITY JAM

SLICED BANANA AND RUNNY HONEY

A SPOONFUL OF NUTELLA

HAM AND MUSTARD

A POACHED EGG

… BUT THERE ARE NO RULES!

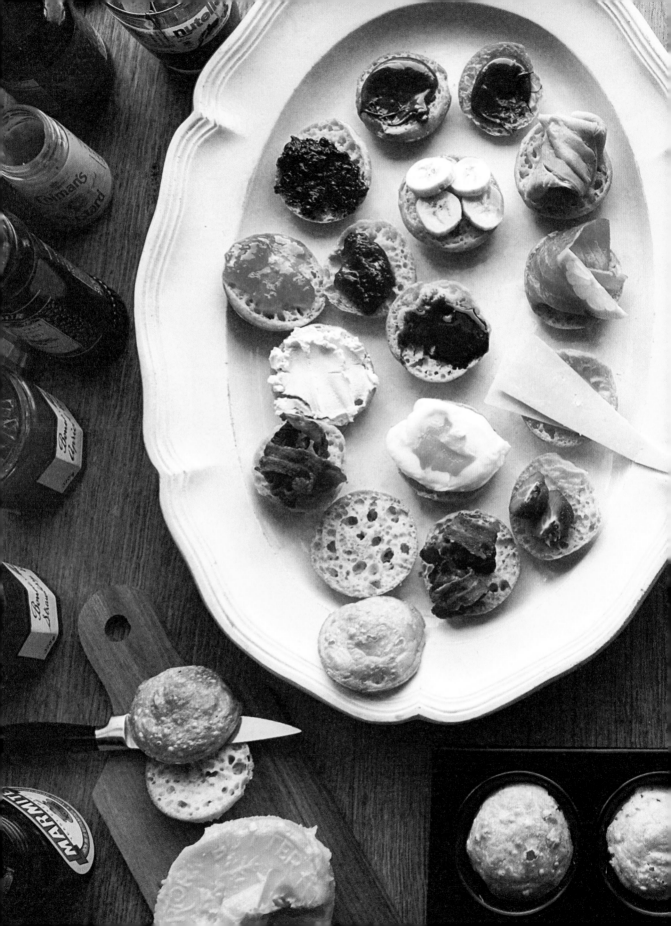

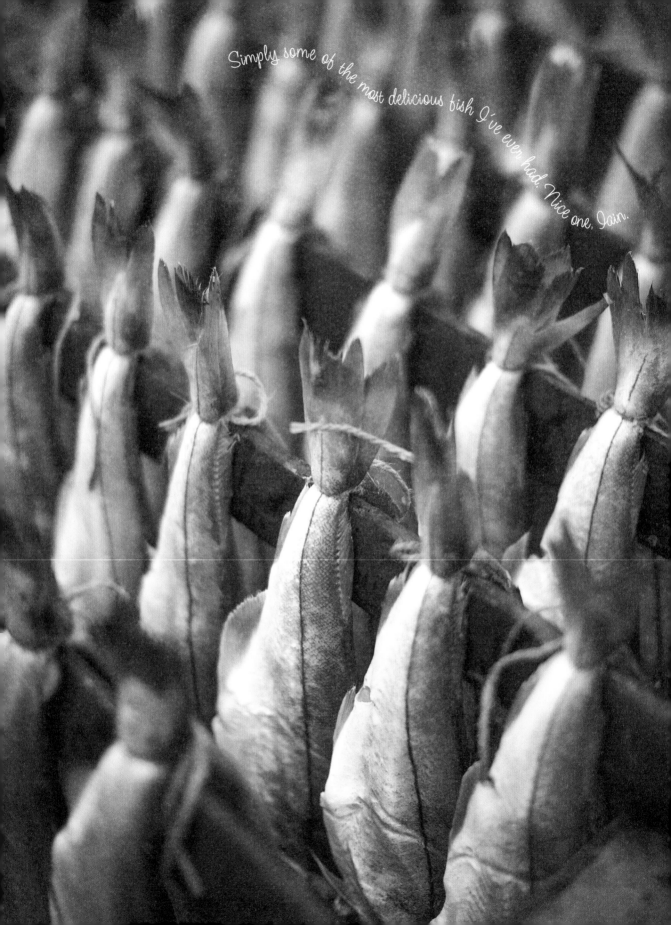

Simply some of the most delicious fish I've ever had. Nice one, Iain.

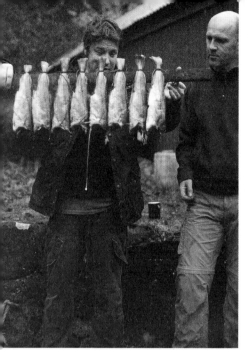

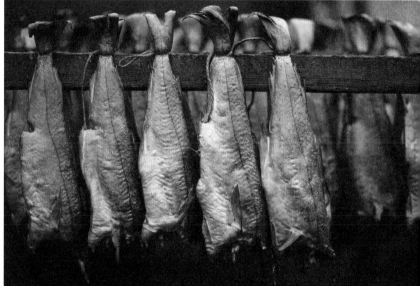

Arbroath Smokies

Historically, hot smoking was necessary to preserve fish, but it's survived because we love the flavour. Iain Spinks makes 'Arbroath' smokies (hot-smoked haddock) the traditional way, and, best of all, he's mobile so he's able to show up anywhere with his oak barrels and hessian sacks. Look out for Arbroath smokies in good supermarkets. If you're having a party and want something different ... he's your man.
www.arbroathsmokies.net

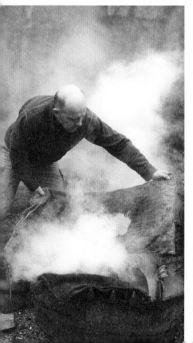

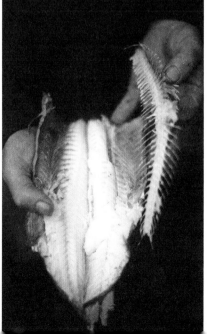

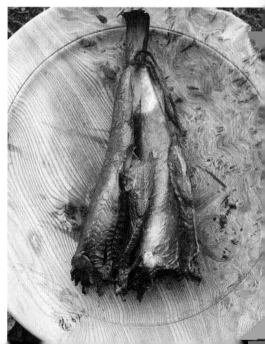

DELICIOUS SMOKED HADDOCK
POACHED EGG • SPINACH ON TOAST

For me this is the fish equivalent of a kind of eggs Benedict. It eats so well and always puts a smile on people's faces. Smoked haddock is the classic fish to use here, and Arbroath smokies, from Scotland, are about the best I've ever had. But if you can't get your hands on quality smoked haddock you can easily use trout or herring or kippers in exactly the same way. Whatever type of fish you go for, look for that all-important labelling.

Your job is simply to make sure all the elements come together at the same time – hot toast, beautiful poached eggs, lovely fish and deep, intense spinach. If you can do that, this will be heavenly. It's all about multitasking, hence doing it for two people rather than four, at least until you get the hang of it.

SERVES 2

- 4 fresh bay leaves
- 10 black peppercorns
- 1 lemon
- 1 x 250g undyed smoked haddock fillet

- 2 large free-range eggs
- a knob of unsalted butter
- 1 teaspoon Gentleman's Relish
- 1 level teaspoon mustard powder

- 1 whole nutmeg, for grating
- 200g baby spinach
- 2 thick slices from a bloomer loaf
- sea salt and ground pepper

Put a large, wide pan of water on a high heat, add the bay leaves, peppercorns and the juice of half the lemon, and bring to the boil. Turn down to a simmer, then add the fish and let it simmer for 4 minutes before cracking in the eggs to poach and cook to your liking. A soft poached egg will take around 3 minutes, and a slightly firmer egg will need around 4 minutes. The fish only needs about 8 minutes to cook, so by the time your eggs are done, it should be perfect.

Put a frying pan on a high heat and add the butter, Gentleman's Relish, mustard powder and about 10 gratings of nutmeg. Once the butter has melted and is starting to bubble, mash up the Gentleman's Relish a bit and squeeze in the juice of the remaining lemon half. Add the spinach and use tongs to gently turn it and move it around the pan for a few minutes, or until it's wilted. Push the spinach to one side of the pan, lean the pan the other way so all the moisture flows out, then let that evaporate over the heat until you've got fairly dry, intense, dark spinach.

Pop your bread into the toaster and keep an eye on the eggs and haddock while your spinach continues to cook. Pop a slice of toast on each plate and divide the spinach and juices between them. Use a slotted spoon to carefully scoop a poached egg on to each toast, sprinkle with salt and pepper, then flake over the fish, discarding the skin. Now you get to enjoy the best bits: busting open the lovely egg and smearing it all over the toast. Lovely.

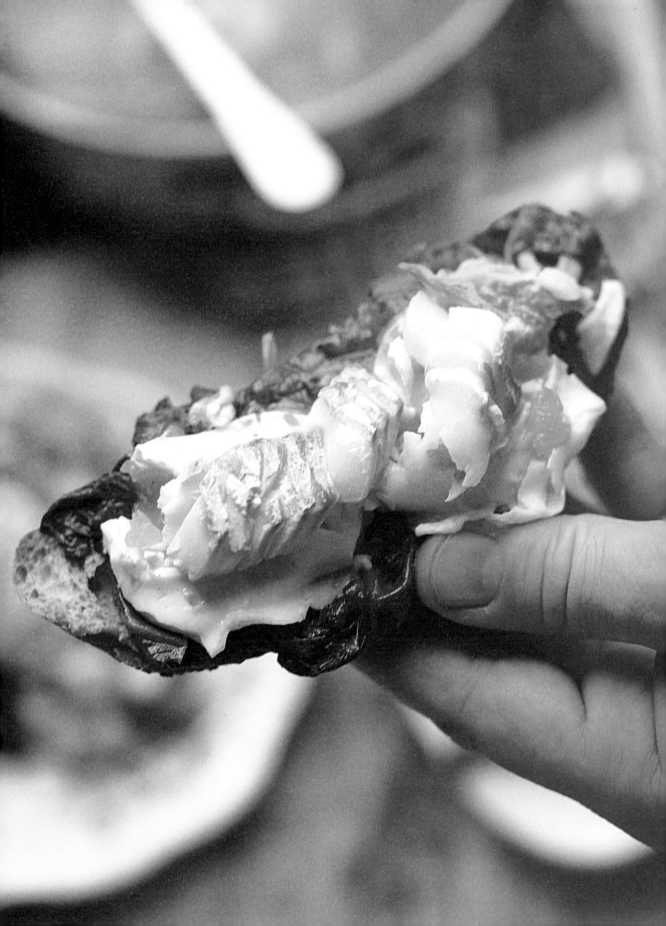

LIGHT & SPICY KEDGEREE

Kedgeree is quite possibly one of my favourite things to eat, but weirdly, I only tend to make it a few times a year; usually for a New Year's Day breakfast, when I look and feel a bit the worse for wear, but need to snap out of it! If you're suffering, this is great served with a pint of Guinness (with a splash of port in it), or a Bloody Mary. Then again, it's also lovely with a simple cup of Earl Grey tea for a posh breakfast, or with wine for a late lunch or dinner. Over the years I've discovered that this is a great dish to give visitors to the UK. When you put that pan down on the table they'll think you're bonkers for serving curried food first thing in the morning, but as soon as they get a spoonful into their mouth they'll love it.

SERVES 6

- 300g basmati rice
- sea salt and ground pepper
- 6 large free-range eggs
- 2 onions, peeled and finely chopped
- 3 cloves of garlic, peeled and finely chopped
- 50g butter
- 1 heaped teaspoon garam masala
- 1 level teaspoon cumin seeds
- 2 level teaspoons black mustard seeds
- 2 heaped teaspoons grated fresh ginger
- 2 fresh red chillies, deseeded and finely sliced
- a small bunch of fresh coriander
- 600g undyed smoked haddock
- 6 fresh bay leaves
- 6 black peppercorns
- 3 lemons
- 1 level teaspoon turmeric
- *optional:* natural yoghurt, to serve

Cook the rice in a medium pan (roughly 18cm wide and 10cm deep) in boiling salted water, according to the packet instructions. Add the eggs to the pan for the first 6 minutes of the rice's cooking time, then use a slotted spoon to move them to a bowl of cold water. Once they're cool enough to handle, peel and quarter each egg. Drain the rice in a sieve, then run it under the cold tap and put aside to drain again.

Gently fry your chopped onions and garlic with the butter in a large frying pan (roughly 30cm) on a medium heat. Add the garam masala, cumin seeds, mustard seeds, grated ginger, sliced chillies, and a good pinch of salt and pepper. Finely slice all the coriander stalks and add to the pan, keeping the leaves aside. Stir and fry everything for about 10 minutes, or until the onions are soft.

Meanwhile, in a clean, snug-fitting pan, poach the haddock in about 1 litre of water, enough to cover the fish, with your bay leaves and peppercorns. Bring to the boil, simmer gently for 5 minutes, then remove from the heat. Let the fish cool down a little, then get rid of the skin and flake the fish on to a plate, being careful to remove any bones as you go.

Now you've done all the hard work, so your job is to make this incredible-tasting dish look beautiful too. Stir and fold the drained rice into the spiced onions and mix well. Check the seasoning and correct it with salt and pepper and add the juice from 1½ lemons. Stir and cook on a medium heat for around 4 minutes, then have a taste and correct the seasoning again. Sprinkle the turmeric over the rice, followed by half the flaked fish, half the eggs and half the coriander leaves. Stir gently - the turmeric will colour some of the rice but not all of it. Scatter the rest of the fish, eggs and coriander over the top of the kedgeree, then cover with a lid or tin foil so that everything can get lovely and steamy and turn into a tasty pan of deliciousness. Cut the remaining lemons into wedges for serving, put out a little bowl of yoghurt if you like, then get everyone round the table and let them help themselves.

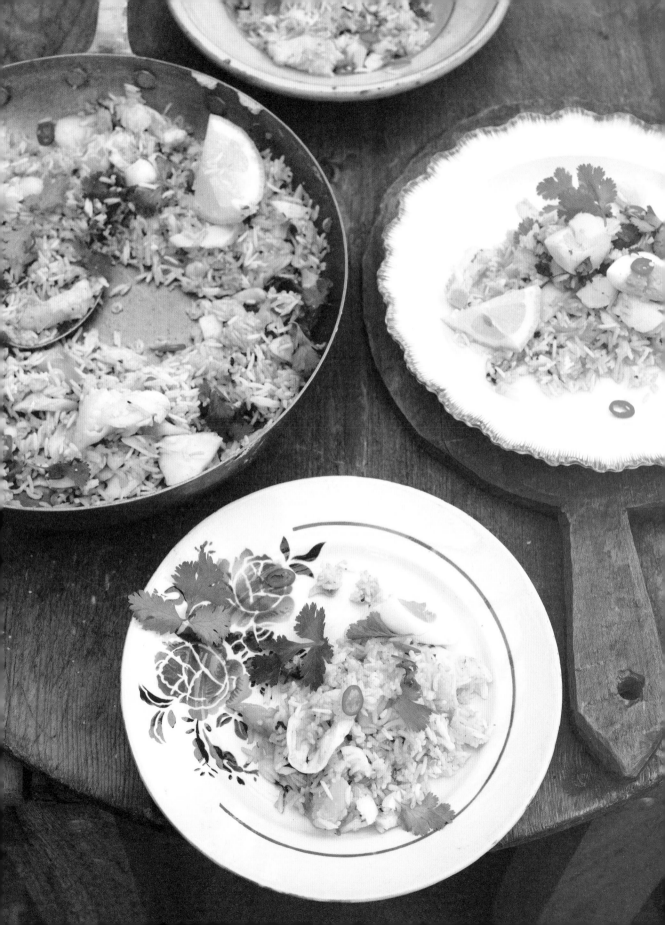

STICKY PRUNE MUESLI
CREAMY YOGHURT • SWEET FRUITY SAUCE

This is a lovely and delicious little breakfast. It's really quick, and the taste of it really takes me back to my childhood and reminds me of being at my nan and grandad's . Even though it's no effort at all, it looks cool and contemporary. If you're making this for kids and they aren't used to eating prunes, just mash the prunes up a bit, ripple them through the yoghurt and they'll clean their plates. Ultimately it's good to grab breakfast in the morning, and we all get stuck in a rut sometimes and need a few new ideas to keep things exciting. There's something quite retro about prunes, and serving them sticky and hot against the cold creamy yoghurt and toasted oats is so yummy. You could easily turn this into a dessert by serving it with a few scoops of good-quality vanilla ice cream instead of yoghurt. Enjoy.

. SERVES 4 ·

- a knob of butter
- 200g jumbo rolled porridge oats
- 3 tablespoons flaked almonds
- 1 heaped tablespoon desiccated coconut
- 1 tablespoon runny honey
- 1 x 410g tin of prunes
- 1 x 500g tub of natural yoghurt, to serve

Get a large non-stick frying pan on a medium heat, add the butter and let it foam, then sprinkle in the oats and almonds. Chivvy it about and toast for around 5 minutes, or until everything is just turning golden. Add the coconut and honey to the pan then toss and toast for 2 more minutes, then move everything to a tray.

Pour the juice from the tinned prunes into the hot pan and bring to the boil over a high heat. Reduce until it's nice and syrupy, then turn down the heat and add the prunes to the pan. Toss them around so they're shiny and coated in that loose, natural, caramelly juice.

Serve up any way you like. I like to divide the oats and almonds between the bowls, then lob some natural yoghurt and prunes on top - simple and delicious. You can use prunes with or without the stones in - just make sure you warn people if you choose the ones with stones!

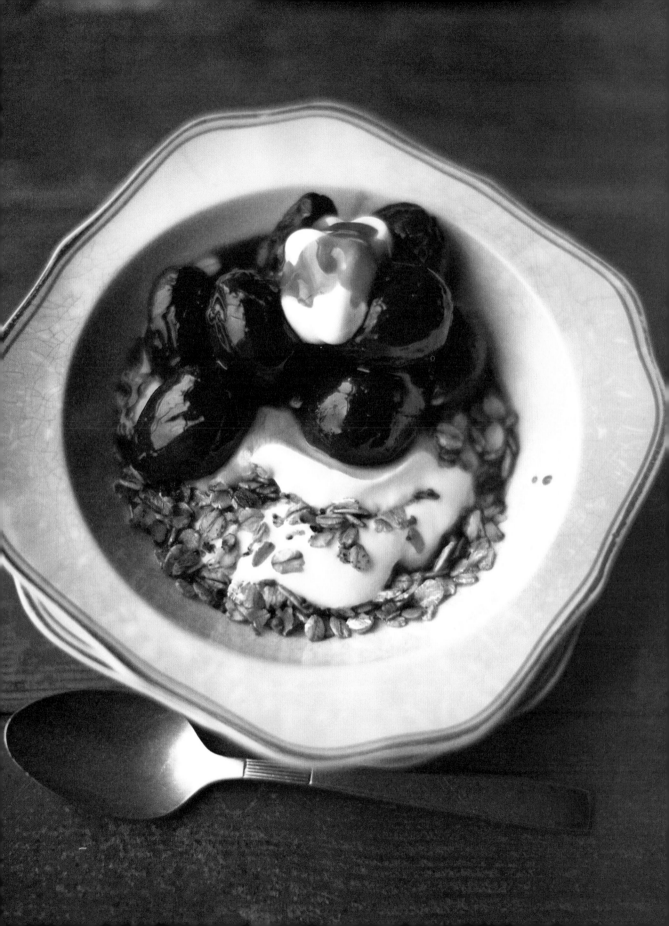

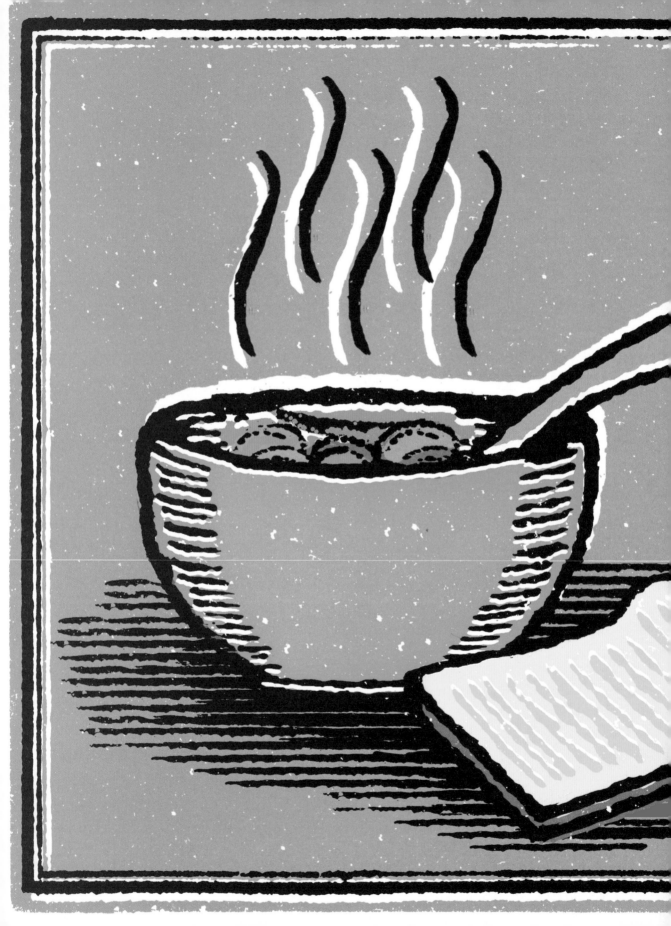

SOUPS

I'm so in love with this chapter. Soups have always been a massive part of our food culture – they're so easy because everything basically goes into one pot, they're warming when it's cold or rainy, and they can be wonderfully refreshing when it's hot. There are a handful of great recipes here, each with a little tweak or kicker to them, whether that's cheesy golden soldiers for dipping, beautiful dumplings or flavoured oils. Without a doubt, soups are one of the cheapest ways to get good nutritious food into your family. It's very easy and convenient to get tinned or pre-packaged soups these days – but there really isn't anything better than making a soup yourself. The flavours are so much more alive, and sometimes certain soups you think you know take on a whole new personality when you make them fresh. So give these a try – you'll get a great reaction.

FRESH TOMATO SOUP
CREAM • LITTLE CHEDDAR SOLDIERS • BASIL

This is a simple end-of-summer cream of tomato soup that celebrates incredible British tomatoes and pays respect to that iconic Heinz tinned soup we've all grown up loving. My version is a little fresher than that tinned soup. Dunk these little cheesy soldiers in a bowl of this and it's going to be seriously delish.

It's so important to have soft ripe tomatoes for this soup. The ones they always knock off dead cheap in the market at the end of the day are perfect for this. I know from experience that the true cooks come out of the woodwork fifteen minutes before the markets start clearing up, to scoop up all the bargain fruit and veg. I remember working at a market where this one old dude would turn up at the end of the day and buy up all the fruit and veg just about to turn. I just know he was taking them home and turning them into something amazing.

SERVES 4

For the soup
- 1 large carrot, peeled and quartered
- 3 cloves of garlic, peeled
- 2kg large ripe tomatoes (leave their little green leaves on if they have any)

- a few sprigs of fresh basil
- sea salt and ground pepper
- white wine vinegar
- 5-6 tablespoons single cream
- extra virgin olive oil

For the cheesy soldiers
- a loaf of crusty bread
- a few sprigs of fresh thyme
- 30g freshly grated Cheddar cheese
- Worcestershire sauce
- olive oil

Preheat the oven to 180°C/350°F/gas 4. Put the carrot, garlic, tomatoes and most of the basil (reserve a few smaller leaves for garnishing later) into a liquidizer and blitz up until smooth – you may need to do this in two batches. Pour into a large saucepan, season well, then leave on a medium low heat for around 20 minutes, to tick away and thicken up. Stir occasionally.

While that's happening, cut the crusty bread into finger-sized soldiers (roughly 10cm in length and 1.5cm thick). Spread these around a large baking sheet and scatter over a few bruised and twisted thyme sprigs. Sprinkle the cheese all over, then add a few good swigs of Worcestershire sauce. Drizzle over a lug of olive oil, toss and cook in the oven for around 10 to 15 minutes, or until the bread is crisp and golden and the cheese has melted all over it.

Meanwhile, bring the soup to the boil, have a taste and adjust the seasoning to perfection with a pinch of salt and pepper and a tiny drizzle of white wine vinegar. Stir in half the single cream and serve as is – semi-smooth – or liquidize one last time for silky smooth soup. Serve it right in the pan surrounded by the croutons, like the picture. Swirl and drizzle the rest of the cream on top, scatter over the reserved basil leaves, add a drizzle of extra virgin olive oil, and get everyone to help themselves.

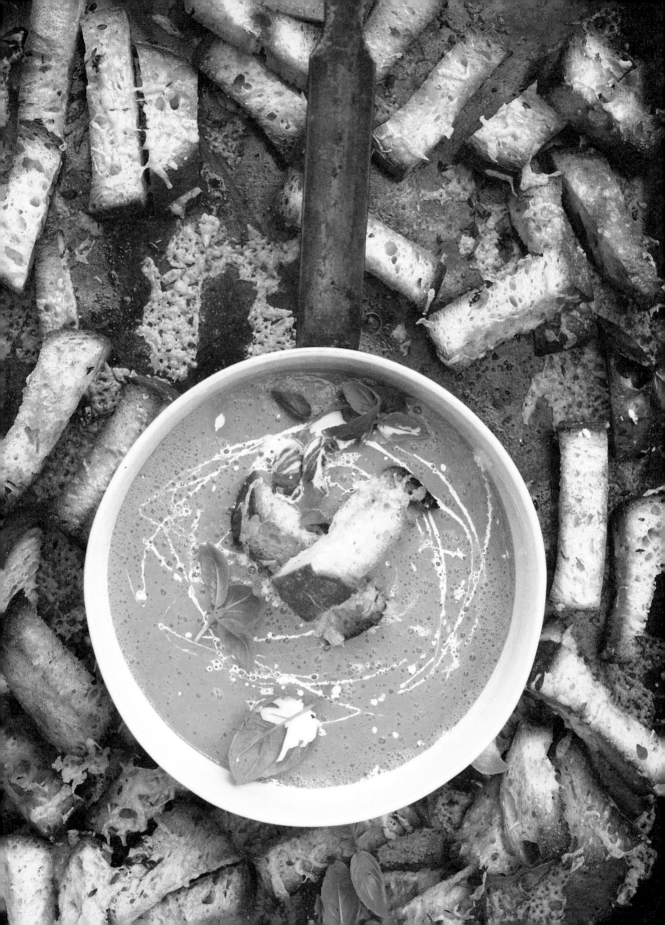

CREAMED MUSHROOM SOUP
WILD MUSHROOMS • DOORSTEP TOAST

Wild mushrooms grow in abundance in Britain, and this soup is a real celebration of this incredible ingredient. When I wrote the recipe I'd had beef stroganoff the day before and just loved the scent and the flavours, so I decided to go with that and take our wonderful wild mushrooms in a slightly different direction. It worked out really well, and the result is this aromatic soup. The meaty intensity of the mushrooms, especially on the sweet little toasts, makes this dish really special, particularly for those colder autumnal days. Give it a try.

SERVES 6

- 1 tablespoon butter
- olive oil
- 3 cloves of garlic (2 peeled and finely sliced, 1 halved)
- 600g mixed wild mushrooms, brushed clean
- 250g field mushrooms, brushed clean
- sea salt and ground pepper

- 1 red onion, peeled and diced
- 2 sticks of celery, trimmed and finely chopped
- 2 fresh bay leaves
- 25ml/a shot of brandy
- 100g white rice, rinsed
- 2 litres organic chicken or vegetable stock
- 6 teaspoons soured cream

- 1 lemon
- 6 slices of rustic bread
- Cheddar cheese, for grating
- a small bunch of fresh flat-leaf parsley, finely chopped
- freshly ground nutmeg
- extra virgin olive oil

Melt the butter with a drizzle of olive oil in a really big, deep non-stick saucepan. Add the 2 sliced garlic cloves and all the mushrooms. Stir and fry on a high heat for 3 to 4 minutes, or until you get some beautiful caramelization happening and any liquid has evaporated.

At this point, taste a mushroom and add a pinch of salt and pepper, if needed. When you're happy with the flavours, move a third of the mushrooms to a little frying pan (preferably non-stick) to reheat later for the toasts. Add the diced onion, celery and bay leaves to the remaining mushrooms and fry for 5 minutes or so on a medium heat, to soften slightly. Pour in the brandy and stir quickly until most of the alcohol burns off, then add the rice and stock and bring to the boil. Once boiling, turn down the heat and simmer gently for about 20 minutes.

While the soup is ticking away, mix together the soured cream and the zest of half the lemon. Add a good squeeze of lemon juice, season, then stir and put to one side until later. After 20 minutes, remove the bay leaves from the soup pan and blitz the soup either in a liquidizer or with a hand-held blender. Taste and correct the seasoning for the last time, adding a little lemon juice to taste. At this point, thin down the soup with a little hot stock, if you like, then put the lid on to keep the soup warm while you make the toasts.

Pop your slices of bread into the toaster while you warm the reserved mushrooms over a medium heat with a swig of water, a squeeze of lemon juice and about 1 tablespoon of grated Cheddar. Once the mushrooms are sizzling hot, rub the garlic halves over each piece of hot toast, then top with the mushrooms. Divide the soup between the bowls, swirl in the lemony soured cream and either put the mushroom toasts next to each soup or on a little platter everyone can steal from. Scatter your bowls of soup and mushroom toasts with some chopped parsley and a pinch of nutmeg, drizzle with extra virgin olive oil, and tuck in.

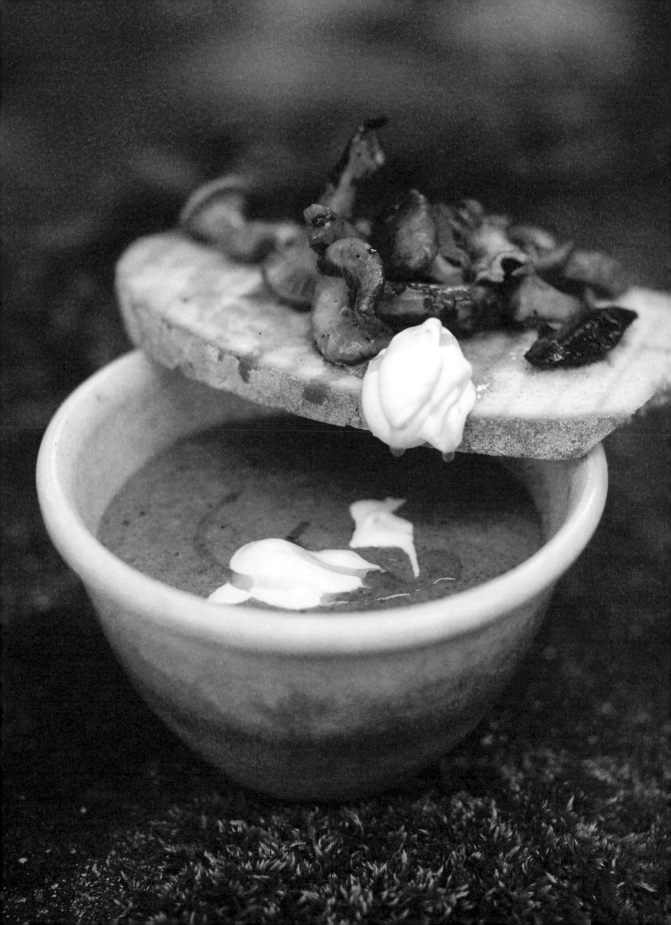

CHILLED SPRING SOUP
MINT • CRUMBLY GOAT'S CHEESE • LEMON

The great British spring and summer really are worth celebrating – and this baby is a great way of doing exactly that. It's excellent in May, June and July, when all our sweet small peas and broad beans are available. The Spanish have their gazpacho, which is all about simplicity and refreshment, and the French have their vichyssoise – lovely chilled potato and leek soup; this is a British riff on those things and I absolutely love it. When the sun shines, and the spring veg are still small, they are at their absolute peak, in every way possible. This is pure goodness, unadulterated by any cooking (though there is a splash of gin for good measure).

SERVES 4

- ½ a cucumber
- 1 stick of celery, trimmed, leaves reserved
- 2 handfuls of freshly podded peas (roughly 75g)
- 1 handful of fresh or frozen (defrosted) broad beans, skins removed (roughly 50g)

- 4 asparagus spears
- 1 large handful of watercress or baby spinach
- a small bunch of fresh chives
- a small bunch of fresh mint, leaves picked
- 100g goat's cheese
- extra virgin olive oil

- 3 lemons
- a splash of cider vinegar
- 1 thick slice of bread, crusts removed, diced up
- 25ml/a shot of gin
- sea salt and ground pepper
- *optional:* ice cubes
- *optional:* Tabasco sauce, to serve

Peel the cucumber, then chop and clank it up with the stick of celery. Put into a liquidizer (not a food processor) with most of the peas, broad beans, asparagus, watercress, chives, mint leaves and goat's cheese – save the rest of those ingredients in a cup of cold water for later. Add a drizzle of extra virgin olive oil, squeeze in the juice of 1 lemon, add a swig of vinegar, the bread, gin and a really good pinch of salt and pepper, then blitz everything together until smooth.

To serve straight away, add a handful of ice cubes and around 50ml of water to the blender to help chill it, then whiz again. But if you're making it in advance, like I do, blitz it with around 150ml of cold water and chill in the fridge along with your reserved ingredients until needed.

All of the ingredients vary in sweetness and acidity, so once it's thick and smooth, have a taste and really have a think about what you need to do to balance the flavours. Do you want it to be more herby? Fresh? Lemony? Season, whiz again, and keep tasting, tweaking and whizzing until you get it just right. Feel free to add a bit more water if you prefer a thinner soup. When you're happy, put some ice in a clean tea towel, then really bash it up with a rolling pin and put on a serving tray. Divide the soup between glasses or bowls and serve over the smashed ice. Drizzle a little extra virgin olive oil over each portion and sprinkle some of the reserved ingredients on top – it's nice to tell the story of what's in it. Put some salt, pepper, lemon wedges and Tabasco on the table so people can pimp their own rides. Delicious.

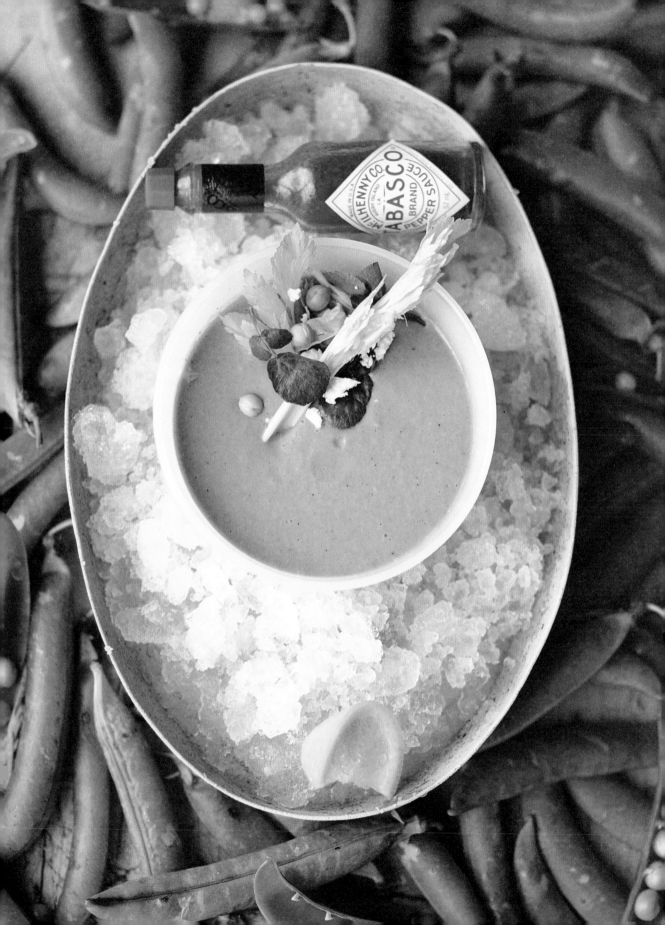

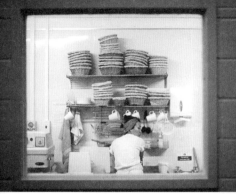
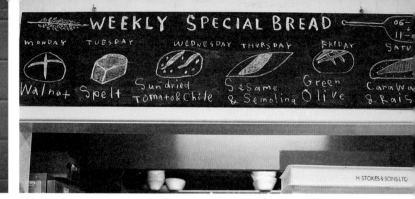

WEEKLY SPECIAL BREAD

MONDAY — Walnut
TUESDAY — Spelt
WEDNESDAY — Sundried Tomato & Chile
THURSDAY — Sesame & Semolina
FRIDAY — Green Olive
SATU — Caraway & Rais

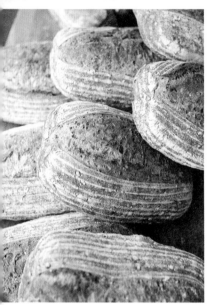
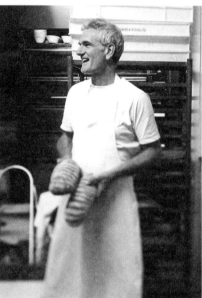
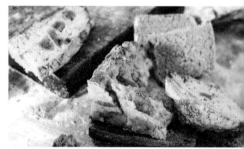
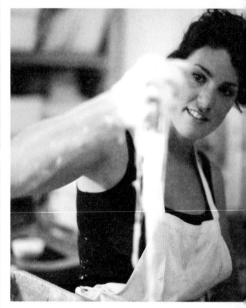

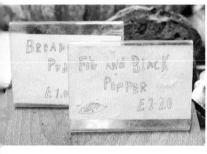

BREAD
PUD
£1.0

FIG AND BLACK
PEPPER
£2.20

Mark's Bread

Mark's Bread is a wonderful little bakery in Southville, Bristol, with brilliant bread and the cutest, most adorable girls baking with him, all full of passion. He was given a bread-making lesson for his fiftieth birthday, ditched his career in IT and opened a bakery shop. He's a brave man, but has made a success in a recession and that's got to deserve respect. *www.marksbread.co.uk*

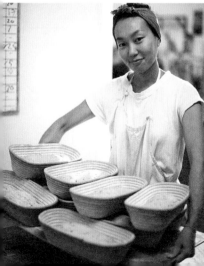
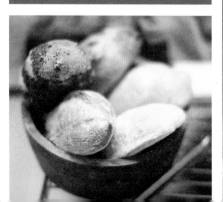
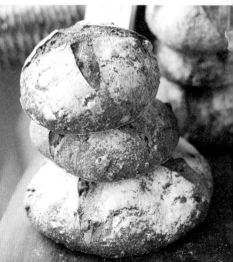

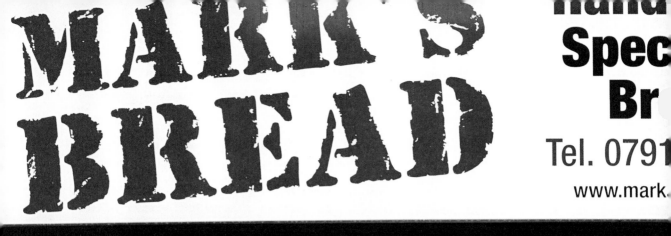

MARK'S BREAD

hand
Spec
Br
Tel. 0791
www.mark.

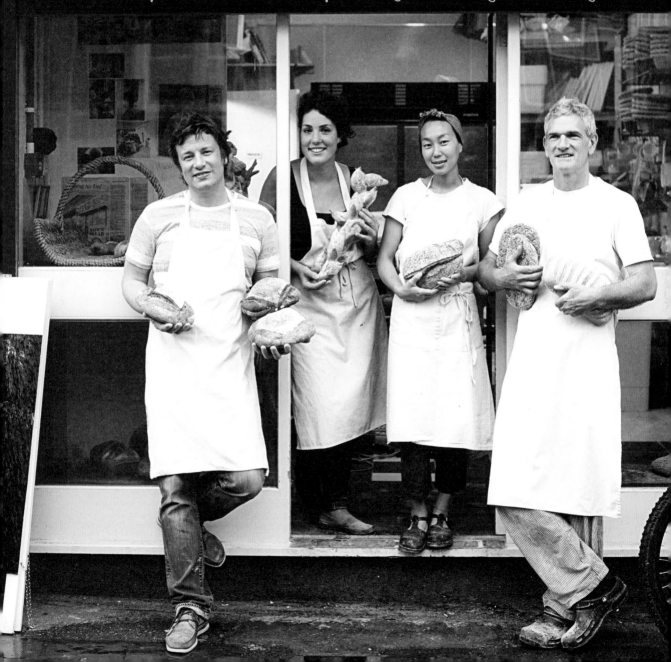

Mark's Bread is proof that with faith and passion anyone can change career at any time.

MY SCOTCH BROTH
... WITH PULLED LAMB ON GRILLED TOASTS

I'm a massive lover of Scotch broth, and I wanted to give it my own little spin by using lamb shanks to add delicious flavour to the broth, then pulling and tearing the tender meat over rustic little toasts to serve next to it. I think you're definitely going to enjoy this; it's a supercharged classic and I love it. It works all year round: you can make it in the middle of winter and it will put a big smile on your face; and then in the height of summer, as you take the lamb shanks out to make the toasts you can throw in handfuls of fresh peas, broad beans, asparagus and random seasonal baby greens to add little pops of freshness.

SERVES 8

- olive oil
- a knob of butter
- 2 rashers of quality smoked streaky bacon, finely sliced
- 2 sprigs of fresh rosemary, leaves picked and finely chopped
- 3 sticks of celery, trimmed
- 3 large carrots, peeled
- 3 onions, peeled

- 3 leeks, trimmed and washed
- I large swede, peeled
- 4 baby turnips, peeled
- 2 lamb shanks (roughly 350g each)
- 2.5 litres organic chicken stock
- 100g pearl barley
- ½ a small Savoy cabbage, tough stalks removed

- 8 small slices of rustic bread, Icm thick
- I heaped teaspoon wholegrain mustard
- 2 teaspoons runny honey
- I tablespoon mint sauce
- a very small bunch of fresh flat-leaf parsley, leaves picked
- sea salt and white pepper

Put a very large pan with a lid (roughly 25cm wide and 20cm deep) on a medium heat with a lug of olive oil, the butter, sliced bacon and rosemary leaves. Starting with the celery, carrots and onion, cut all the veg (except the cabbage) into rough 1cm chunks. It might take 5 minutes to cut them all up, but throw them into the pan as you go so things can get started. Once all the veg is in, add in the lamb shanks, then pour in 1.5 litres of stock and simmer gently, on a low heat, for 3 to 3½ hours with a lid on. It's ready when the lamb is falling off the bone. Add a splash more water if you think it needs it.

After 3 hours, add the pearl barley to the pan and cook for another half an hour. The lamb should be tender and falling off the bone by now, so chop your cabbage into 1cm chunks and add it to the pan, along with the remaining litre of stock, leaving the lid off. Turn the grill in your oven to medium high. Lay the slices of bread on a tray and grill on both sides till lightly golden. Remove the lamb to a plate and use 2 forks to shred it apart into little strands, discarding any bones, fat and gnarly bits. Stir in the mustard, honey, mint sauce and roughly chopped parsley leaves to the meat, mix in and add a little salt and pepper, if needed. Put little piles of meat on the toasts and pop back under the grill for just 2 or 3 minutes, or until the lamb is crispy. Importantly, have a final taste of the broth to check the seasoning. I like to serve the broth in the middle of the table and put the pulled lamb toasts on a nice platter, so that everyone can help themselves, then slurp and crunch away.

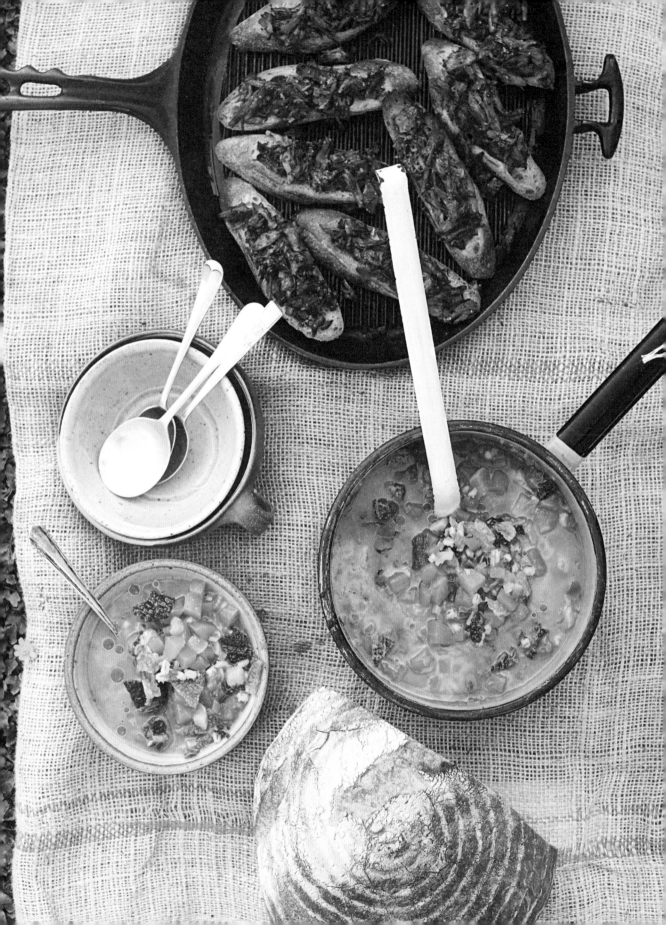

HUMBLE PEA & HAM SOUP
... A DOZEN FLUFFY LITTLE DUMPLINGS

Even though this soup is fairly quick to make, the flavours aren't compromised in the slightest because the gammon gives the broth a beautiful smoky depth. The other ingredients are ever so humble, and a bit frumpy, so I think popping the sweet peas in right at the end with the simple dumplings adds contrast and brightness. In the past I've made almost exactly this soup recipe but have just added a few swigs of cream and a few handfuls of clams and sweetcorn at the end, rather than peas and dumplings. That turns it into a kick-ass New England clam chowder. Not the most British recipe in the world, but equally tasty.

SERVES 10 WITH LEFTOVERS

For the soup
- 600g free-range smoked gammon
- 3 onions, peeled
- 3 sticks of celery, trimmed, yellow leaves reserved
- 3 large carrots, peeled
- 3 fresh bay leaves
- ground pepper
- 500g frozen peas
- 3 sprigs of fresh rosemary, leaves picked and chopped
- ½ a lemon

For the dumplings (makes 12)
- 200g self-raising flour, plus extra for dusting
- sea salt
- 100g unsalted cold butter
- 1 whole nutmeg, for grating

Cut the gammon into long slices roughly 2cm thick, discarding any fat and skin. Put the slices into a very large, deep pan (at least 25cm wide). Finely chop the onions and celery, roughly chop the carrots, add to the pan and throw in the bay leaves. Cover with 3 litres of water, add a good pinch of pepper and place over a high heat. As soon as it starts boiling, put the lid on, turn down the heat and leave to simmer for 1½ hours, skimming away any foam or froth from the top every now and then as it cooks.

Meanwhile, put the flour for the dumplings into a bowl with a pinch of salt, then grate in your chilled butter and add a few good scrapings of nutmeg. Add about 60ml of cold water, then push and squash everything together into one doughy piece (it should be fairly firm and malleable). Divide into 12 equal-sized pieces and roll them into balls. Place on a generously floured tray, cover with clingfilm and put into the fridge until needed.

When the cooking time is up, taste the broth. The smoked meat should have seasoned the soup really nicely already, but this is your opportunity to correct it if not. Use tongs to move the meat to a board, then shred and tear into irregular pieces and return them to the broth. Bring it back to the boil, add the peas and chopped rosemary, and grate over the zest from the lemon half before plopping in the dumplings. Turn the heat down to medium and leave to simmer for another 15 to 20 minutes, or until the dumplings have plumped up and are a pleasure to eat. When you're ready to serve, get everyone around the table, tear any reserved celery leaves over the top, and serve straight away.

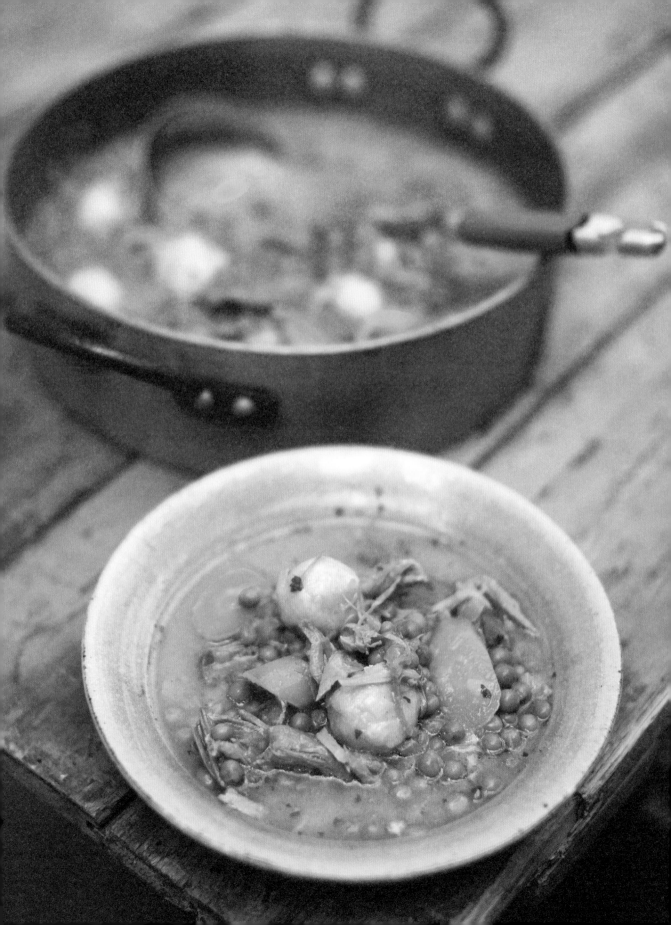

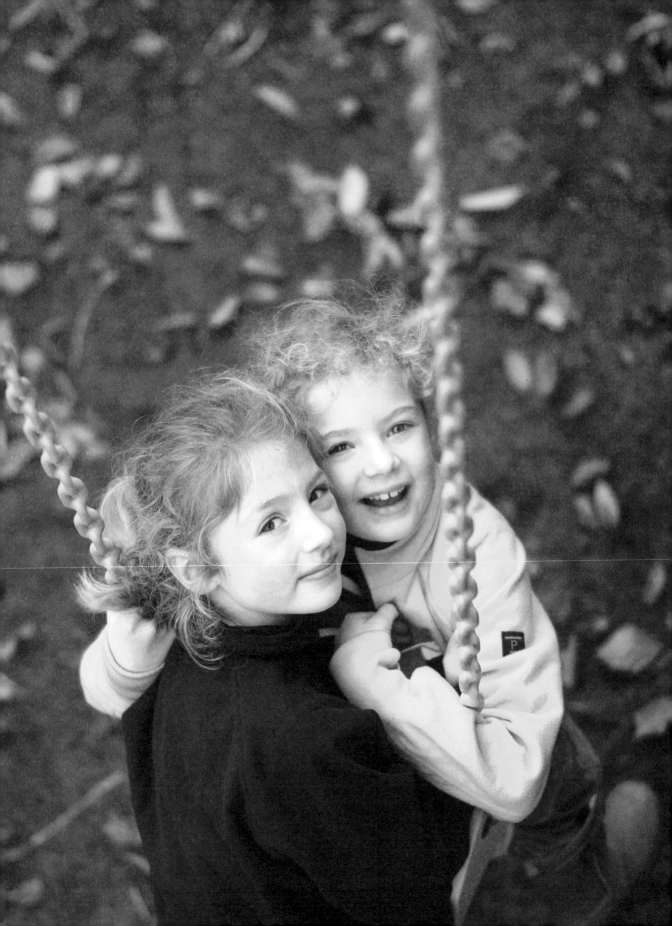

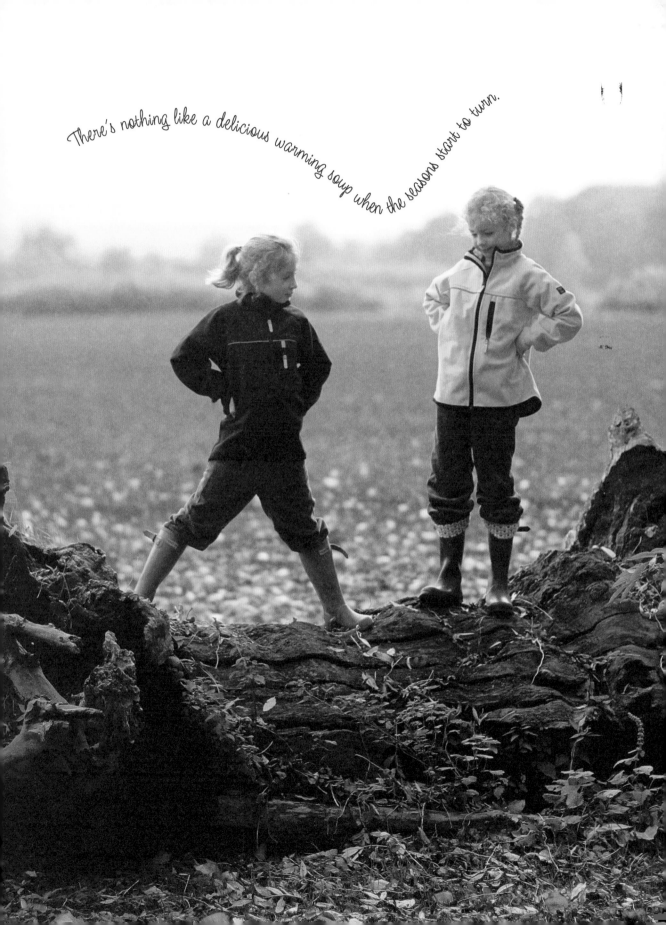

There's nothing like a delicious warming soup when the seasons start to turn.

ROASTED APPLE & SQUASH SOUP

On my travels around Bristol I spent an afternoon with Leona, who runs the Boiling Wells café in the allotment gardens. She's a lovely young lady and a real food activist in many ways. What's more, she's a great cook, and I'd rather eat food made by a great cook than a great chef any day of the week. The food she makes is clearly a reaction to the wonderful ingredients she gets from the allotments, which are a stone's throw from her café. She knocked out this soup for me, which I've tweaked slightly. I genuinely love it.

SERVES 4 TO 6

- 1 butternut squash (roughly 1kg)
- 3 good eating apples, such as Cox's or Braeburn
- 1 large onion
- 1 or 2 fresh red chillies
- 4 cloves of garlic, unpeeled and bashed
- olive oil
- sea salt and ground pepper
- a pinch of coriander seeds
- a few sprigs of fresh rosemary, leaves picked and finely chopped
- 3 heaped tablespoons pumpkin or mixed seeds
- a pinch of sweet cayenne pepper
- 800ml organic vegetable or chicken stock
- 150ml single cream
- *optional:* edible flowers or flowering herbs, to serve

Preheat the oven to 200°C/400°F/gas 6. Very carefully(!) slice the squash lengthways and scoop out the seeds. Cut into 2.5cm chunks and put them into your largest roasting tray. To see how to safely cut up butternut squash, go to *www.jamieoliver.com/how-to*.

Peel the apples, then quarter them and remove the core. Peel and roughly chop the onion and add the apples and onion to the roasting tray. Halve and deseed the chillies and add to the tray with the unpeeled and bashed garlic cloves. Drizzle over a good amount of olive oil and add a good pinch of salt and pepper – I also like to add a pinch of coriander seeds and a little chopped rosemary because I think it brings out the best flavour. Toss everything together so all the veg is nicely coated, season one more time, then whack into the oven and cook for around 45 minutes, or until everything is cooked through, intensely golden and delicious.

Toss the pumpkin seeds with salt, pepper, olive oil and the cayenne. Spread on a baking tray and roast in the oven for 10 to 15 minutes until nice and toasted, then put aside for later.

Put some of the roasted veg into a liquidizer, making sure you squeeze the garlic flesh out of its skin first. Add a swig of stock, then place a tea towel over the lid and gently blitz until smooth and lovely. Put this into a large pan while you blitz the rest. Pour in most of the cream and bring to a simmer over a medium to low heat. Have a taste, season to perfection and either add another splash of stock, or carry on simmering until you've got it to the consistency you love.

To serve, divide between warm soup bowls and add an 80s swirl of cream and a sprinkling of toasted seeds. If you're as creative as Leona, you can also grab some flowering herbs or edible flowers to sprinkle over the top and make it extra beautiful. Serve with warm crusty bread.

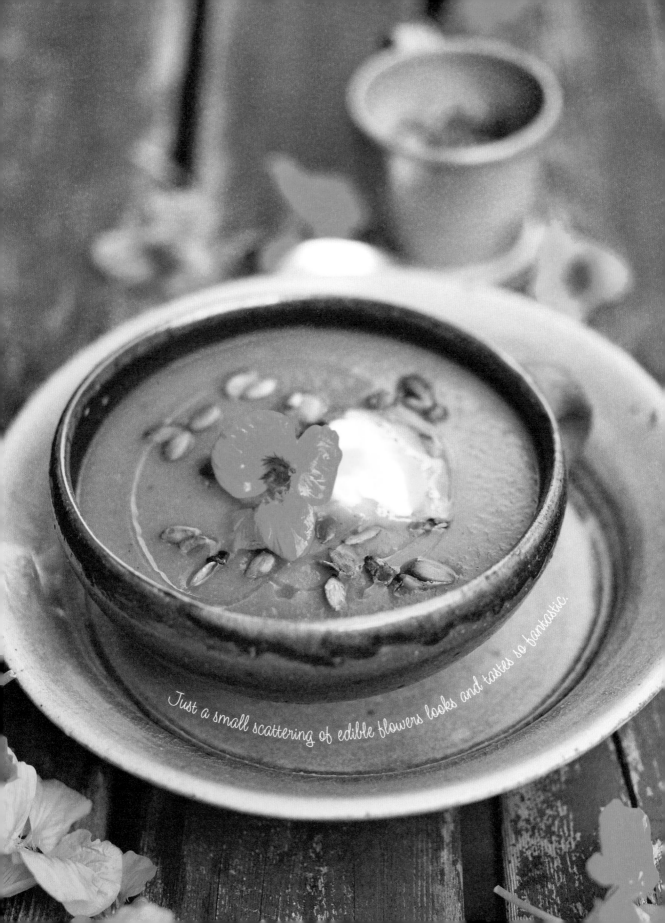

Just a small scattering of edible flowers looks and tastes so fantastic.

MINTED COURGETTE SOUP

This might not sound like the most epic of soups, but it really is absolutely delicious, fresh, and very straightforward to make. If you can, try to make use of the different coloured courgettes you can often get in good supermarkets or farmers' markets, and make sure you go for courgettes that are no bigger than twelve or fifteen centimetres long and are firm to the touch; spongy ones are never that great.

SERVES 4 TO 6

- 6 spring onions, trimmed
- 1kg green courgettes (or yellow, if you can get them)
- olive oil
- a knob of butter
- sea salt and ground pepper
- 1 lemon
- 8 sprigs of fresh mint
- 1.4 litres organic chicken or vegetable stock
- 5 heaped tablespoons soured cream
- 150g good-quality Cheddar cheese, freshly grated
- extra virgin olive oil

Finely slice the spring onions and courgettes by hand or in a food processor using the fine slicing attachment. Put them into a large pan on a medium low heat with a lug of olive oil, a knob of butter and a good pinch of salt and pepper. Grate in the zest of half the lemon, and pick in the mint leaves from 2 or 3 sprigs to get the flavours going. Give it all a good stir and cook for 40 minutes, stirring every 5 minutes or so. Make sure you control the temperature and don't let any courgettes catch. By slowly cooking down the courgettes like this you bring out an incredible sweetness – the trick to amazing flavour is slow frying and time.

When the 40 minutes is up you should have a soft, green-yellow courgette mush. Turn the heat up, pour in the stock and bring everything to the boil. Remove the pan from the heat and add 3 tablespoons of soured cream, the grated cheese, and the juice of the zested lemon half. Pick in the rest of the mint leaves, but put a few of the small ones into a cup of cold water and keep for garnish. Carefully pour the soup into a blender or liquidizer (you might need to do this in batches), or use a hand blender to purée it until smooth. Have a taste and correct the seasoning with salt, pepper, mint or lemon juice if required, and add a splash of water if the soup is a little too thick for your liking.

Feel free to reheat the soup gently, but don't boil it again because the cheese won't like it. If you're serving it cold, you'll probably need to add a little more water to thin it down because the cheese will start to thicken as the soup cools. Divide between your bowls, then let down the remaining soured cream with a splash of water until you get a good drizzling consistency and drizzle over the portions. Sprinkle over the reserved baby mint leaves and serve with a drizzle of extra virgin olive oil.

PS: Towards the end of summer, when it's getting a bit colder and nearing the end of the courgette season, it's quite nice to throw a handful of chickpeas or rice into this soup and just cook until everything is hot and lovely.

PPS: And also, if you're lucky enough to grow or have courgettes with flowers, a few of those flowers, torn into strips and added a few seconds before serving, is also really lovely.

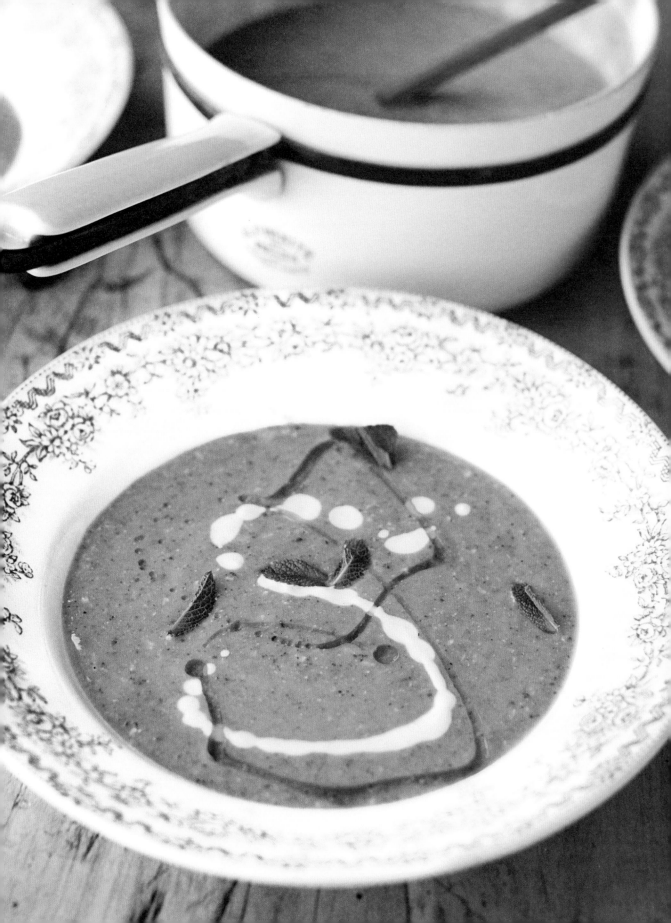

CAULIFLOWER CHEESE SOUP
CREAMY STILTON • BACON BITS • COUNTRY BREAD

You can create incredible, deep cauliflower flavour by stewing down the stalks first, then adding the florets later so they stay bright and delicious - by cooking one part slowly, and another quickly, you're getting the best of both worlds. I've used Stilton cheese in small quantities so there's a lovely hum of flavour, but if you're not really into it, another great British blue cheese or melting cheese will be lovely. There is an element of French onion 'soupiness' about this, but if you use brilliant British ingredients you'll find it's got a totally different personality. Give it a go; you'll love it.

SERVES 8

- a knob of butter
- olive oil
- 6 rashers of quality smoked streaky bacon
- 2 large onions
- 1 teaspoon Gentleman's Relish

- a small bunch of fresh thyme, leaves picked
- a few sprigs of fresh sage, leaves picked and finely sliced
- 1 large cauliflower
- sea salt and white pepper

- 2 litres organic chicken stock
- 9 big slices of rustic sourdough bread, 1cm thick
- a small bunch of fresh rosemary
- 100g Stilton cheese

Put a large pan on a medium heat and add a knob of butter and a drizzle of olive oil. Thinly slice the bacon and add it to the pan, then peel and finely chop the onions. The bacon should have good colour by now, so throw in the onions, Gentleman's Relish, thyme and sage leaves and give it all a good stir.

Cut the cauliflower in half, then cut off the florets and put them aside. Finely slice the stalk and any nice outer leaves. Throw the stalks and leaves into the pan with a good splash of water and a generous pinch of salt and pepper. Cook with a lid on over a medium low heat, stirring occasionally, for 40 minutes, or until really soft and intense. Mash up a bit to thicken it up, then cut the cauliflower florets into bite-sized pieces and add them to the pan with the stock. Turn the heat up, bring to the boil, then cover and reduce to a simmer for 10 to 15 minutes, or until the cauliflower florets are cooked through. Taste the broth and season to perfection with a pinch of salt and lots of pepper. Preheat the oven to 180°C/350°F/gas 4.

Meanwhile, start toasting your bread. As it comes out golden and hot, rub each piece of toast hard on both sides with the bunch of rosemary. Find a nice, deep, appropriately sized casserole dish or pan, or an earthenware soup terrine, around 25 x 20cm (whether round or rectangular, you want it about the size of an A4 sheet of paper). You're going to make three layers of soup, toast and cheese. Add a third of the soup, then lay or roughly tear 3 pieces of toast over the top and crumble over some of the cheese. Repeat the layers twice more, finishing with a final layer of 3 slices of toast to give a good covering. Spoon over any remaining broth and gently push the top layer of toast down so it sucks up the broth. Flick over any random bits of cheese or leftover rosemary, and drizzle with a little oil. Pop into the oven for around 25 minutes, or until golden and bubbling. You'll get a beautiful baked croutey-like top and when you cut into it you'll find softer chunks of bread and cauliflower underneath - which will be heavenly.

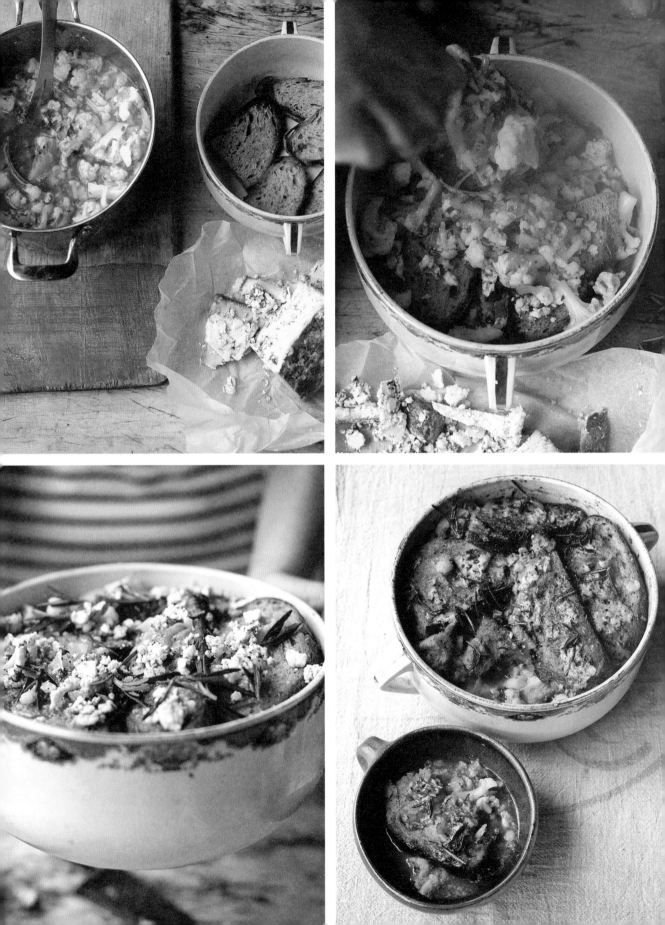

MIGHTY MULLIGATAWNY

This is a mighty, mighty soup with loads of personality. Ultimately, it evolved from a thinned-out stew-slash-curry cooked by Tamils during the years of the British Raj – after British soldiers stationed in India fell in love with it and asked for it to be tweaked to their tastes. When the soldiers came back home, this recipe came with them. Fast-forward 150 years and you'll find it on the shelves in your local corner store. I love the way recipes can evolve and travel to the other side of the world, so here is my version of this beautiful soup – evolved, yet again.

SERVES 6

- olive oil
- 250g quality minced beef
- 1 red onion, peeled and finely chopped
- 2 carrots, peeled and finely chopped
- 4 cloves of garlic, peeled and finely sliced
- 1 red pepper, deseeded and finely chopped

- a 3cm piece of fresh ginger, peeled and finely chopped
- 1 or 2 fresh red chillies, deseeded and finely chopped
- a small bunch of fresh coriander
- 1 heaped tablespoon Patak's Madras curry paste
- 1 tablespoon tomato purée
- sea salt and ground pepper

- 1 heaped tablespoon HP sauce
- 1.5 litres organic beef stock
- ½ a butternut squash (roughly 350g)
- a couple of sprigs of fresh thyme, leaves picked
- a couple of pinches of garam masala
- 1 cup basmati rice
- natural yoghurt, to serve

Put a large pan on a high heat and add a splash of olive oil and the minced beef. Cook for about 7 minutes, stirring occasionally and breaking up the mince, until it starts to turn golden and caramelize. Stir in the onion, carrot, garlic, red pepper, ginger and most of the chillies, and add a splash more oil, if needed. Cut the top leafy section off of the coriander and put aside in a cup of cold water for later. Finely chop the stalks and add to the pan. Cook and stir for around 10 minutes on a medium heat, or until the veg have softened.

Stir in the curry paste, tomato purée, a good pinch of salt and pepper and the HP sauce. After a few more minutes, when it smells fantastic, pour in the stock. Leave to blip away with the lid on over a medium heat for 40 minutes, stirring occasionally.

Meanwhile, cut the butternut squash into 1cm chunks, getting rid of any seeds and gnarly bits (there's no need to peel it). Put a smaller pan on a high heat. Add a lug of olive oil and the squash. Stir in the thyme leaves and the garam masala. Pop a lid on the pan and cook for around 10 minutes on a medium heat, stirring every few minutes, until softened and golden. Add a cup of rice to the pan with 2 cups of water (use the same cup for both measures) and a good pinch of salt and pepper. Replace the lid and cook for around 8 minutes on a medium heat, then turn the heat off and leave to steam for 8 minutes with the lid on.

Fluff up the rice and tip it into the soup. Have a taste, and season if needed. Gently mix together, then divide between your soup bowls with a good dollop of natural yoghurt. Scatter over the coriander leaves and add a sprinkling of fresh chilli, if you like.

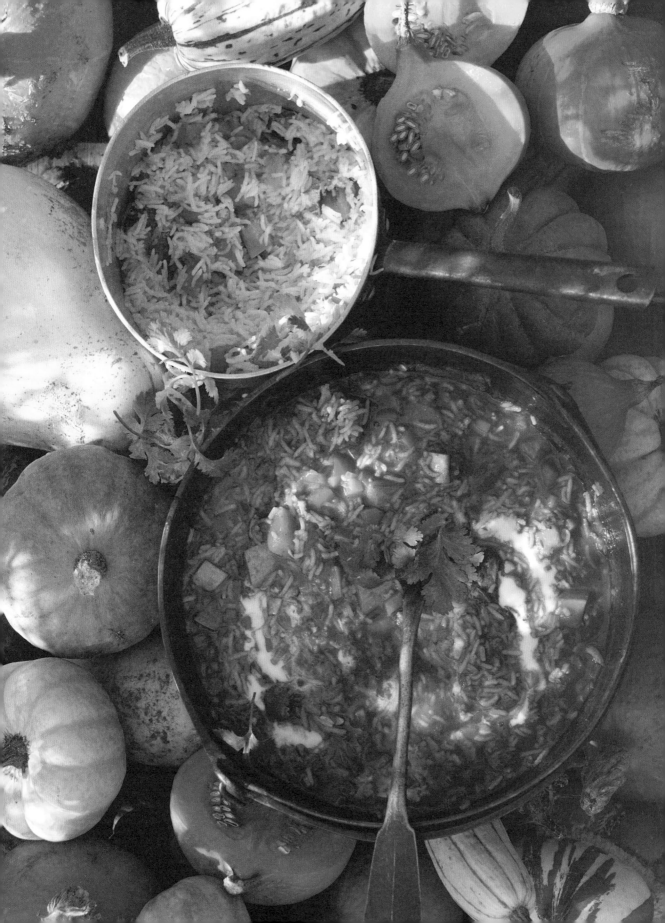

CHESTNUT PUMPKIN SOUP
DRIED PORCINI MUSHROOMS • HOT SAGE BREAD

A bowl of this spectacularly delicious soup feels like a cuddle from your granny. Fresh chestnuts are so easy to slit, roast and peel, and they create a really nutty sweet flavour in this soup. But you can also buy them already peeled and vac-packed, which makes this dish smooth and lovely, not to mention convenient. I love them both, so it's your choice.

SERVES 6 TO 8

- 2 rashers of quality smoked streaky bacon
- 2 red onions, peeled
- 1 butternut squash (roughly 1kg)
- a few sprigs of fresh rosemary, leaves picked
- 50g dried porcini or mixed wild mushrooms
- olive oil
- 400g fresh roasted and peeled, or vac-packed chestnuts
- 1 dried chilli
- a handful of pearl barley or rice
- 1.2 litres organic chicken stock
- 1 loaf of rustic country bread
- a bunch of fresh sage
- salt and ground pepper

Roughly chop the bacon and onions into 1cm pieces, and do the same to the butternut squash after you've sliced it in half lengthways and deseeded it (be careful – I'll show you a fast, safe way to do this if you go to *www.jamieoliver.com/how-to*). Finely chop the rosemary leaves. Soak the porcini mushrooms in a cup of boiling water, and after about 5 minutes stir with a fork so any bits of grit sink to the bottom.

Put the bacon into a large casserole-type pan on a high heat with a swig of olive oil. After a minute, when it starts to get golden, add the rosemary, crumble in the chestnuts, and add half the dried chilli. Stir and fry for 3 to 4 minutes; while that's happening, pull out the porcini mushrooms from the cup (keep the liquid) and add them to the pan with the onions, squash and pearl barley (if using wild mushrooms, tear them into the pan now). Cook and stir for around 10 minutes, then pour in about three-quarters of the mushroom water, discarding the rest. Just cover with hot stock. Bring to the boil, then reduce the heat and simmer for around 40 minutes. Turn the oven to 180°C/350°F/gas 4.

Use a serrated knife to crudely cut 8 deep scores in your loaf of bread, stopping before you cut through the base so the loaf still holds together. Get your whole bunch of sage, rip off the stalks, then scrunch up the leaves to get the oils going. Drizzle the bunch all over with olive oil and a good pinch of salt, toss it around, and when every leaf is coated, quickly stuff the sprigs into all the cut sections of the bread. Put to one side. When your soup has 15 minutes to go, pop your bread into the oven to crisp up, remembering to keep an eye on it.

When the time is up on your soup, check that the squash is cooked through, then have a taste and correct the seasoning. If you want a bit more heat, crumble in a little more of your dried chilli. At this point, you can leave the soup crude and brothy, which I sort of love; or blitz a quarter of it up in a blender and return that to the pan for a mixture of chunky and smooth; or whiz up the whole lot in a liquidizer so it's silky and smooth. Serve with warm hunks of that hot crispy sage bread and it will be absolutely delicious.

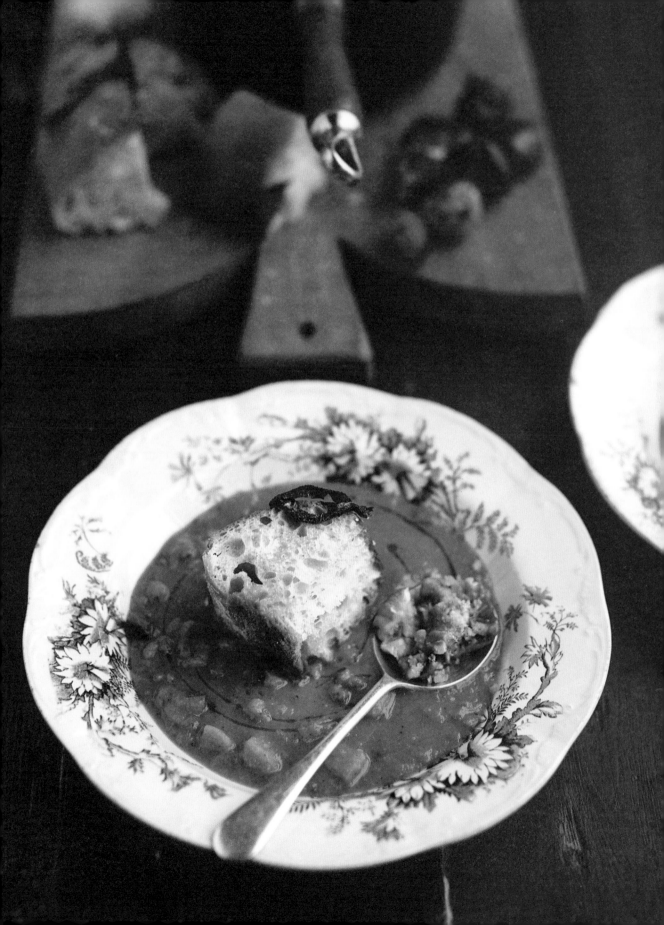

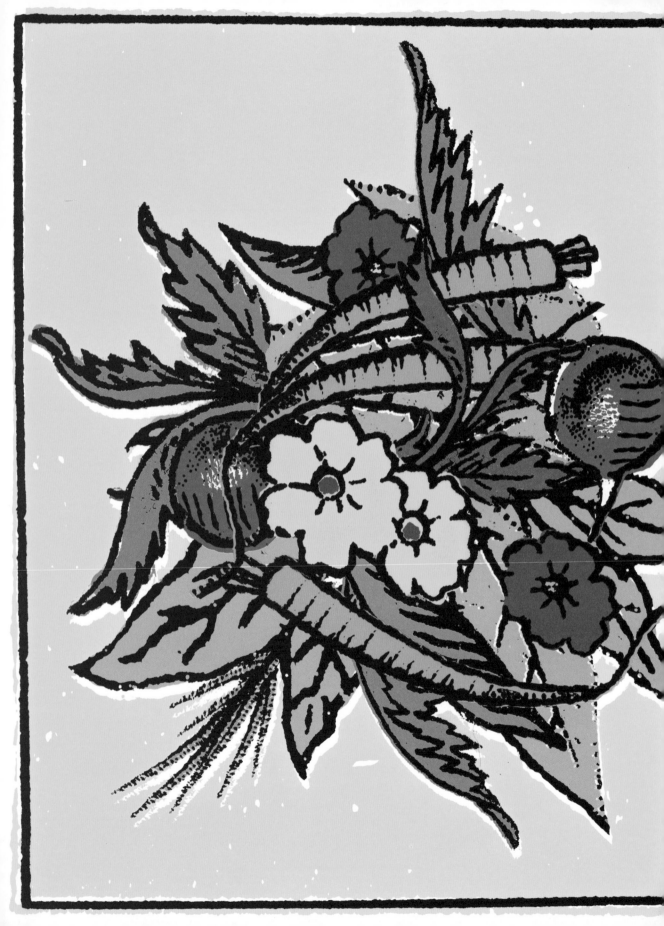

SALADS

Salads are something I've always been passionate about. I love dreaming them up, making them and eating them. Historically, salads were mainly eaten by the upper classes because they weren't filling enough to keep the workers going all day in the fields and factories. But now of course, they're much more accessible, not to mention incredibly diverse. In this chapter you'll find exciting side salads, quick salads you can have for lunch or stuff inside sandwiches, and hearty salads like the roast chicken bread salad, which is filling enough to have for a lunch or dinner. All of them make use of our beautiful seasonal ingredients, and some mix hot crispy meaty elements with cold beautiful veggies. Some of the brilliant flavoured vinegars I've done on page 388 would set these salads off brilliantly, so have a look at those and enjoy.

APPLE & WATERCRESS SALAD
BLUE CHEESE DRESSING • CRUSHED WALNUTS

All these ingredients are quintessentially British, and this salad is best when it's assembled at the last minute. It's lovely as a starter, or as part of a picnic or potluck dinner, and works a treat with a crispy bit of pork. The combination of watercress, crunchy apples and mild blue cheese is a classic through and through. The joy in eating this is having perfect thin round slices of apple, so if you don't already have a mandoline slicer, it's worth adding one to your kitchen kit. It will make life so much easier and make you look so much better – you can pick one up for around 15 quid.

SERVES 4

For the dressing
- 1 spring onion, trimmed
- 50g mild blue cheese, plus extra for crumbling over
- 3 tablespoons natural yoghurt
- 3 tablespoons cider vinegar
- a pinch of sea salt and pepper
- extra virgin olive oil

For the salad
- 2 nice eating apples, red and green if you can get them
- a handful of whole shelled walnuts
- 2 x 100g bags of watercress, washed and ready to eat

Blitz the dressing ingredients in a liquidizer with a few lugs of extra virgin olive oil, then have a taste to make sure the dressing is really good and delicious and the salt and acidity is slightly too much. Once you are happy with it, set aside.

Wash the apples, remove their stalks, then carefully slice them, core and all (this is the best bit), ideally using a mandoline slicer with a finger guard. If you don't have a mandoline, either slice as thinly as you can, or use the thin slicer of a food processor. Slice, chop, or bash up your walnuts. Put big pinches of watercress all over a serving platter and arrange the thin slices of apple on top. Sprinkle over the walnuts, then drizzle over your dressing. Some apples won't go brown because they have a higher acidity level – others will. If yours do, just squeeze a little lemon juice over them to slow this down. Drizzle over a little extra virgin olive oil, crumble over a little blue cheese, and serve with a pint of beer.

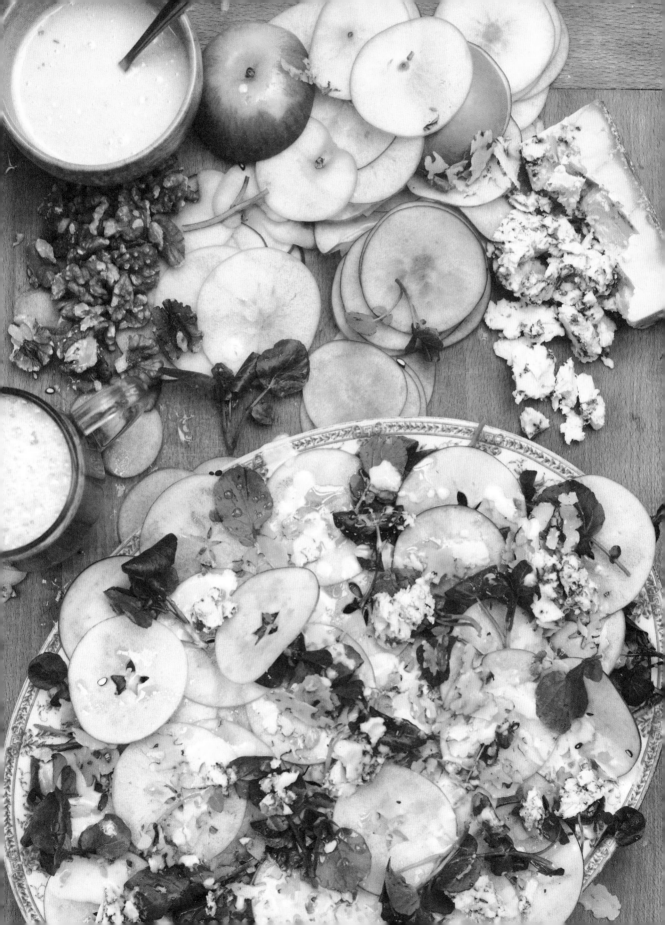

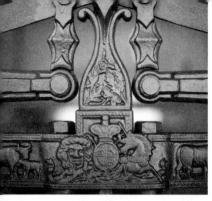

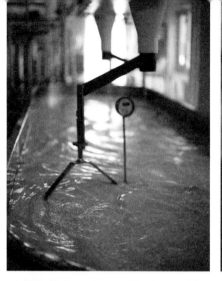

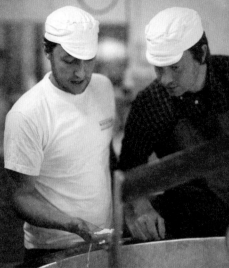

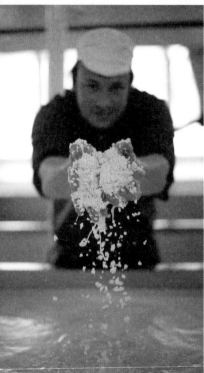

Westcombe Dairy Farm

I had the complete pleasure of making the famous Westcombe Cheddar with its young and enthusiastic owner, Tom Calver. The cheese is fantastic, and it's so reassuring to see young Brits pushing through and sustaining really high standards of British cheese by bringing new ideas to our old traditions, and by their attention to detail. Well done, Tom.

www.westcombedairy.com

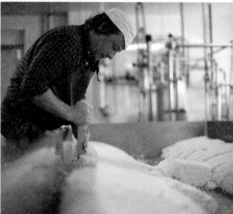

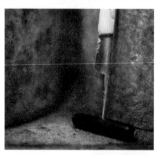

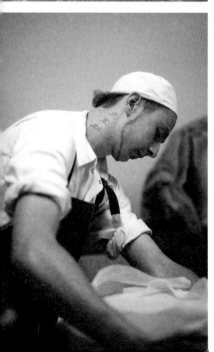

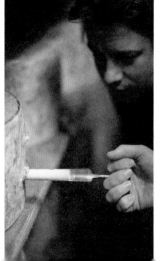

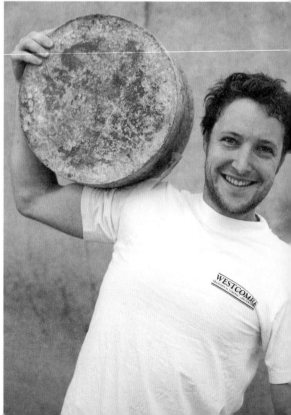

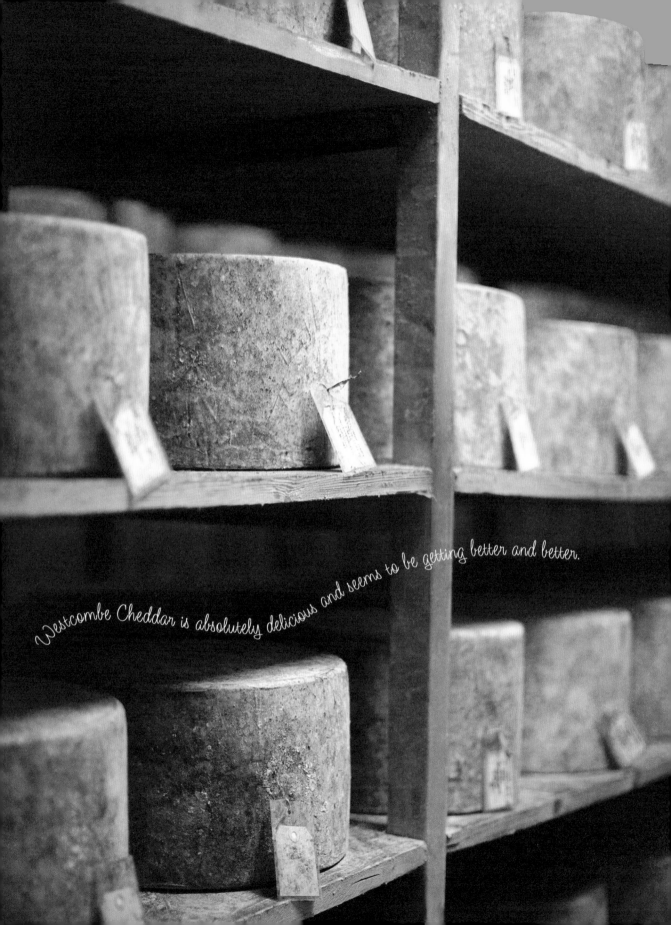

Westcombe Cheddar is absolutely delicious and seems to be getting better and better.

BABY BROAD BEAN SALAD
APPLE MATCHSTICKS • CRUMBLY CHEESE

I realize it's unusual to ask you to eat whole broad beans raw, but they are so unbelievably good if you catch them just before they're fully grown, when the beans are 1cm big (between May and June in the UK). When you pick them just before they are fully grown, the protective body around the bean itself hasn't become stringy and tough – so you get this amazing grassy sweetness of the baby beans and the cucumbery watermelonyness of the pod that surrounds it. I know this little window of time is a bit limiting, but just stick a note in your calendar to remind you when they're in season and pull this book off the shelf when early summer rolls around.

Saying that, if you miss this window and your beans have grown bigger, you can take them out of the pods and skins and still serve them this way with a bit of rocket, or use baby spinach and fresh peas instead. So at the beginning of the season, get a bean and bite into it – pod and all. If it's a pleasure, you're rocking and rolling. If not, pod the rest of them and go to page 90.

SERVES 2 AS A MAIN OR 4 AS A SIDE

- 1 or 2 large handfuls of fresh unpodded young broad beans
- 1 crunchy red apple
- 4 sprigs of fresh mint
- 1 lemon
- extra virgin olive oil
- sea salt and ground pepper
- *optional:* 1 fresh chilli, halved and deseeded (added to your taste)
- a 50g wedge of crumbly cheese such as Lancashire or a good Cheddar

Wash the broad bean pods and trim the stalky ends, then carefully slice them about 1cm thick at a fairly steep angle to give you long beautiful slivers of green broad bean, delicate fluffy insides and outer pod. Put them into a nice salad bowl. Cut the apple into thin slices, about 0.25cm thick, then cut these into delicate matchsticks as finely as you can and add them to the bowl too. Cutting fruit and veg into matchsticks isn't hard, but if you want to watch a video and learn how to do this easily go to *www.jamieoliver.com/how-to*.

Pick the mint leaves, roll them up, then finely slice them and add them to the salad bowl. Squeeze in the juice of the lemon, and the same amount of good-quality extra virgin olive oil, add a pinch of salt and pepper, then toss and mix well together. Have a taste – it should be seasoned and slightly too lemony, because by the time the cheese has been crumbled on top it will be perfection. Sometimes I'll finely chop up some chilli at this point and sprinkle it over, but that's up to you. Put the dressed salad on a large platter to share between two people, or divide between two plates. Use a knife to slice and crumble the cheese into a few nuggets over the top. It's heavenly and delicious – especially with pork chops or roast chicken.

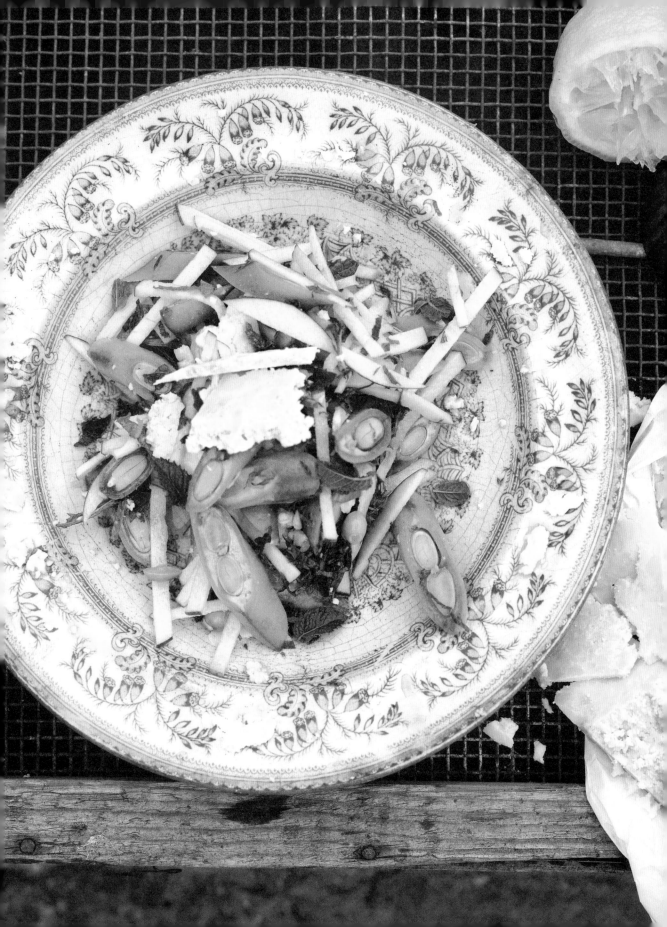

BIG BEEFY TOMATO SALAD

The dressing on this salad seems to make the tomatoes taste even sweeter, while delicately pickling and dressing them at the same time. When you grow your own tomatoes, the flavour is absolutely incredible. There are so many shapes and personalities of tomato and it's those home-grown ones that are really going to wow people in a salad like this, so you should definitely check out the websites below for some ideas or simply go to Homebase, where I've got some crackers.

You don't need to have loads of land to successfully grow a crop of your own; tomatoes are robust and really will grow pretty much anywhere with sun, soil and water. I've grown them in windowboxes, in buckets, on roofs, and my mate has grown them on the 36th floor of a tower block, so it can be done.

SERVES 4 TO 6 AS A SIDE

- 750g ripe large or beef tomatoes, mixed colours if you can get them
- sea salt and ground pepper
- 1 heaped teaspoon dried dill
- 4 tablespoons extra virgin olive oil
- 2 tablespoons red wine vinegar
- 1 level teaspoon caster sugar
- ½ a clove of garlic, peeled
- *optional:* 1 teaspoon fresh or jarred horseradish

Cut the tomatoes into random big chunks, around 2.5cm, and put them into a large bowl with a good pinch of salt and pepper. Add the dried dill, extra virgin olive oil, red wine vinegar and sugar, then finely grate over the garlic (a few gratings of fresh horseradish or a little jarred horseradish [see page 383] at this point can also be amazing).

Toss everything together and leave for 5 minutes to give the flavours a chance to really get in there. Using clean hands, serve on a large platter and let everyone help themselves. Any leftovers can be kept in the fridge, then blitzed up with a cucumber, watercress and some mint leaves for an English gazpacho.

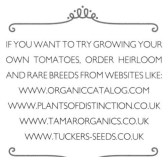

IF YOU WANT TO TRY GROWING YOUR OWN TOMATOES, ORDER HEIRLOOM AND RARE BREEDS FROM WEBSITES LIKE:
WWW.ORGANICCATALOG.COM
WWW.PLANTSOFDISTINCTION.CO.UK
WWW.TAMARORGANICS.CO.UK
WWW.TUCKERS-SEEDS.CO.UK

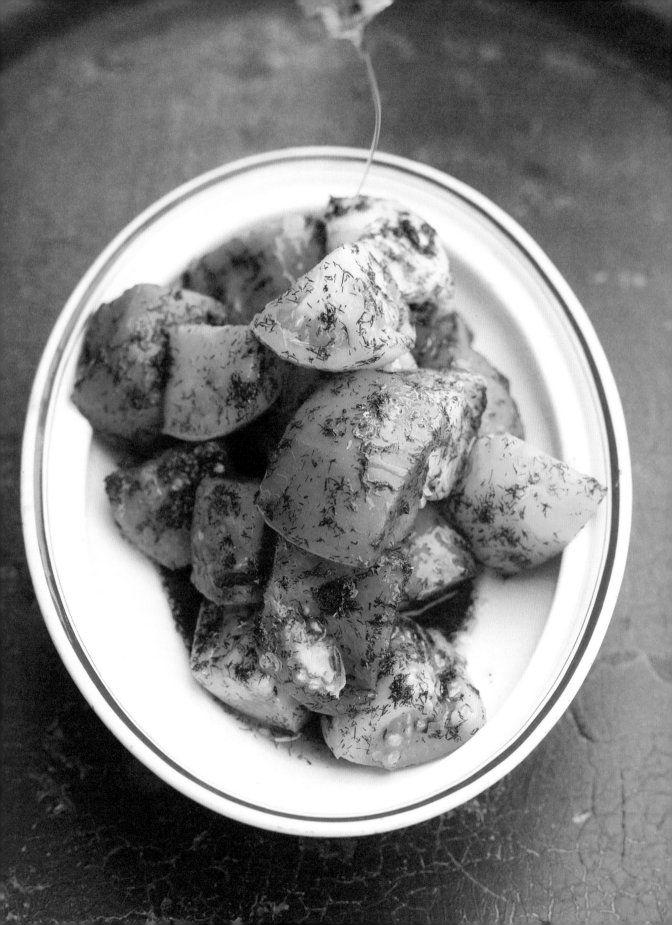

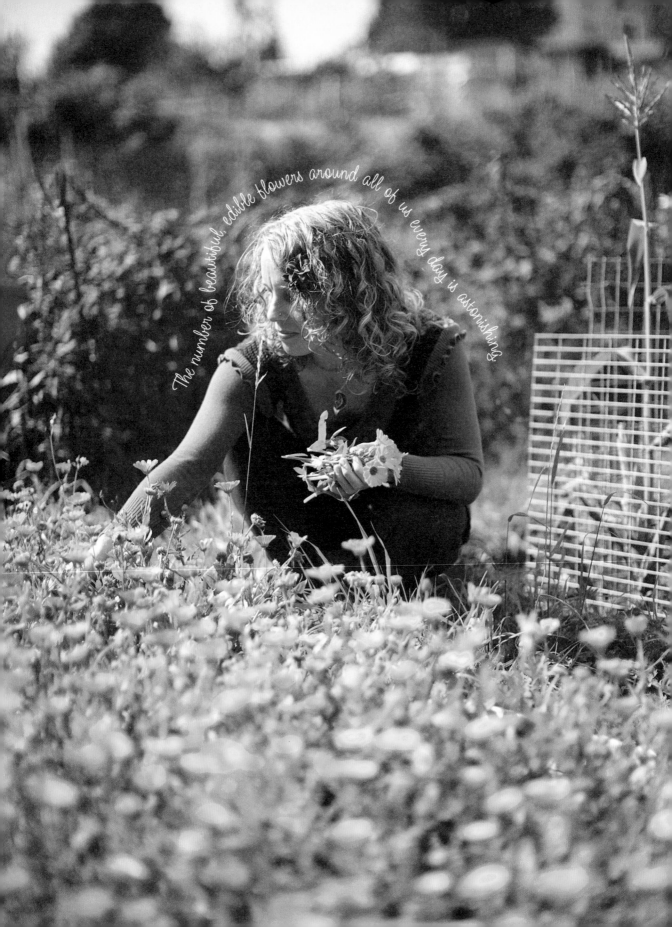

The number of beautiful, edible flowers around all of us every day is astonishing.

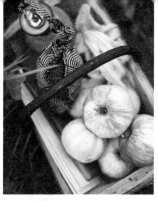

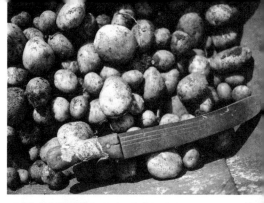

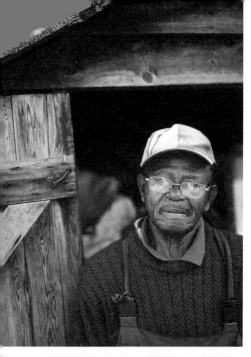

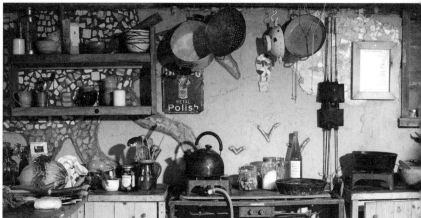

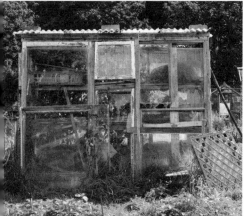

Bristol Allotments

Leona is a lovely young lady who works at the Boiling Wells café in Bristol. She is a true foodie, and she always cooks with food picked in the urban allotments. Allotments have been part of British culture for many years, and local authorities are obliged to make more space available as allotments run out, but I'm sure they won't do it without a push, so if you want one, go fight for it.

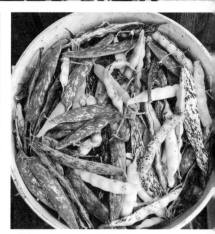

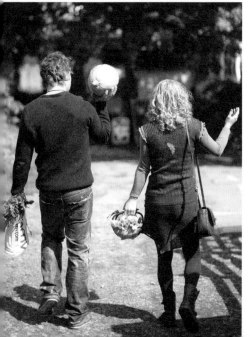

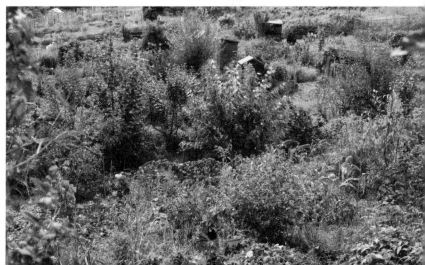

CRUNCHY ALLOTMENT SALAD

I adore this recipe. It transforms vegetables that some people might consider boring into something exciting, crunchy and stylish. It will complement almost anything, whether you have it with roast chicken, a beef burger or between slices of crusty bread with nice cheese. There are no rules - basically any crunchy colourful veg will work - so try all colours of beets and carrots, radishes, mouli, celeriac, kohlrabi, fennel, baby courgettes, cucumber … a gesture of fruit like apples or pears will rock too - just mix it up, baby!

SERVES 4

- 1 beetroot
- 1 carrot
- 1 bulb of fennel
- ¼ of a cucumber
- a small bunch of radishes, or other crunchy veg
- sea salt and ground pepper

- 4 tablespoons cider vinegar
- a handful of mixed fresh soft herbs, such as mint, tarragon, flat-leaf parsley and basil, leaves picked
- extra virgin olive oil

Peel and trim vegetables such as beets and carrots, then slice everything thinly, or just do what I do and whack them through a food processor with a thin slicing attachment (it's so easy, why wouldn't you?). There's no right or wrong way, you just want to make everything delicious to eat. If the tops of your radishes are nice and small, feel free to leave them on.

Put all the prepped veg into a bowl, add a really good pinch of salt and pepper and the cider vinegar, and toss everything together about five or six times over a 10-minute period. This is a light pickle-style dressing that will amplify the wonderful natural flavours of the vegetables. You can either serve the salad straight away, or pop it into the fridge until needed.

Before serving, finely chop or slice the leaves of your soft herbs and add them to the bowl with a good lug or two of extra virgin olive oil. Give everything one last toss, then have a taste to check the seasoning. Use your fingers and thumbs like a basket to pick it all up and pile it on a plate. Drizzle over a little more extra virgin olive oil and serve.

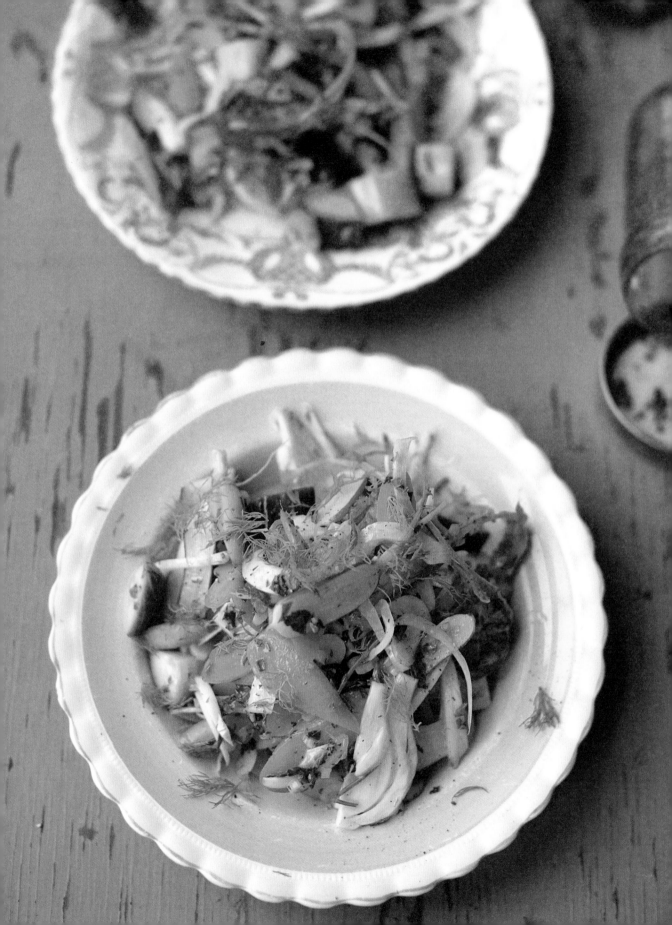

SHREDDED RAINBOW SALAD

This is probably one of the nicest and quickest salads you could ever make. I think my record is about 40 seconds thanks to the magic of food processors. They turn the everyday veg and cabbage that might be sitting in your fridge right now into something light, pretty and wonderful. It's amazing with meat, fish and all sorts of other dishes. I never want to be presumptuous about what you have or what you've seen, but there are incredible varieties of beetroot and carrot available: white, yellow, pink, candy-cane … and the greater the variety of colours of the vegetables you use, the more beautiful it will be. If you make a big batch like this, it will keep for a day in the fridge and still be crunchy and lovely. You do need a large food processor bowl for this, so if yours is a bit small make two smaller batches instead.

SERVES 8 AS A SIDE SALAD

- 2 raw beetroots (different colours if available), scrubbed hard, tops cut off, quartered
- ¼ of a red cabbage, quartered
- 2 large carrots (it's really nice if you have different colours), scrubbed and trimmed
- ¼ of a white cabbage, quartered
- 2 pears, stalks removed, quartered
- 2 handfuls of curly parsley or fresh mint
- 2 big handfuls of shelled walnuts

To serve
- mayonnaise
- English mustard
- cider vinegar
- extra virgin olive oil
- sea salt and ground pepper
- Worcestershire sauce
- Tabasco sauce

Put the coarse grater attachment into the food processor and push through all the ingredients in the following order, so that the juice from the red cabbage and beets doesn't stain everything else: beets, red cabbage, carrots, white cabbage and finally pears. Turn the contents of the bowl out on to a platter so you get a pile of rainbow colours.

Finely chop the parsley and sprinkle it on top of the vegetables. Roughly bash up the walnuts in a pestle and mortar and serve on the side with the dressing condiments.

I like putting the platter down in the middle of the table so one person can dress it for everyone. A tablespoon of mayo, a few teaspoons of mustard, 2 or 3 tablespoons of vinegar and then double that amount of extra virgin olive oil should do the trick once tossed through and seasoned well. Add a few drips of Worcestershire sauce, and a tiny drip of Tabasco if you like. Sprinkle over some of the bashed nuts, then grab a big pinch of the salad and place it on top. Toss and mix everything together until you get a big beautiful plate of dressed veg. Taste to check the seasoning, and tuck in. Or let everyone make their own so they can tweak the seasoning to their own specific tastes.

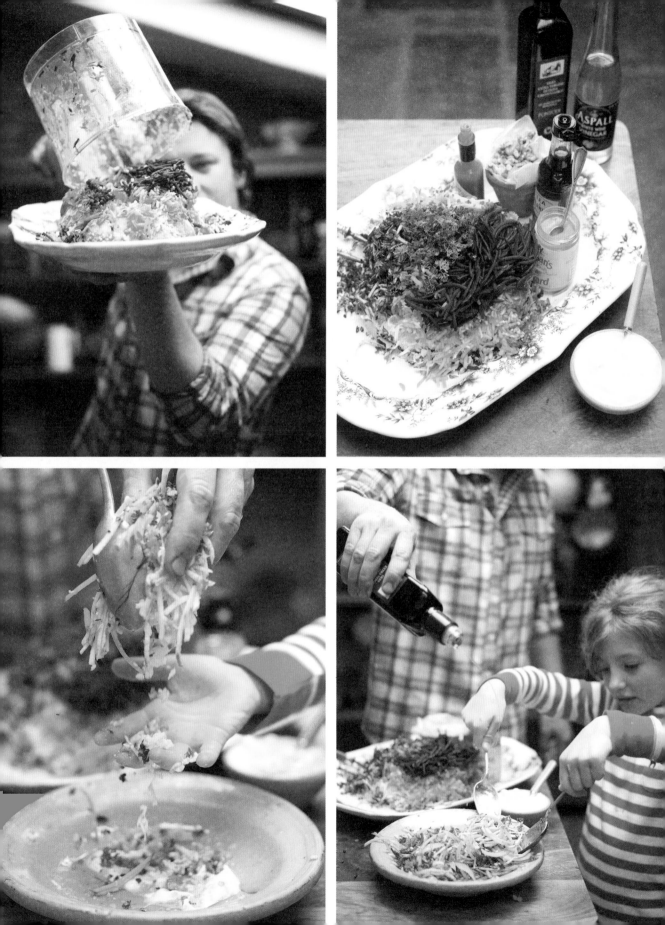

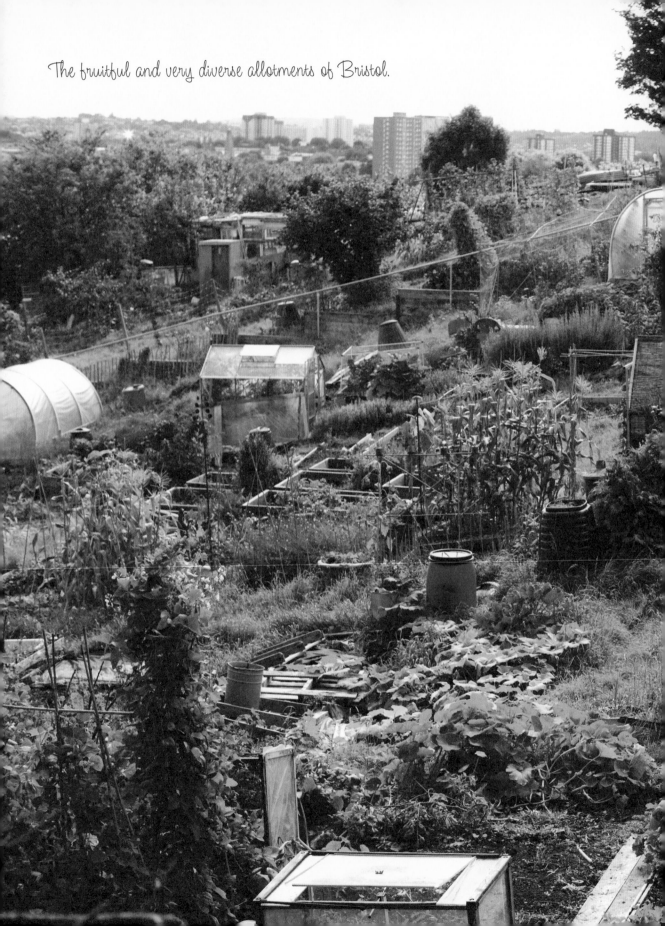

The fruitful and very diverse allotments of Bristol.

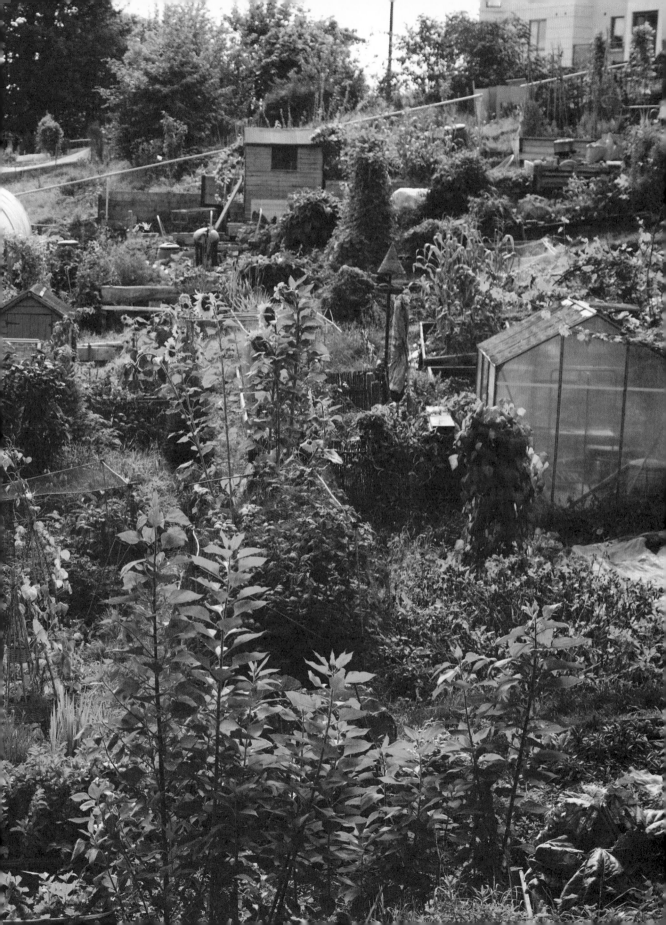

WARM CRISPY DUCK SALAD
GIANT TOASTS • CLEMENTINE DRESSING

Two giant toasts, a robust winter salad and crispy duck; this really is a heavenly dish. It's a cross between a warm salad and an open-faced sandwich. Just put it in the middle of the table and let everyone rip and tear it up - I can promise you there'll be nothing left.

SERVES 6

- 1 duck
- olive oil
- sea salt and ground pepper
- 1 tablespoon five-spice, or 1 teaspoon each of ground spices such as nutmeg, cinnamon, cloves, ginger

- 50g dried sour cherries
- 1 loaf of sourdough bread or a bloomer
- red wine vinegar
- 2 cloves of garlic
- 2 sprigs of fresh rosemary
- 6 clementines or 4 blood oranges

- a little runny honey
- 4 tablespoons extra virgin olive oil
- 2 red chicory
- 2 white chicory
- 4 handfuls of washed watercress
- 4 sprigs of fresh mint

Preheat the oven to 180°C/350°F/gas 4. Put the duck into a roasting tray and rub it all over with a good drizzle of olive oil, a good pinch of salt and pepper and the five-spice, or the mixed ground spices, then roast in the oven for 2 hours, or until tender and crispy skinned. Put the dried cherries into a bowl and just cover them with boiling water to rehydrate them.

After 2 hours get the duck out of the oven and move it to a board. Cut the bread into 2cm slices lengthways. Very carefully, pour most of the fat from the roasting tray into a clean jam jar, leaving about 4 tablespoons behind (that jar of fat will keep brilliantly in the fridge for a couple of months and be great for roast veg). Add a few splashes of vinegar to the tray to help pull up all the sticky bits, then use a garlic crusher to crush in the garlic cloves. Pick in the rosemary leaves, then use the bread to wipe up all those flavours. Lay the slices juicy side up in the tray, sprinkle over the rehydrated sour cherries, and whack into the oven for around 10 minutes.

To make the dressing, zest 2 of the clementines into a small bowl and squeeze in the juice of 3. (If you're using blood oranges, zest 1 orange and squeeze in the juice of 2.) Mix in 4 tablespoons of red wine vinegar, a good pinch of salt and pepper, a drizzle of honey and the extra virgin olive oil. Have a taste - this dressing should have attitude and be slightly too acidic and salty.

Halve the chicory, finely slice the stalk end and take apart the leaves. Put them into a large bowl with the watercress. Peel the remaining clementines and slice them into rounds, then pick the mint leaves.

Pull all the crispy skin off your duck. Take the tray of bread out of the oven. At this point it should be golden, but still soft in the middle. Quickly pull the duck skin apart over the bread and return the tray to the oven for 4 to 5 minutes, while you use two forks to pull and shred every last bit of duck meat off the carcass, getting rid of any bones or wobbly bits. Spoon a few tablespoons of the salad dressing over the pile of shredded meat to stop it drying out.

Once you've got perfect crispy toasts, place them crisscrossed on a serving platter. Add the shredded meat to the bowl of salad leaves along with the remaining dressing and quickly toss everything together, then scatter the salad over the croutons with the clementine slices and mint leaves. Eat before the warm meat wilts the salad.

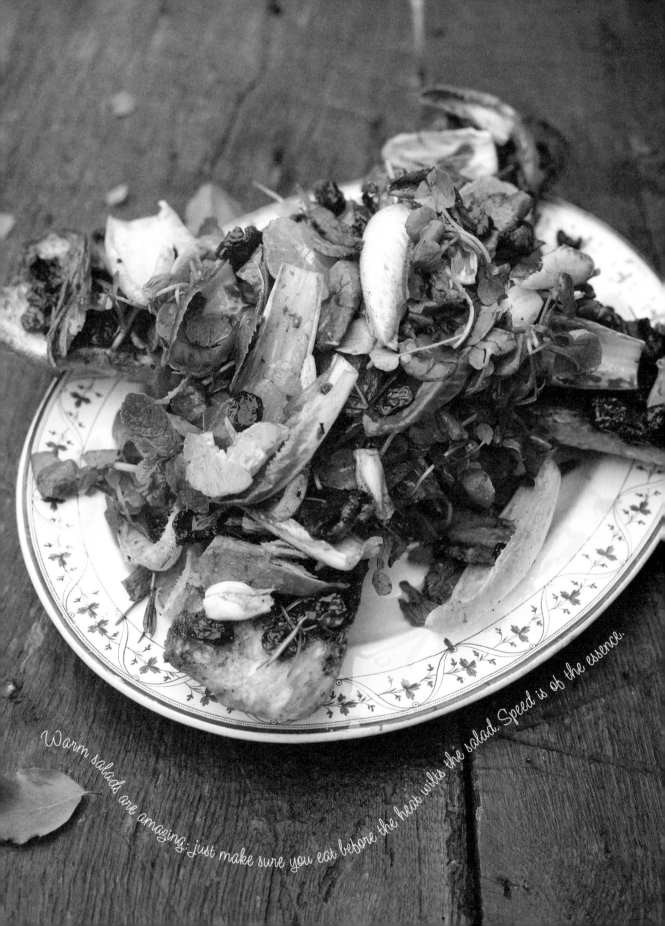

Warm salads are amazing; just make sure you eat before the heat wilts the salad. Speed is of the essence.

SUPER-QUICK SALADS

Grated Apple and Beetroot Salad

Wash 2 large **beetroots** and a nice **red eating apple**, then use the coarse side of a box grater to grate them, one after the other, on to a platter. Drizzle over a couple of tablespoons of **cider vinegar** and the same amount of **rapeseed/extra virgin olive oil**. Season with **sea salt** and **ground pepper**, then sprinkle over some chopped **chives** or **chive flowers**, and any small **beetroot leaves** if you've got them. Toss together just before serving, adjusting the dressing if need be.

Pickly Cucumber and Red Onion Salad with Loads of Dill

Scratch a fork down and all around the length of a **cucumber**, then slice it on an angle into 1cm slices and put the slices into a bowl. Grate over half a peeled **red onion**, using the coarse side of a box grater. Add a few generous splashes of **white wine vinegar** and a pinch or two of **sea salt**. Pick and roughly chop a very small bunch of **fresh dill** and sprinkle over. Leave for about 30 minutes to get cold and to marinate, if you can, before serving with a drizzle of **rapeseed/extra virgin olive oil**, to intensify the pickled flavours.

Broad Bean and Bacon with Mint and Lemon Juice

Fry 4 rashers of **quality smoked streaky bacon** until lovely and crisp, then allow to cool. Take 4 large handfuls of young **broad beans** (if you end up using older beans, gently squeeze them out of their pods and their skins), and place in a serving bowl. Add a tiny pinch of **sea salt** and **ground pepper**, then snap over your crispy bacon, tear over a few little **mint leaves**, and add 1 or 2 drizzles of **rapeseed/extra virgin olive oil** and a few good squeezes of **lemon juice**. Have a taste, adjust the seasoning if necessary, and serve.

Crunchy Radish and Tarragon Salad

Scrub a bunch of **radishes**, then, depending on their size, halve, quarter or slice them, leaving a few of their tender leaves on, and put them in a serving bowl. Roughly chop a handful of **tarragon leaves** and sprinkle all over the radishes. Dress with a splash of **red wine vinegar**, the same amount of **rapeseed/extra virgin olive oil**, a pinch of **sea salt** and **ground pepper**, and serve. Also delicious with a few chopped grapes and a sprinkling of feta cheese if you fancy.

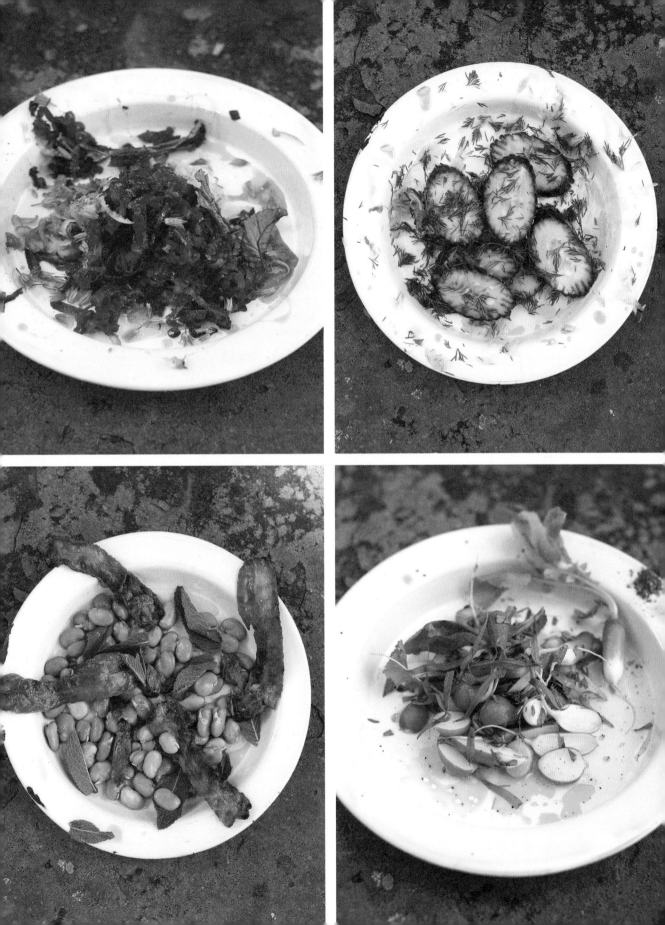

SHAVED FENNEL SALAD
ANCHOVIES • CELERY HEART • LEMON

This is an absolutely delicious salad. It's beautiful with grilled meat, fish and cheese, and lovely in both winter and summer … basically whenever you can get your hands on a nice fat bulb of fennel with herby tops. On the day I made this I created a strange frozen plate to serve it on (don't ask why). I simply poured water into a round tray, threw in a few lavender flowers and herbs for prettiness, then whacked it into the freezer. A few hours later it had set, so I turned it out and used it for a plate. It sounds like a funny thing to do, but everyone loved it and most importantly, it amplified the freshness of the fennel by making it crunchy and cold. It's a bit camp and a bit Martha Stewart, but life is short - so viva la Martha!

SERVES 4 AS A GENEROUS SIDE

- 8-10 salted anchovy fillets in oil
- 1 lemon
- 1 large fennel bulb, or 2 smaller bulbs, with herby tops
- 1 head of celery, with leaves
- extra virgin olive oil
- sea salt and ground pepper

Finely slice your anchovies lengthways (save the oil from their jar or tin in the freezer, to use when roasting lamb or cooking pasta sauces, greens or stews another day). Put the sliced anchovies into a mug, squeeze in the lemon juice and leave to sit for 10 minutes to calm down their strong flavour. If you aren't an anchovy fan, you have to trust me that they will get lost in this salad and act as a seasoning element, rather than something fishy.

Get your fennel bulb and pick off the nice fennel tops. Trim and discard the bare ends from the base, then finely slice the fennel using either your good knife skills, a mandoline slicer, a speed-peeler to peel the fennel into slices, or the fine slicing attachment of a food processor, which is what I do. Put the sliced fennel into a large bowl with the delicate leafy tops.

Click off the outer sticks of celery and put them into the fridge for another time. You only need the bottom part of the celery for the heart, so cut off the top half and put that in the fridge too. Trim the stalk and bare ends of the heart. Wash well and pick off any yellow leaves to use later, then finely slice or speed-peel the celery heart and throw it into the bowl with the fennel.

By now your anchovies should be perfect, so stir in a generous lug of extra virgin olive oil to balance out the lemon. Have a taste and adjust the seasoning so it's slightly too lemony and too salty. Quickly toss the dressing and salad together and serve immediately on a lovely platter. For me, the best results come from serving this cold and crunchy, with other things that are hot for contrast, like slices of toasted bread or a piece of grilled fish.

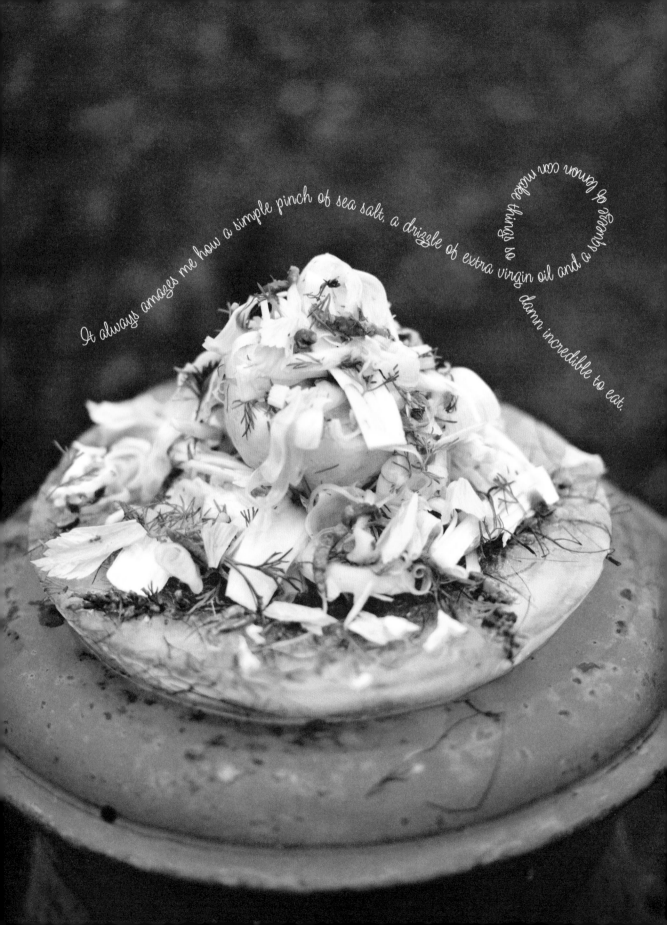

It always amazes me how a simple pinch of sea salt, a drizzle of extra virgin oil and a squeeze of lemon can make things so damn incredible to eat.

HEAVENLY SALMON SALAD
LOVELY NEW POTATOES • FRESH CUCUMBER DILL DRESSING

Salmon and new potatoes is a combo that works every time, but only on the proviso that you don't overcook the salmon, as many people often do. This salad is fresh, zingy and simplicity itself. Eating a plate of this makes you feel clean and healthy, so it's a brilliant lunch or dinner. Of course you can make this at any time of year, but it really is beautiful in the summer when the best new potatoes are in season and you've got a chilled glass of white wine nearby.

SERVES 4

For the salad
- 700g fillet of salmon, skin on, scaled and pin-boned
- sea salt and ground pepper
- a small knob of butter
- olive oil

- I lemon
- 600g baby new potatoes, scrubbed clean
- a small bunch of fresh mint
- a small bunch of fresh dill

For the cucumber dressing
- extra virgin olive oil
- I cucumber
- 2 lemons
- 4 heaped tablespoons thick Greek yoghurt

Preheat your oven to 180°C/350°F/gas 4. Get a large square of tin foil and put your salmon, skin side down, in the middle of it. Rub your fish with salt, pepper, a knob of butter, a drizzle of olive oil and a small squeeze of lemon juice. Fold the tin foil up into a bag, make sure the ends are sealed, then pop it on to a tray and cook in the hot oven for exactly 12 minutes. Once the time is up, remove and leave to cool in the bag.

Meanwhile, put the new potatoes into a large pan with enough boiling, generously salted water to cover. Hold the mint and dill bunches together, rip the top 5cm of each bunch off and put aside, then tie up the stalks and add to the water with the potatoes.

How fast your potatoes will cook depends on how 'new' they are. The fresher they are, the faster they'll cook, so after 8 to 10 minutes taste one. If it eats well and is tender, they're done. Drain the potatoes, remove and discard the herb stalks, then tip the potatoes back into the pan. If they are small, leave them whole, if they are larger, use your fingers to squash them or halve or quarter them, then put them on a nice serving platter. Season well with a pinch of salt and pepper and a good squeeze of lemon juice.

Quickly make your dressing. Get a mixing bowl and put in a good lug of extra virgin olive oil and a pinch of salt and pepper. You can finely chop the reserved dill and mint leaves and grate the cucumber by all means, but what I like to do is cut into the cucumber lengthways, but not all the way through, so it stays in one piece, then stuff the dill and mint into the cut and grate it on the coarse side of a box grater. It's a Japanese technique that really bruises the herbs and gets great flavours out of everything. Grate it on to a board, then add to the mixing bowl. Use the fine side of the grater to zest in a lemon (save a little bit for garnish), then squeeze in all the juice from one lemon. Stir in the yoghurt, and season really well to taste.

Once the salmon has cooled, simply flake it into nice lobes and chunks over the new potatoes, discarding the skin and any bones you come across. Spoon over the cucumber dressing. Sprinkle over a pinch of salt and pepper, grate over some more lemon zest if you like, and squeeze in a little more lemon juice. Scatter over any leftover dill, and serve. What a joy.

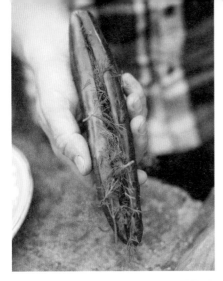

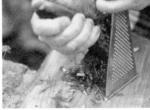

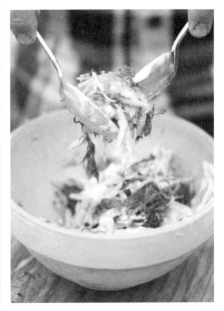

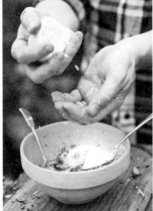

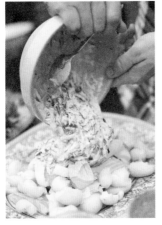

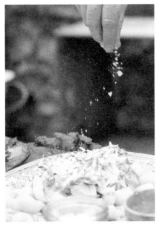

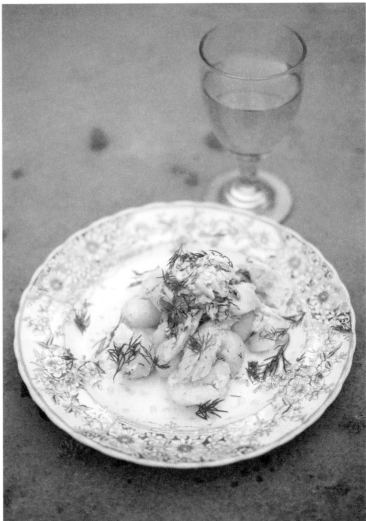

GRANNY SMITH'S PORK & RICE SALAD

The great Caribbean classic, rice and peas, inspired me to create a really exciting rice salad of my own, because when done well, it's a truly wonderful thing. The flavours in this one are like a roast pork dinner meets a rice salad. By cutting the belly into small pieces, you're helping it cook quickly and get crispy, before adding that roast-dinner feel with the honey, apple and herbs. Tossing the pork with the rice helps lighten the dish up a little – so it's perfect hot, or cold for a more summery vibe.

SERVES 6 AS A MAIN OR 8 AS A LIGHT LUNCH

- sea salt and ground pepper
- 750g free-range pork belly
- olive oil
- 2 fresh bay leaves
- 2 sprigs of fresh rosemary
- 3 Granny Smith apples
- a handful of shelled walnuts (roughly 50g)
- 2 tablespoons runny honey
- 1 tablespoon fresh thyme leaves
- 1 orange
- 300g pre-mixed basmati and wild rice
- 2-3 tablespoons cider vinegar
- a large bunch of fresh flat-leaf parsley, leaves finely chopped
- 2 spring onions, trimmed and finely sliced

Preheat the oven to 200°C/400°F/gas 6. Get out one large ovenproof frying pan and one large saucepan. Fill the saucepan with salted water and put both pans on a high heat. Use your sharpest knife to slice the pork belly into about 1.5cm slices then across into 1.5cm chunks, or lardons. Put a couple of good lugs of olive oil into the frying pan, followed by the diced pork and the bay and rosemary. Season well. Fry and stir fairly frequently, for around 25 minutes, or until the pork is dark golden and crispy. When the bay and rosemary are crispy, remove them from the pan. At this point, pour most of the fat into a jam jar for roast potatoes another day.

Quarter the apples, then carefully remove and discard the cores. Cut the apples into rough chunks about the same size as the pork and add to the frying pan with a few lugs of olive oil, the walnuts, honey, thyme leaves and the juice squeezed from the orange. Stir well. Place the pan in the oven for around 20 minutes or until the mixture turns gorgeous and dark golden – keep a close eye on it and take it out as soon as it's perfect. Basically you want to be almost getting nervous that it's going to burn and then you're at exactly the right point.

Meanwhile, cook the rice in the boiling salted water according to the packet's instructions. Drain the rice in a colander and leave to steam dry. Take the frying pan out of the oven and carefully tip the pork, apples and walnuts on to the rice. Add a couple of tablespoons of vinegar to the hot pan to allow you to scrape all those lovely sticky pork bits off the bottom – that's where all the flavour is.

Once you've got it all looking sticky and delicious, tip the rice and pork mixture back into the frying pan, add the parsley and spring onions and toss together well. Have a taste, adjust the seasoning and add a little more vinegar, if needed. Serve it straight away, at room temperature, or leave to cool, then cover it and put into the fridge to have cold the next day.

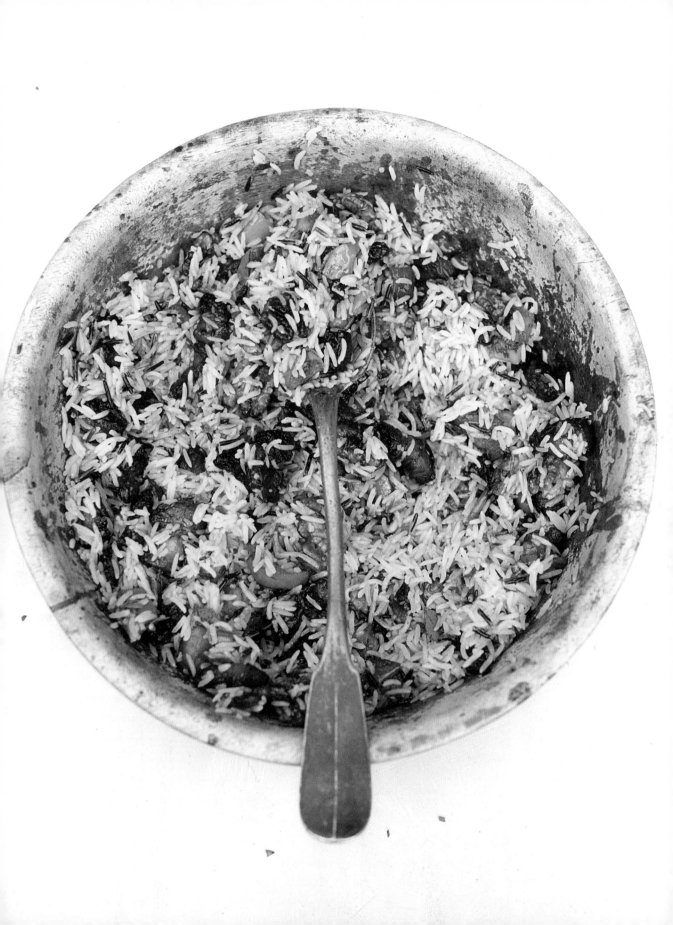

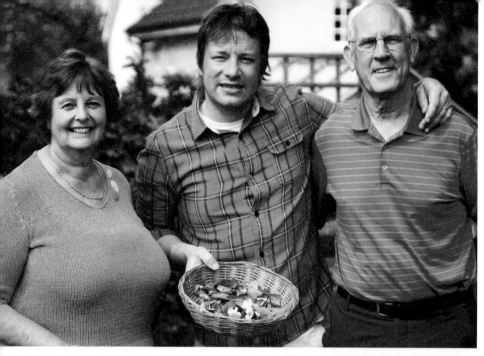

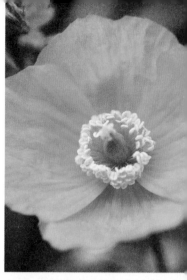

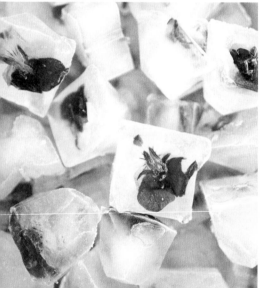

English Country Garden

Margaret and Vic have such a wonderful garden, packed with edible flowers, and Margaret loves using them across all sorts of cooking. She does it beautifully, for garnish and for flavour. Her passion began when she went on a course after she got married, and she told me that one day the wind blew some apple blossoms into her dinner and she's been eating them ever since, which shows how adventurous she is. Her garden is small, proving that, with a guidebook, and fairly basic knowledge, you'll learn what's good to eat too.

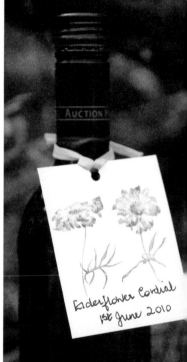

Elderflower Cordial
1st June 2010

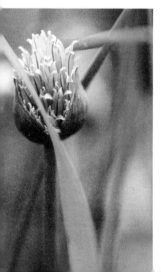

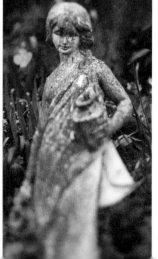

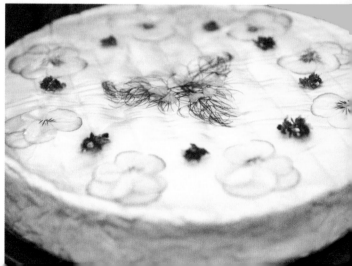

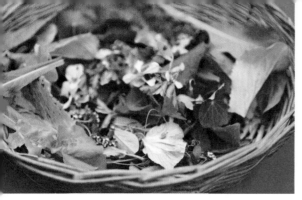

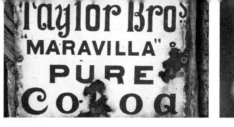

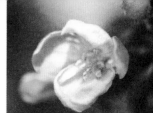

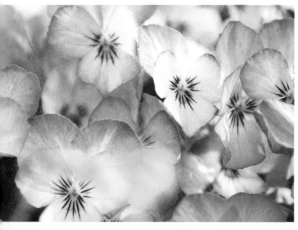

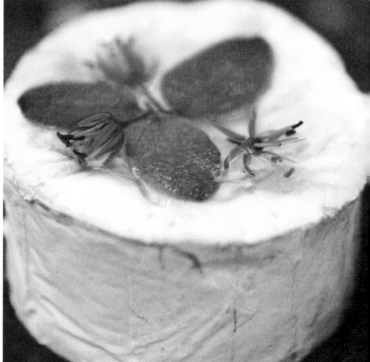

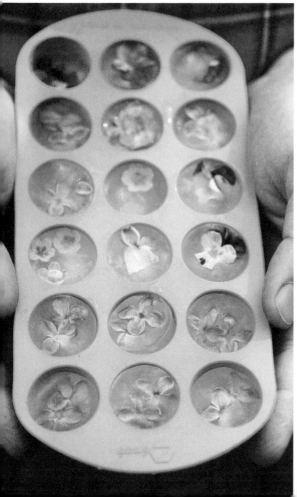

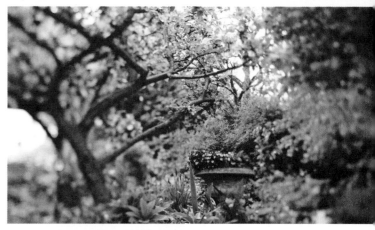

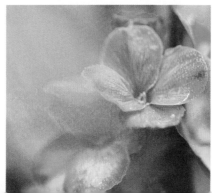

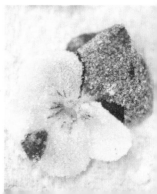

ARISTOCRAT'S SALAD
... WITH A CRUSHED RASPBERRY VINAIGRETTE

You might not think salads are necessarily British, but it turns out we've had a soft spot for them for hundreds, if not thousands, of years. In 1689 John Evelyn wrote a book singing the praises of different leaves, shoots, vegetables and herbs: *Acetarium: A discourse on sallets*. And this salad is really a homage to the delicate flowering salad of that time, made popular by Queen Catherine of Aragon and then by rich Englishmen using things from their impressive gardens. It's a really loose recipe, but the whole point of it is taking you away from the supermarket veg shelf and getting you thinking about embracing things that are soft, pretty and represent new growth, from pea shoots and the soft leafy tops of vegetables, to edible flowers. So go for it. These salads make a lovely start to a meal and are also great with smoked fish, on little toasts with nice cheeses, next to leftover roasted meats, or as the base for a warm salad with chicken livers and sherry … You name it. A little philosophy: Start by creating a base for your salad. Take a small handful of soft leaves (one per person is about right) and put them into a large and beautiful bowl. You can use watercress, lamb's lettuce, rocket, baby spinach, pea shoots, broad bean leaves or beetroot leaves, then let your palate guide you as you add little pinches and sprigs of other delicate herbs (and use their flowers, if flowering), like torn-up leaves of mint, tarragon, parsley, oregano or marjoram, dill, fennel tops, chives or different mustard cresses. A few pinches of lemon or orange thyme tips, borage flowers or even hyssop could also be really exciting. **The flowers:** Once you're happy with the flavours in your base salad, you can move on to the delicate flowers, which are an absolute must for this salad. You can usually buy edible flowers in farmers' markets, but if you can't get to one, feel free to look in your window-boxes or gardens. All my suggestions below are safe and delicious, but please make sure you look online, or know what you're picking (not all flowers are edible! But don't let this put you off because it's very easy to learn what's good!). Taste as you pick, and have a sense of what will brighten your salad. If anything tastes a little bit bitter, it's good to add just a few petals, as a gesture. Marigolds, violas, pansies, a few pinches of lavender, flowers from rosemary, chives or thyme, and allium flowers all look and taste beautiful, but nasturtiums are one of my favourite edible flowers because they have a mustardy, peachy flavour that I just love. **The dressing:** Using berries in the dressing gives this salad a real plumminess that makes it rock. Use a fork to mash up a large handful or two of fresh raspberries or brambles in a nice serving bowl. Add a good swig of white wine vinegar, roughly three times as much rapeseed/extra virgin olive oil, and pick in a few thyme leaves if you have them. Drizzle in about 1 teaspoon of runny honey and add a good pinch of sea salt, then mix up, taste and adjust with a little more salt, vinegar or honey if needed. Drizzle this all over the salad, use your fingers to delicately toss and mix everything together, and serve right away. If you like, you can add a bit more excitement by sprinkling over some crushed nuts, or by taking a good British cheese – like Montgomery Cheddar or Lincolnshire Poacher - and using a knife to twizzle off little nuggets to scatter over the top. The whole point of this is that whether you're an inner-city liver buying from a market, or a country dweller walking the long way home, you should be able to seek out these delicate, exciting ingredients. So get busy with it, and eat like an old-school aristocrat.

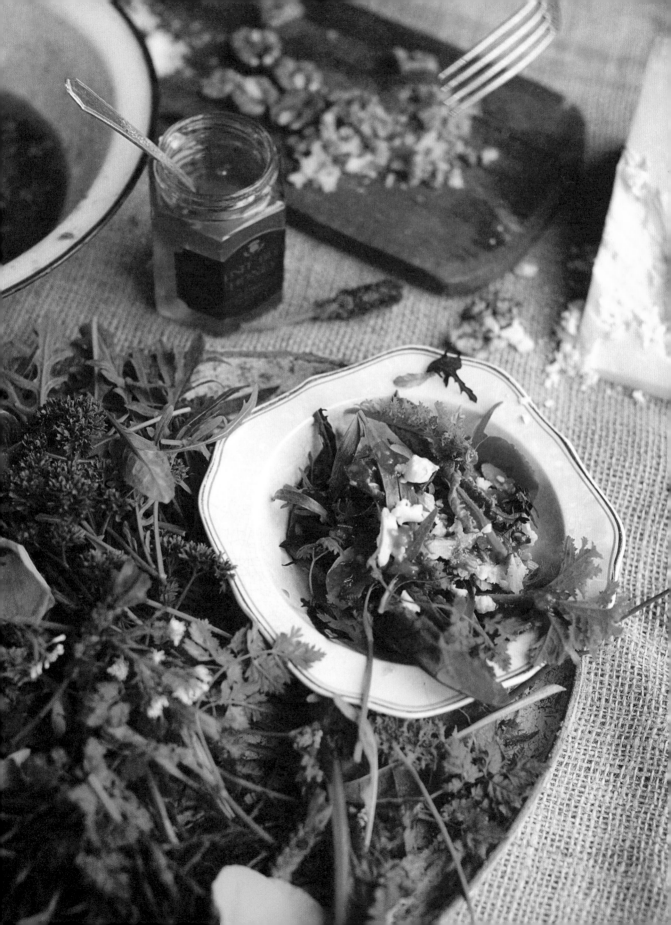

WARM TOMATO SALAD

CRISPY BLACK PUDDING • WORCESTERSHIRE DRESSING

Just when you thought there were only a few ways to make tomato salad, along comes this bad boy. If you're one of those people who dismiss black pudding, please, please give it a chance. It's always best to get it from a quality butcher. Ask if they've got one made with rice or barley, because that's really nice.

To offset the crunchy black pudding and sweet tomatoes, I'm making a gorgeous sticky cooked vinegar using Worcestershire sauce and sugar. It's a beautiful combo, and by the way, this salad jammed into a bap or sandwich makes a brilliant lunch.

SERVES 4 AS A MAIN OR 6 AS A SIDE

- 3 or 4 handfuls of mixed ripe tomatoes, such as heirloom, cherry, orange, red and green
- 150g good-quality black pudding
- olive oil
- 1 heart of celery, yellow leaves reserved
- sea salt and ground pepper
- 2 heaped tablespoons demerara sugar
- 3 tablespoons Worcestershire sauce
- 3 tablespoons cider vinegar
- extra virgin olive oil
- a few sprigs of fresh thyme

Put a medium frying pan on a high heat. While it's getting hot, slice the tomatoes into erratic wedges, halves or quarters depending on their size. You want them to look interesting, so let the size and shape of each tomato guide you. Put the tomatoes on a platter or into a serving bowl.

If the black pudding has an outer skin, remove it, then cut the pudding into 1cm slices. Put these into the hot frying pan with a drizzle of olive oil and cook on a medium to high heat, turning every few minutes, for around 5 or 6 minutes, or until the black pudding is dark and crispy. Click off the outer sticks of celery and pop them into the fridge for another day. Wash the inner yellow celery heart, then trim off the top few centimetres and the base, leaving the root intact. Finely slice the heart lengthways into very thin strips, and sprinkle these and any yellow celery leaves over the tomatoes. Add a really good pinch of salt and pepper and toss.

Once the black pudding is nice and crisp, pour away any fat in the pan and tip the pudding slices on to some kitchen paper to drain. Put the pan back on a low heat and add the sugar, Worcestershire sauce and cider vinegar. Let this mixture come to a gentle bubble, then cook and reduce for a few minutes until it's thick and shiny. Carefully drizzle this all over the tomatoes, then drizzle over the same amount of extra virgin olive oil. Sprinkle over a few fresh thyme tips, toss well, then have a taste and adjust the seasoning if need be. Quickly clean up the sides of the bowl so it looks presentable; I garnished it with some flowering thyme because it was to hand, but you certainly don't have to. Crumble over that crispy black pudding and serve with a hunk of nice bread - pure heaven.

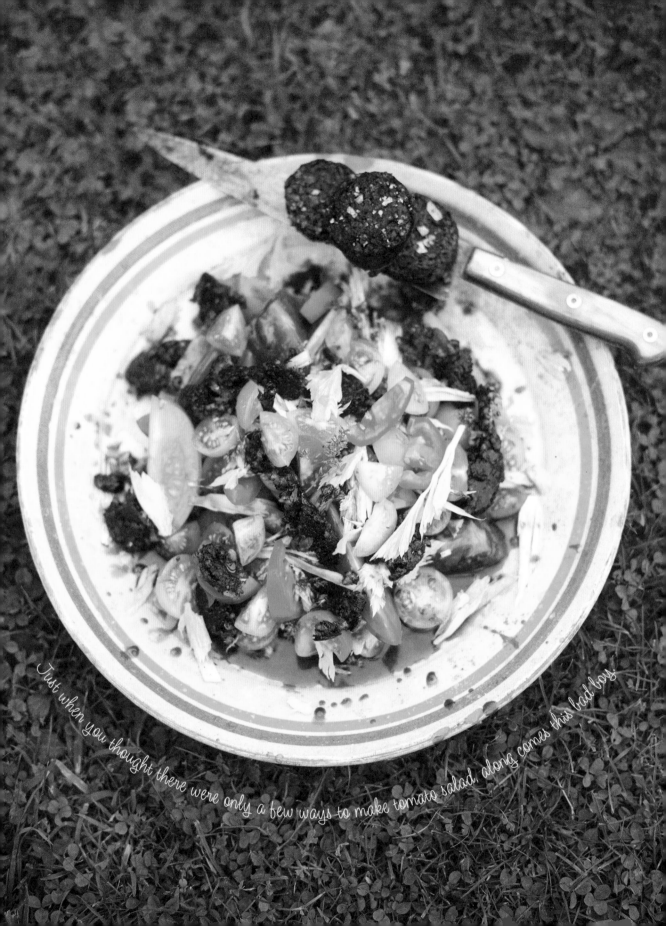

Just when you thought there were only a few ways to make tomato salad, along comes this bad boy

EPIC ROAST CHICKEN SALAD
GOLDEN CROUTONS • GREEN BEANS • SWEET TOMATOES

I could tell you that this is a wonderful way of using leftover chicken, and it would be true, but it's fully worth cooking a whole chicken to perfection to make this beautiful salad.

SERVES 6

For the roast chicken
- olive oil
- 1 x 1.2kg free-range chicken
- sea salt and ground pepper
- a small bunch of fresh thyme
- 1 lemon
- 400g mixed cherry tomatoes
- 1 bulb of garlic

For the salad
- 1 country loaf (roughly 300g)
- 6 rashers of quality smoked streaky bacon
- 200g green beans, topped
- extra virgin olive oil
- 1 tablespoon wholegrain mustard

- cider vinegar
- a bunch of fresh flat-leaf or curly parsley, leaves picked
- a bunch of fresh mint, leaves picked
- 6 spring onions

Preheat your oven to 200°C/400°F/gas 6. Drizzle olive oil all over the chicken and sprinkle it with salt and pepper. Pick and scatter over the thyme leaves (reserving the stalks). Rub the flavours into the skin, then halve the lemon and put it inside the cavity along with the thyme stalks. Pop the chicken into a large roasting tray (roughly 25 x 32cm) and cook in the oven for 1 hour. Meanwhile, halve the cherry tomatoes, then smash up your garlic bulb and discard the papery white skin. After about 30 minutes, throw the tomatoes and garlic into the chicken tray, ideally holding the chicken up with tongs while you slush everything around and coat the tomatoes in the juices underneath. Put the chicken back on top, then return it to the oven for the remaining 30 minutes, or until the chicken is golden and the juices from the thigh run clear when pricked with a knife.

Transfer the roasted chicken to a plate, cover with tin foil and leave to cool. Tear the bread into the roasting tray in thumb-sized croutons, then toss them in all the cooking juices. Spread the croutons out in the tray and lay the rashers of bacon on top. Pop back in the oven for around 15 to 20 minutes, or until everything is crispy, golden and gorgeous.

Meanwhile, remove all the chicken skin and set aside, then use two forks to strip every last bit of meat off the bone. Pile the meat into a large bowl and drizzle over any resting juices from the plate. Cook your green beans in boiling salted water for 5 to 6 minutes, until cooked but not squeaky when you bite them. Quickly drain and add them to the bowl of shredded meat, with 5 to 6 tablespoons of good-quality extra virgin olive oil, the wholegrain mustard and a few good swigs of cider vinegar. Chop up the parsley and mint leaves and finely slice the spring onions. Add them to the bowl. Toss everything together, then have a taste and adjust with more vinegar or seasoning if you like.

Once the croutons are golden, quickly tear the chicken skin into the roasting tray (skip this if you want a healthier salad) and put back into the oven just until it crisps up again. When it's looking lovely, tip everything from the bowl into the tray or on to a large serving platter. Toss everything together and serve in the middle of the table.

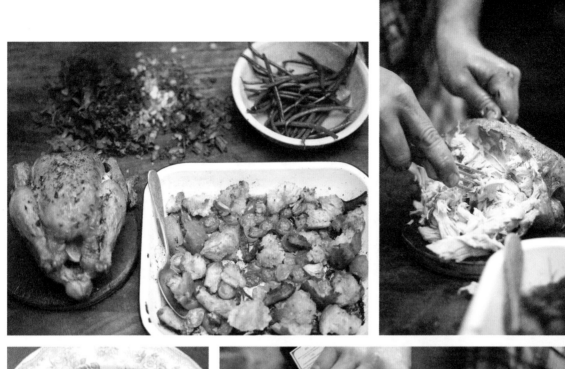

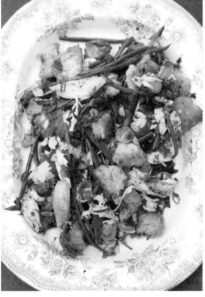

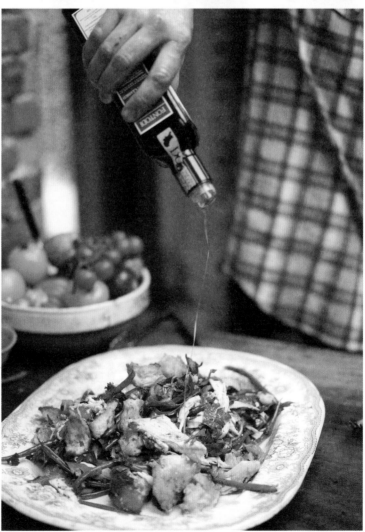

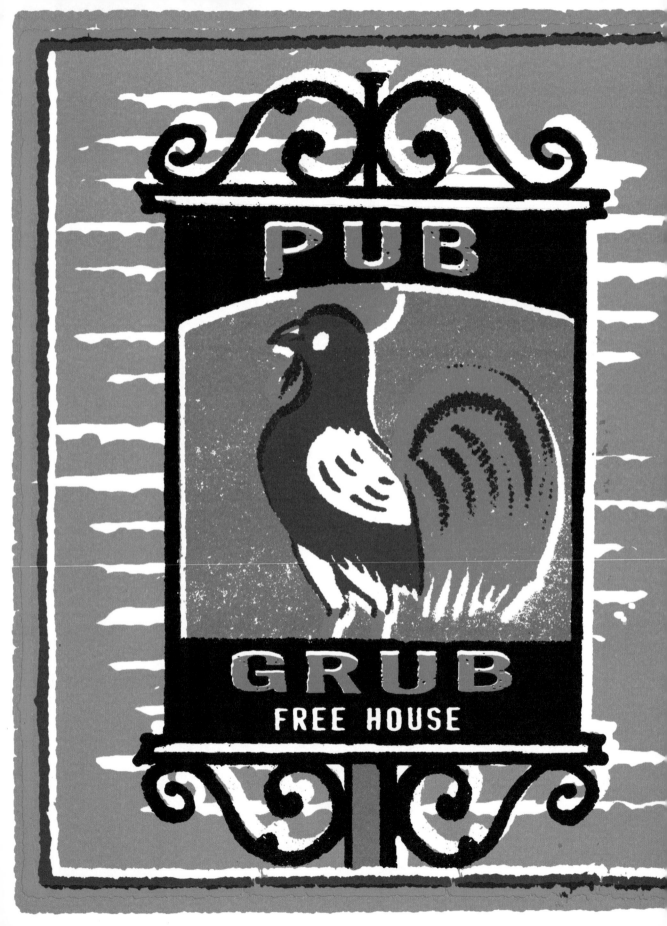

I grew up in my parents' pub, so obviously this chapter is close to my heart. Over the years, I pretty much worked at every job in the pub, from cleaner, to pot-washer, to cook. And I loved it. It's not hard to see why British pubs are the envy of the drinking world. They're quirky, cosy and so much a part of the British landscape it's impossible to imagine Britain without them. Food has always been a big part of pub culture. Hundreds of years ago, horse-drawn coaches would pull up for the night to eat and rest at local taverns. And back when food was really very regional, this would have been the first time someone from one part of the country tasted the food of another, so that network of taverns and travellers really helped to spread our food and recipes around the country. To this day, food served in pubs is best when it is local, honest, and represents the surrounding area or countryside. There are some wonderful pub classics in this chapter – some are new, some are updated versions of things I've been making since I was a boy. But a plate of any of these things, with a pint of beer, all your mates around you and some decent banter, sums up everything I love about our pub culture. Cheers.

BABY YORKSHIRE PUDS

...CREAMY SMOKED TROUT & HORSERADISH PATÉ

I can't lie: this dish has become one of my new favourite things. Each mouthful is an outrageously delicious bit of heaven that anyone sensible won't be able to resist. The contrast of hot crispy soft Yorkshire pudding and cold creamy smoky trout with a good hit of horseradish is unbelievable. You can put the creamy smoked fish in one big serving bowl if you like, but I think it's quite sweet to make up a few individual servings in little teacups. Around May and June you'll start to see flowering chives around, and those are beautiful for decorating the top of the potted fish if you're out to impress. This is dead quick, so easy and absolutely perfect for a starter – just whack it right in the middle of the table so everyone can help themselves. Your guests will be fighting over it, I promise.

SERVES 6 TO 8

For the creamy smoked fish
- 125g cream cheese
- 2-3 heaped teaspoons jarred horseradish
- 1 lemon
- a small bunch of fresh chives, finely chopped

- sea salt and ground pepper
- 125g hot-smoked trout, skin removed
- rapeseed oil

For the Yorkies
(makes 16 baby Yorkies)
- vegetable oil
- 2 large free-range eggs
- 100g plain flour
- 100ml milk
- lemon wedges, to serve

Put the cream cheese into a mixing bowl with the horseradish, the zest of 1 lemon and the juice from half, and mix together. Mix in most of the chopped chives, then have a taste and add a pinch of salt and pepper. It's very important that this mixture has a bolshie attitude – it should be hot, smoky, salty, so add more horseradish or lemon juice if needed. Flake in the trout, removing any skin and bones, then use a spatula to fold the mixture together gently so you have smaller bits and nice chunks. Decant into a single nice serving dish or several little bowls or cups, then drizzle over a little rapeseed oil and sprinkle over a few more chopped chives. Cover with clingfilm and put into the fridge to get nice and cold.

When you're nearly ready to eat, preheat the oven to full whack (about 240°C/475°F/gas 9) while you make your Yorkshire pudding batter. Get yourself a mini muffin tin (you can buy these easily online or in cooks' shops) and pour a little thimble of vegetable oil into the 16 compartments of the tin, so you have a thin layer covering the bottom of each. Pop the tray on to the top shelf in the hot oven for around 10 to 15 minutes, so the oil get so hot that it smokes. While you're doing that, aggressively beat the eggs, flour, milk and a pinch of salt and pepper together, either by hand or in a food processor, until light and smooth. Transfer the mixture into a jug.

Carefully take the tray out of the oven and quickly and confidently pour the batter into the hot tin so it nearly fills each well. Return the tray to the top shelf of the oven to cook for around 10 to 12 minutes, or until the Yorkies are puffed up and golden. Whatever you do, don't open the oven door! Get your cold cups and bowls of potted fish out of the fridge and serve on a board with those sizzling hot little Yorkies and some lemon wedges.

To. Die. For.

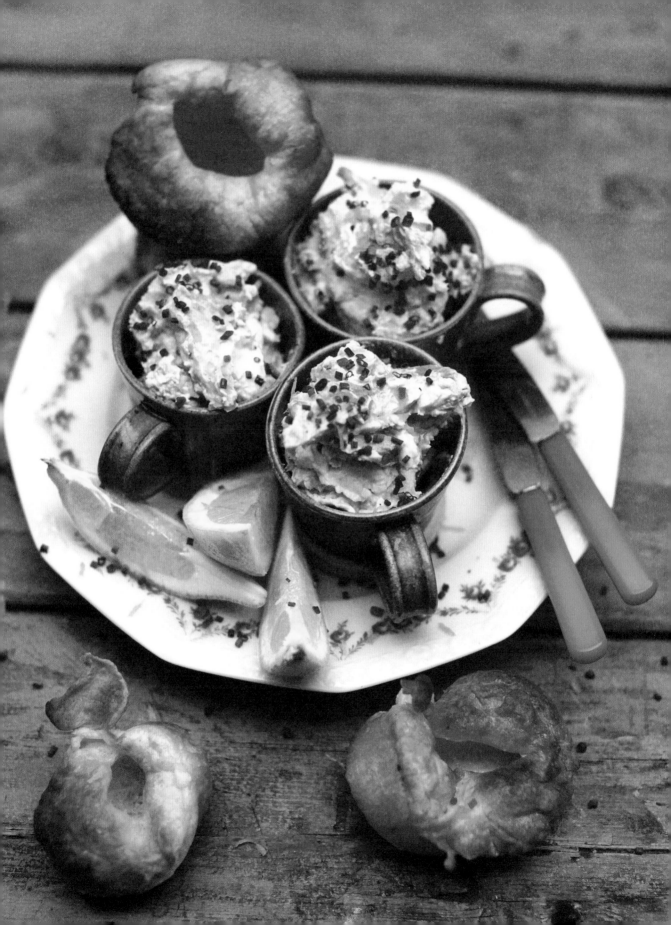

MY PRAWN COCKTAIL

This is an absolute classic; it's old school, retro, and just a tiny bit naff, but in a brilliant way. It's the kind of thing I grew up seeing on the menu at my mum and dad's pub in the 80s. Revisiting things that have become a bit uncool is great - I love the idea of bringing this dish back, approaching it with all the enthusiasm of that decade but using today's better-quality ingredients. And speaking of great ingredients, it's worth keeping in mind that prawns can be a dicey area when it comes to ethics and sustainability - look for labelling that tells you yours are from responsibly sourced areas.

SERVES 4

For the Marie Rose sauce
- 8 tablespoons quality mayonnaise
- 3 teaspoons ketchup
- cayenne pepper
- a swig of brandy
- ½ a lemon
- sea salt and ground pepper

For the prawn cocktail
- olive oil
- 1 clove of garlic
- cayenne pepper
- 12 large unpeeled raw tiger prawns
- ½ an iceberg lettuce
- a handful of mixed tomatoes
- ½ a cucumber

- 2 sprigs of fresh mint
- 1 small punnet of salad cress
- 1 x 180g pack of quality smoked salmon
- 100g peeled little prawns
- *optional:* 100g brown shrimps, or little prawns if you can't get them
- 1 lemon, for serving

Heat a large pan on a high heat, add a lug of olive oil and crush in a clove of garlic using a garlic crusher. Sprinkle in a good pinch of cayenne pepper and add the whole prawns, which you can butterfly if you like (this isn't hard to do, go to *www.jamieoliver.com/how-to* and watch how it's done). Toss the prawns around for 3 to 4 minutes, or until cooked through and smelling delicious. Take the pan off the heat and put to one side.

Make the Marie Rose sauce and put it to one side. Finely slice the lettuce, slice the tomatoes into delicate pieces and dice up your cucumber. Pick the mint leaves, snip the cress leaves and get your smoked salmon and prawns out. Layer up all those lovely ingredients in the middle of plates, bowls, or even in Kilner jars, which I've used here because they are nice for picnics and travel well in a coolbox. Dollop Marie Rose sauce over the prawns and finish with a few slices of smoked salmon, prawns and brown shrimps if you've got them. Add a pinch of cayenne from a height, and hang a lovely hot prawn or two off the side of the jar or plate. Serve with wedges of lemon for squeezing over. With some nice buttered bread, the job's a good one!

PS: I like to fry off some breadcrumbs in olive oil and salt so they're nice and crispy, and sprinkle them over the prawns for a bit of crunch and contrast.

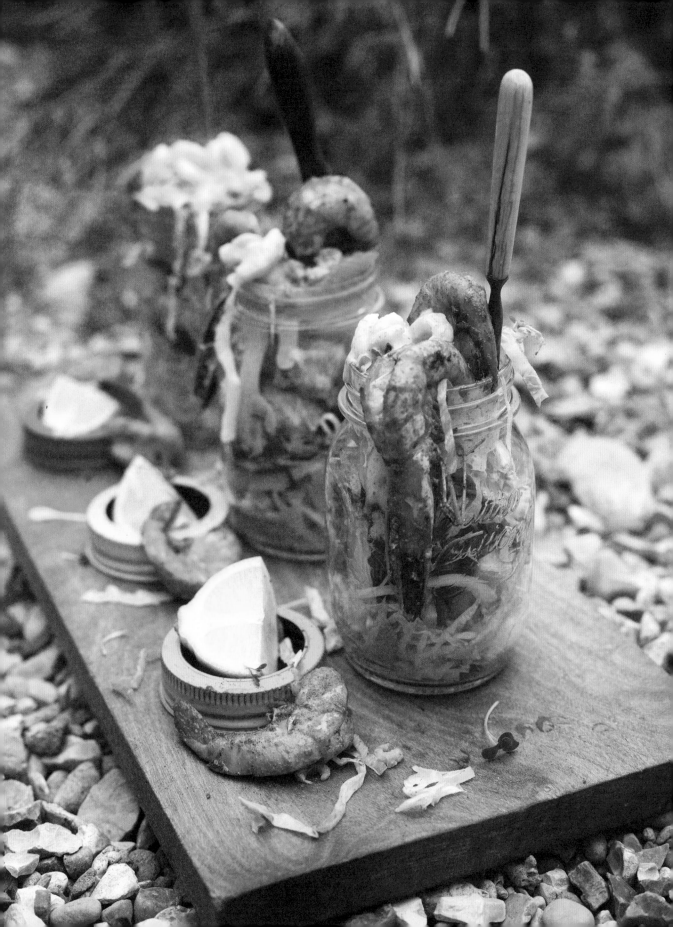

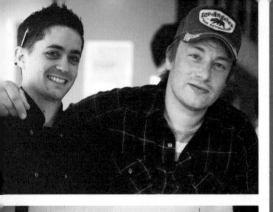

Today's British Pub

The pub industry has taken a hammering over the past thirty to forty years for various reasons, and sadly many have closed. But offering quality, value and good local beer and food has never been more important. It's great to see young blood coming through, like Sam and Michael from the Midnight Bell, in Holbeck, Leeds. They work with their talented master brewer, Venkatesh, from Mumbai, to make several really quality beers. Their chef, Jimmy Black (now that's a name!), is also doing a great job and using it all sorts of ways across their menu.

www.midnightbell.co.uk

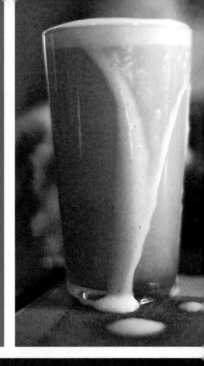

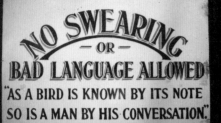

NO SWEARING — OR — BAD LANGUAGE ALLOWED

"AS A BIRD IS KNOWN BY ITS NOTE
SO IS A MAN BY HIS CONVERSATION."

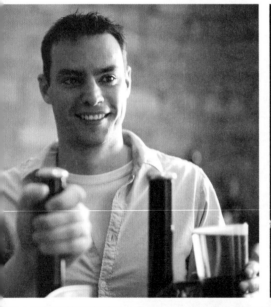

* ONION & MIDNIGHT BELL ALE SOUP WITH WENSLEYDALE CROUTON £4.25

* MUSSELS STEAMED IN LEEDS BREWERY PALE ALE STARTER £6.00 MAIN £ WITH HANDCUT

* PUY LENTIL & SPRING ONION BURGER (v) WITH HANDCUT CHIPS £8.50

* MIDNIGHT BELL CHEESECAKE WITH LEEDS BREWERY ALE SYRUP £4.50

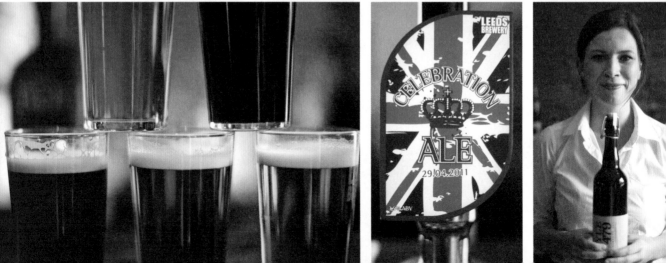

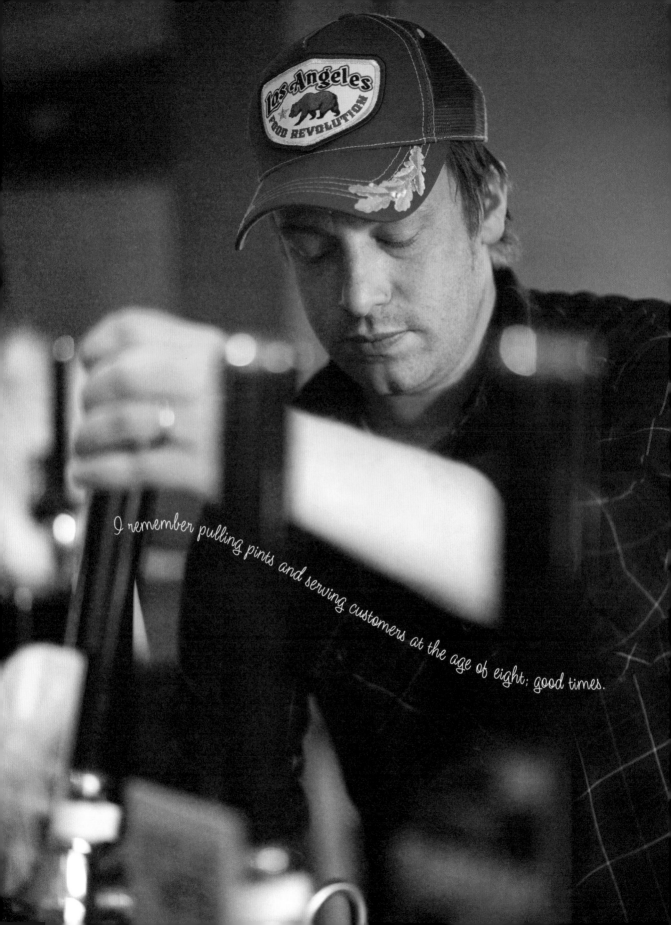

I remember pulling pints and serving customers at the age of eight; good times.

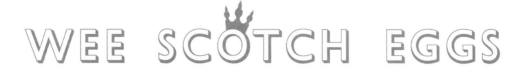

WEE SCOTCH EGGS

Although it's not hard, this recipe does have a few stages - but bloomin' hell, it's worth it. Bizarrely, it's not much more effort to make 30 than it is to make 12. Once you are set up, you're ready to go. Eat these while they are hot, crispy and still oozy in the middle, or if you want to go down the picnic route, just boil the eggs for an extra minute.

MAKES 12 LITTLE SCOTCH EGGS

- 4 quality Cumberland sausages (roughly 300g)
- ½ teaspoon sweet paprika
- 1 sprig each of fresh rosemary and sage, leaves picked and very finely chopped
- 1 whole nutmeg, for grating
- sea salt and ground pepper
- 3 handfuls of plain flour
- 2 free-range hen's eggs, beaten
- 125g white breadcrumbs
- 12 free-range quail's eggs
- vegetable oil (roughly 2 litres)
- 1 new potato, for testing

Put the kettle on to boil. Meanwhile tear open the sausages and squeeze the meat on to a plate. Season with the paprika, the chopped herbs, a few gratings of nutmeg and a little salt and pepper, then use a fork to mash it all up. Put out your bowls of flour, beaten egg and breadcrumbs.

Carefully put the quail's eggs into a small pan. Once the kettle boils, pour in the boiling water straight away and cook for 2 minutes, no longer. Move the pan to the sink and run cold water over the eggs for 2 to 3 minutes. Tap, roll and - ever so gently - peel the shells off them. Do it under running water if it helps. You'll get quicker at peeling them as you go.

We've got a video up on *www.jamieoliver.com/how-to* with the whole assembling process, so check that out if you want to rattle through this bit really efficiently. Take a marble-sized piece of sausage meat and flatten it out in the palm of your clean hand until it's about 6cm in diameter. Pop an egg into the middle, then carefully shape and mould the sausage meat up around the egg with your floured hands. You need to get into the routine of pulling up the sides, gently squeezing, moulding, patting and very gently squashing the meat around the egg. Repeat with all 12 eggs, then coat them well with flour. Transfer them to the bowl of beaten egg and coat well, then roll them in the breadcrumbs. They'll be more robust to hold now, so pat and hug them into shape. When they're all done, put them into a container and pop them into the fridge until needed.

When you're ready to cook, put a deep casserole-type pan on a medium high heat and fill it about 8cm deep with vegetable oil. Make sure you never fill a pan more than halfway up. Add a piece of potato to help you gauge the temperature - it's ready once the potato turns golden and floats (or when the oil reaches 180°C on a thermometer). Carefully lower one wee Scotch egg into the pan. After about 4 minutes it should be golden and perfectly cooked through, so take it out of the pan and cut it in half to see if you should have cooked it for less or more time - once you know where you stand, you can cook the rest, in batches of 6 or less.

Transfer the cooked Scotch eggs to a plate lined with kitchen paper to drain, and serve scattered with a pinch of sea salt, alongside a pot of English mustard and a cold beer.

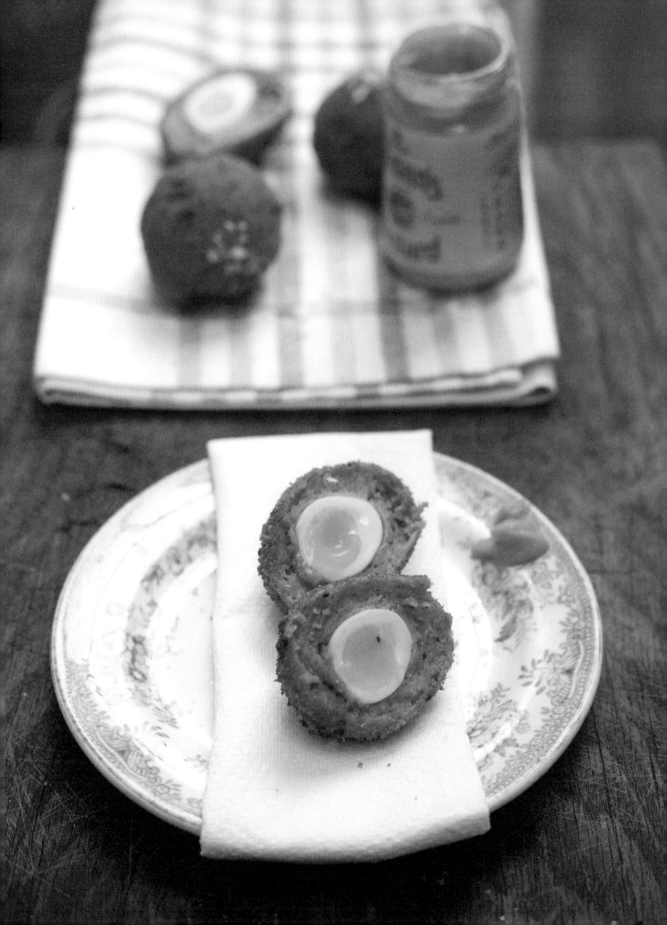

ROOT VEGETABLE CRISPS

Look, I know what you're thinking: why are you making crisps when you can buy packets of them in every flavour in every supermarket up and down the country? But sometimes it's the simplest things, done really well, that make people truly happy about food. This isn't something I do often, it's more for parties or special occasions. I love how excited everyone gets. If you've got a mandoline slicer in your kitchen you'll be able to rattle these out so quickly. A decent mandoline is something I think every serious cook should have, and a good one will last a lifetime and give you bigger, more beautiful crisps than you'll ever get in a packet. Use different coloured root veg if you can, to up the excitement. A big pile of these with a bottle of Sarson's vinegar at a family get-together is joyous.

SERVES LOTS

- vegetable oil
  (roughly 2.5 litres)
- 1 new potato, for testing
- 3 potatoes, washed

- 3 parsnips, washed,
  stalks removed
- 4 beetroots, washed,
  stalks removed

- 3 sweet potatoes, washed
- sea salt (or flavoured salt)
  and ground pepper
- Sarson's vinegar, to serve

Fill a large sturdy pan halfway up with vegetable oil and put it on a high heat. Make sure you keep your eye on the pan and don't let anybody run around the kitchen, because hot oil is very dangerous and can burn badly.

Add a chunk of potato to the pan to act as a temperature gauge or use a thermometer. While the oil heats up (it needs to reach around 180°C), prepare all your vegetables, keeping them in separate piles. If you have a mandoline with a finger guard, very carefully slice the vegetables really thinly, about 1mm thick. If you don't have a mandoline, a food processor with a nice fine slicer attachment could also work well here.

Once ready, lower a small batch of one vegetable into the oil using a slotted spoon and gently move it around if they stick together. Cook each batch for around 3 to 4 minutes (depending on the thickness and the vegetable you're cooking). Potatoes and sweet potatoes will be pretty good in around 3 minutes, parsnips around 3½, beetroots maybe 4. Just play it by ear, you know when a crisp looks like a crisp. Once cooked remove them to a tray of kitchen paper with your slotted spoon and lower in the next batch. Keep doing this until you've used up all of your vegetables, then transfer them to a lovely big bowl, sprinkle over a pinch of salt or flavoured salt of your choice, and serve, with the Sarson's vinegar on the side.

Once the oil in the pan has cooled, pass it through a sieve to remove any bits and pour it into a jar with a lid to use another time.

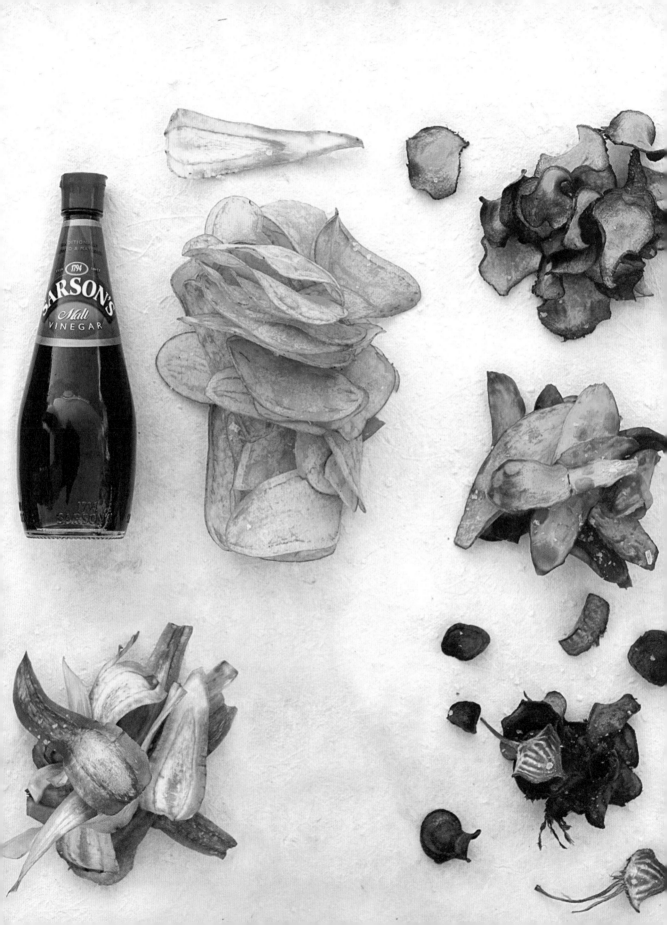

BREADED SCAMPI BITES
HOMEMADE TARTARE SAUCE • LEMON WEDGES

Back in the 60s and 70s, before pubs started cooking lots of different things and developing their menus, like my dad did at his, scampi in a basket really was one of the few things you'd find on pub menus all over the UK. It's a true classic, and as a young cook in my parents' kitchen I can certainly remember crumbing loads of prawns for scampi. The name refers more to the preparation method than it does to the actual seafood itself. It was common to use Dublin Bay prawns or langoustines, but as they became desirable pubs moved on to cheaper fish, like monkfish, until that became desirable, and so on. I guess the point I'm making is that this recipe is really flexible and can be used for pretty much any firm white fish or crustacean – lobsters, prawns, big or small. Just look out for MSC-approved prawns if using them, as prawns can be a bit of a hot potato from a sustainability point of view.

SERVES 4 TO 6 (MAKES AROUND 30 PIECES)

- a few good handfuls of plain flour
- 200g white bread, whizzed to fine crumbs
- 3 large free-range eggs
- sea salt and ground pepper
- cayenne pepper
- 1 lemon
- 800g fresh or frozen scampi or prawns
- tartare sauce (see page 390 to make your own)
- vegetable oil (2-3 litres)
- 1 new potato, for testing

Put the flour into one baking tray and the breadcrumbs into another. Beat the eggs in a bowl with a good pinch of salt, pepper, cayenne and a few good gratings of lemon zest. Put whatever seafood you're using for the scampi into the flour, toss until completely coated, and shake off any excess. Next coat the scampi well in the flavoured egg mix and drop them into the tray of breadcrumbs. Coat well, and shake off the excess. It's quite nice to have someone do the flouring with one hand, the egg part with the other, and you do the breadcrumb part; it's cleaner and quicker than trying to do it all yourself. Put the scampi on a plate, cover, and place in the fridge until needed. In the meantime, make up a batch of tartare sauce (see page 390).

When you're ready to cook, half-fill your largest sturdy pan with vegetable oil so it's about 8cm deep and put it on a high heat. Make sure you don't have any kids running around the kitchen, as hot oil can burn badly. Drop a small piece of potato into the oil to act as your temperature gauge. When it's golden and floats, the oil should be around 180°C (ideally, check this with a thermometer). Use a slotted spoon to lower half the breaded scampi at a time into the hot oil. Cook for around 2 to 3 minutes, until golden and beautiful, then carefully remove to a piece of kitchen paper and season with salt. Simply serve with some tartare sauce, a wedge of lemon for squeezing over and a pinch of cayenne over the top. Sometimes I also like to serve mine with iceberg cups and cress, which in the old days would have been there for a naff garnish, but actually hot crunchy scampi, refreshing cold iceberg lettuce and mustardy cress is delish. All you need to round off the experience is some football, a pint of beer and some 'man talk'.

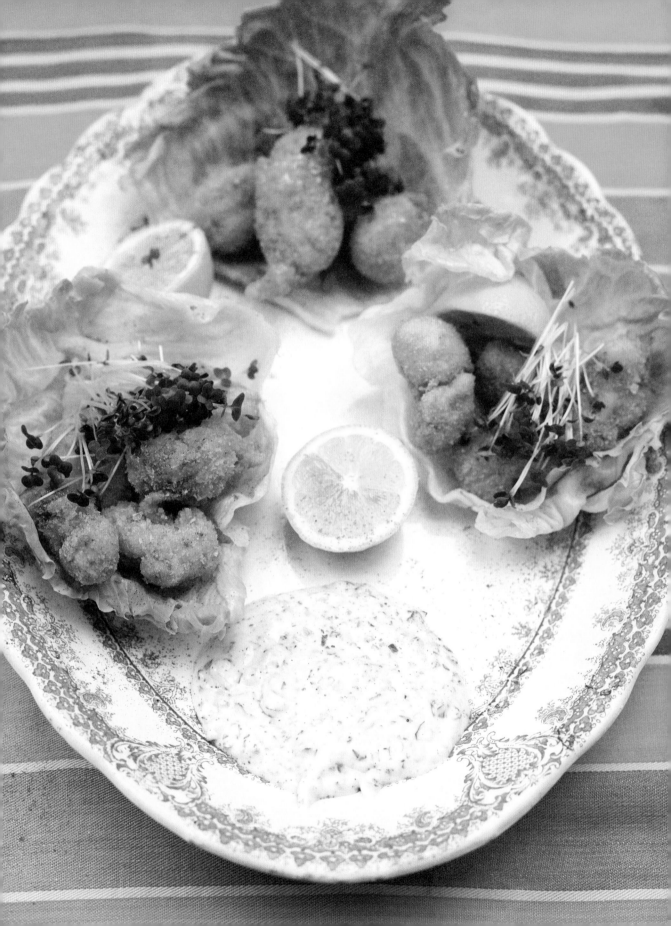

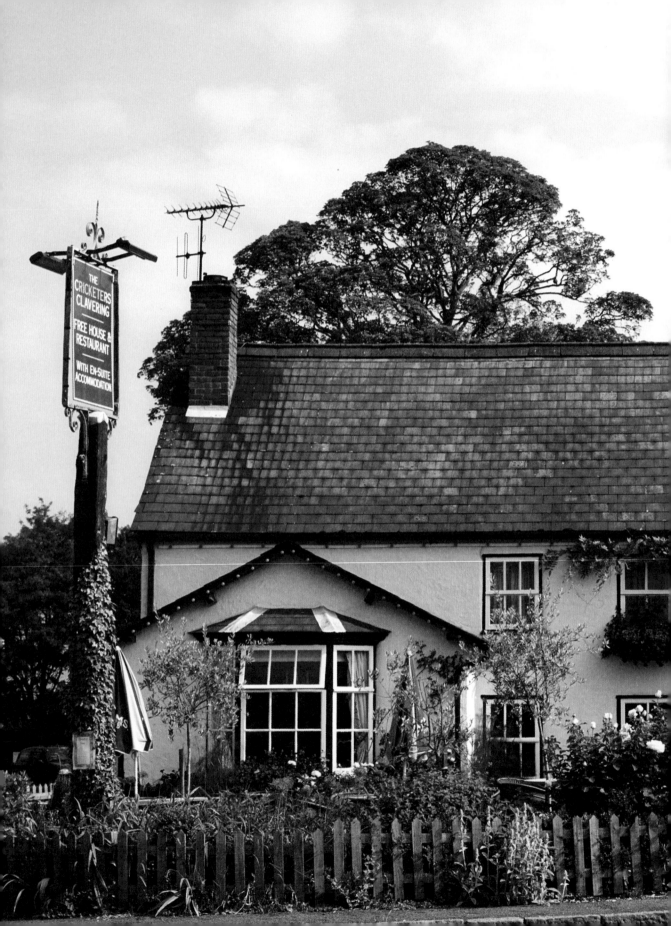

Mum and Dad's pub, where I lived for sixteen years of my life, a true gastropub.

PLOUGHMAN'S LUNCH

Yes, the rumours are true: the ploughman's lunch was actually dreamt up by some bright spark at the milk or cheese marketing board back in the 80s, as a cunning way to shift more cheese. So it's not the historical dish many people assume it is (unless you are so youthful you consider the 80s historical), though that hasn't stopped it becoming a force to be reckoned with on pub menus across Britain. The reality is that the ploughman's lunch really encapsulates the philosophy behind putting a little picnic together. It's a bit like the way you eat on Boxing Day, but you're doing it every day, which is my idea of heaven. It certainly isn't rocket science, but there is a certain frame of mind that, if you can get into it, will make it easy for you or your partner to procure a few handfuls of things and create the perfect little lunch. Of course we've taken the concept of the ploughman's to heart because we've always eaten this way. Working people have always needed food that is portable, and food that doesn't go off quickly like salted or smoked hams, pies, pickles and chutneys. Add a chunk of fresh fruit, a few vegetables and some crusty bread, and it's happy days. Wherever you are in the world, the minute you start putting great ingredients together you're guaranteed good eating. Thankfully, each nook and cranny of Britain has its own great produce, and producers, to draw on for endless combinations of the ploughman's. Most start with quality meat: that might be some thinly carved leftover roast beef, some shaved cured ham, a beautiful little wedge of pork pie or a sausage roll. Next you need a cheese to complement that meat: so do you go with a strong Cheddar? A creamy Stilton? Or maybe a crumbly goat's cheese? After that, it's about choosing elements that are going to lift those flavours, so you're looking at adding smears and spoonfuls of great preserves and condiments, like Branston pickle, piccalilli, mustard or horseradish. And maybe you want a soft crusty roll or some thinly sliced country bread to carry those flavours. A few wedges of crunchy fruit or vegetables for contrast are never a bad thing, and then there's usually a pickled onion or two... just because. Have a look at the picture next door and just make the concept yours. Regardless of who invented the original ploughman's, it's here to stay. And when you can go into a pub or restaurant, or even your own backyard, and have a celebration of beautiful ingredients on one plate, it's never a bad thing.

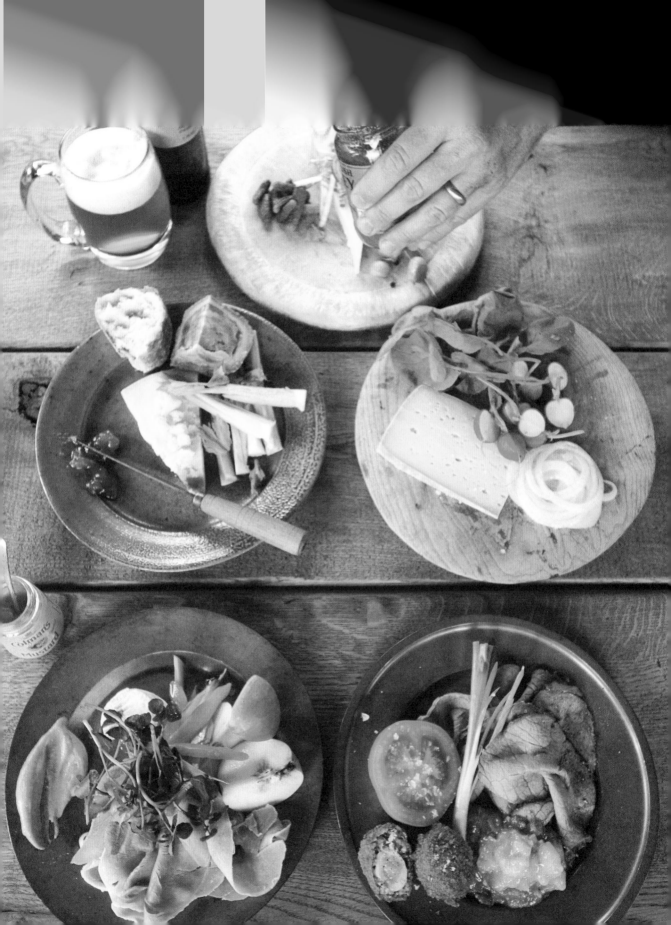

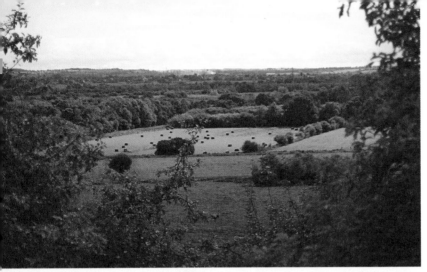

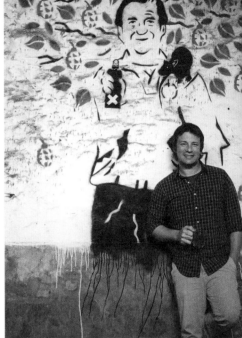

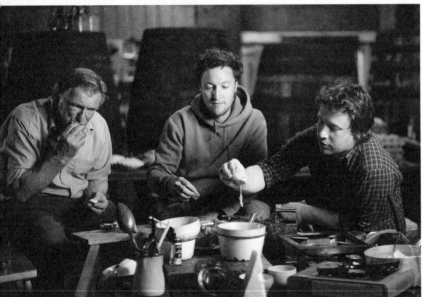

Wilkins Cider Farm

I had a great time hanging out with Roger Wilkins, who has a really humble old-school cider farm in Mudgley, in Somerset, where his family have been running it for nigh on 1000 years, or so he likes to say. People can just drop in, fill up on delicious cider and pick up some lovely local produce. I wish it was just around the corner from where I live. So, if you're on your way to Glastonbury, make sure you stop off there and fill your boot.
www.wilkinscider.com

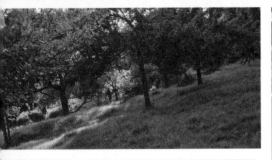

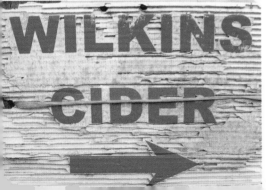

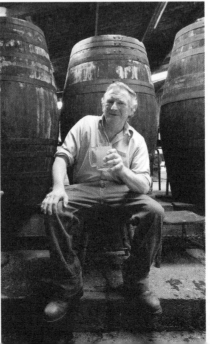

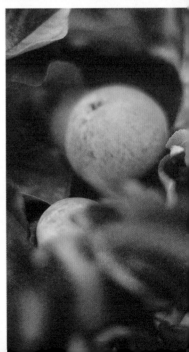

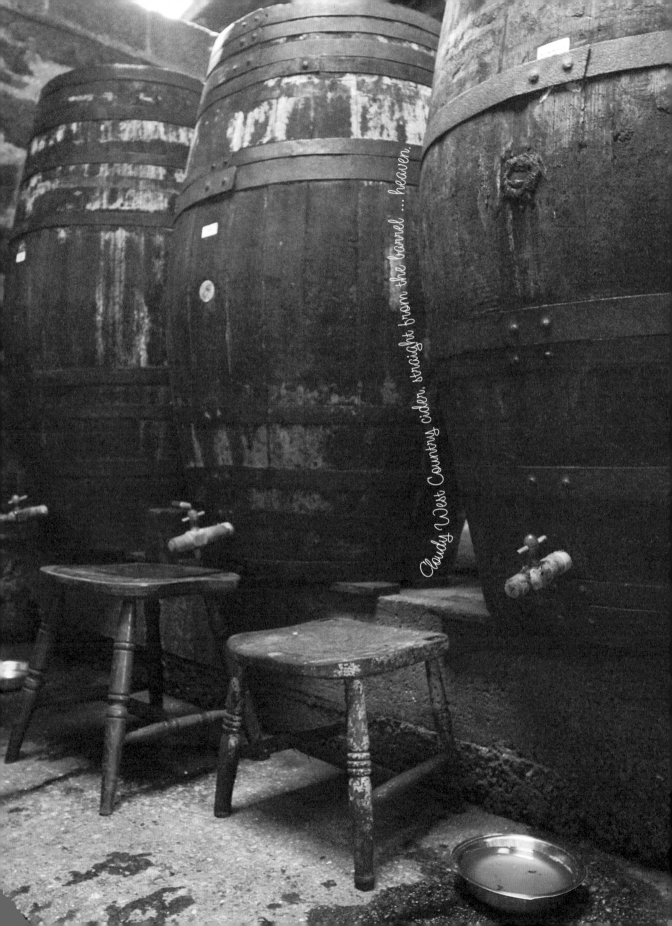

Cloudy West Country cider, straight from the barrel ... heaven.

TOAD·IN·THE·HOLE
... FOR RHYS & KATIE PENDERGAST

Rhys Pendergast made a really kind donation to Help a Capital Child this year, so I'm dedicating this dish to him, in celebration of his wedding to the lovely Katie. I'm told Rhys makes a mean toad-in-the-hole, and I hope they enjoy this version for years to come. In Yorkshire, I learned how real Yorkshire folk approach making a great Yorkie. They aren't into making their batter the night before, instead they focus on getting plenty of air into the batter and achieving a hot consistent temperature in the oven. I truly love this great classic and have only ever had one issue with it: quite often, you end up with half a sausage (the toad) poking out of the Yorkshire (the hole). The bit sticking out is crispy and golden – good times – but the other half of the sausage, inside the batter, is soft, anaemic and boiled – bad times. So in the spirit of family-style sharing and creating a dish that makes everyone go 'Oooh!' I'm separating out the elements so you end up with amazing crispy sausages, a tray of giant Yorkshire to tear up and a wonderful onion and apple gravy. Heaven.

SERVES 6

For the batter
- 3 large free-range eggs
- 100g plain flour
- 250ml semi-skimmed milk
- sea salt

For the sausages and gravy
- 2 large onions, peeled
- 3 eating apples
- a large knob of butter
- olive oil
- 4 sprigs of fresh rosemary
- sea salt and ground pepper

- 2 tablespoons runny honey
- 12 big Cumberland sausages
- 1 heaped tablespoon plain flour
- 250ml good cider
- 250ml organic beef stock
- Worcestershire sauce

Whisk the eggs, flour, milk and a pinch of salt in a bowl, then pour into a jug. Preheat the oven to full whack (about 240°C/475°F/gas 9). Cut your onions into 1cm thick slices, and do the same with the apples - removing the core. Put a large pan on a medium heat. Add the butter, a lug of olive oil, the onions and the apples. Pick in the leaves from 2 sprigs of rosemary. Cook for 20 minutes, stirring occasionally, until soft and golden. Remove the sauce from the heat once soft, season, and add the honey and a splash of water, if needed. Put the sausages into a sturdy roasting tray (roughly 30 x 40cm), toss with a little olive oil and cook in the oven for 20 minutes, or until golden.

Transfer the cooked sausages to a pretty ovenproof dish and toss with half the apple and onion sauce. Cover with tin foil. Remove any excess fat from the roasting tray, replace with a good lug of olive oil and place on a medium heat. Add the remaining rosemary leaves and after 30 seconds, pour in the batter, then put straight into the middle of the oven with the sausages on the shelf underneath. Cook for around 8 to 10 minutes, or until the pudding is fluffy, golden and puffing up at the sides. Whatever you do, do not open the oven door.

Put the pan of apples and onions back on a high heat and stir in the flour. Be brave; let it get really golden before adding the cider, stock and a couple of really good splashes of Worcestershire sauce. Let it boil and bubble away until thickened to your liking. Get your guests to the table, with their knives and forks in their hands. Put the bubbling gravy on a board in the middle of the table. Remove and uncover your sizzling sausages, then slide your Yorkshire pudding on to a nice board. This lovely dish definitely needs balancing, so serve with something green and fresh, like runner beans, greens, salad or dressed chard.

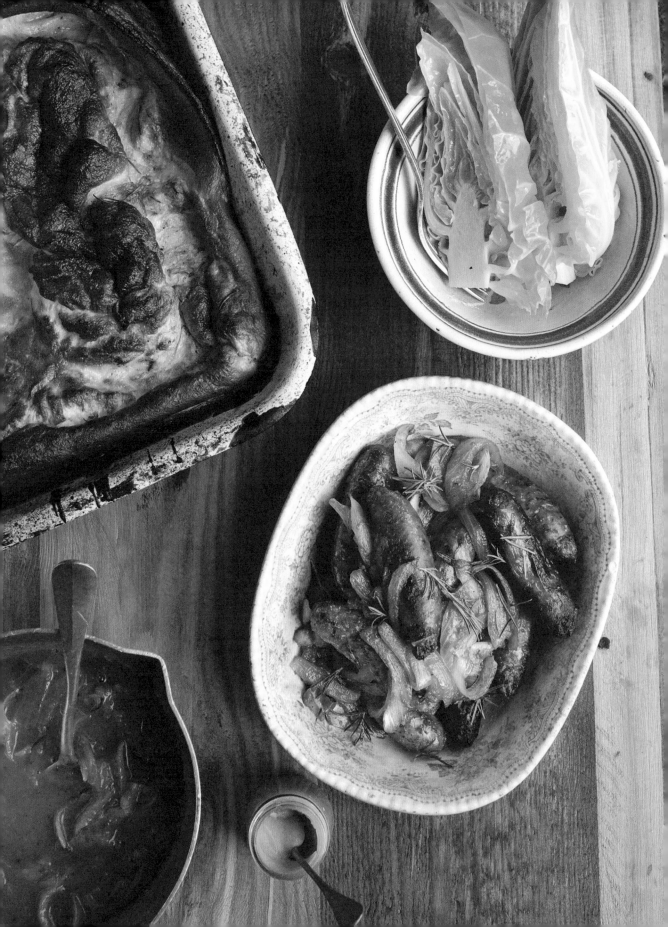

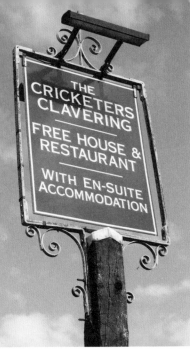

THE CRICKETERS CLAVERING

FREE HOUSE & RESTAURANT

WITH EN-SUITE ACCOMMODATION

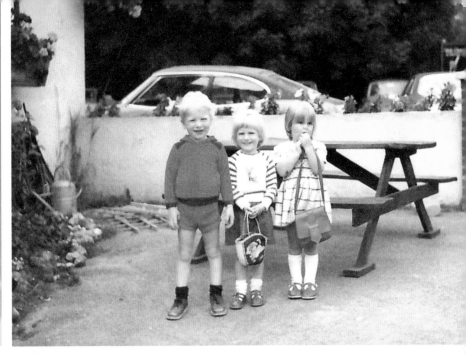

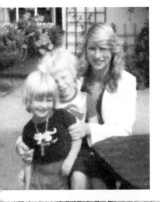

Stylish revamp at The Cricketers

The Cricketers at Clavering opened its doors today on a totally refurbished restaurant, increased bar area and more extensive new bar menu.

Alterations began in January but the public house and restaurant were only closed for a few days for completion work.

The Cricketers, is an established part of Clavering village life, aptly named because cricket is played nearby on the village green.

The premises are 400 years old, beamed and brimful of olde worlde character. There are new, larger tables in the bar area for diners who prefer a quick snack such as steak or lasagne or a choice of buffet meals.

Bar snacks are available lunchtimes and in the evenings and their Botham burger is highly recommended.

An added bonus inside is the family room, which has always proved to be popular. Now it covers a larger area where children can gather with their parents for an enjoyable lunchtime snack or evening out.

"The family room has always attracted customers, and we didn't want to lose it," said Sally Oliver, who jointly runs The Cricketers with husband, Trevor.

Anyone who went to The Cricketers prior to the extensive refurbishment will remember the fantastic display of food in the buffet area, with wholemeal rolls and an assortment of crunchy salads. Plentiful helpings of coleslaw and large slices of turkey or roast beef were included in a clear cabinet full of colourful and tasty foods. Now, it's even better.

Feast your eyes on the delights in the new refrigerated cabinets, you won't be disappointed. Have a little or everything, it's far too difficult choosing between the crisp green salad and the colourful bowls of rice salad.

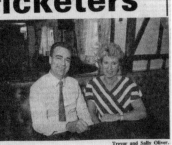

Trevor and Sally Oliver.

Meet the owners

Trevor and Sally Oliver are well-known to local residents and visitors to the area as they have run The Cricketers for the past nine years.

Trevor is experienced in the catering industry, having trained as a chef at the 'A l'ecu de France' restaurant in London. When he heard that the Clavering pub was for sale, he decided to put his energy and catering experience into running his own restaurant and pub.

Both Sally and Trevor take an active interest in the pub and up until last week they were clad in overalls helping with the refurbishment work!

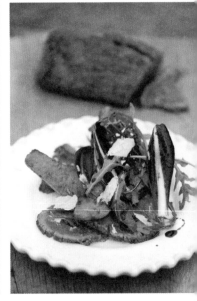

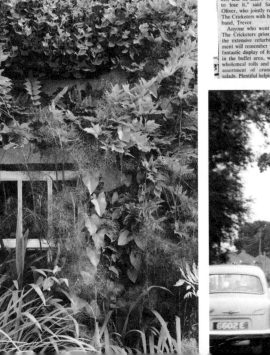

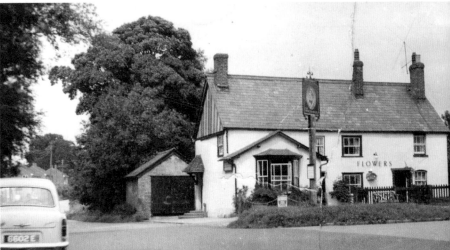

THE CRICKETERS

Christmas 1980.
16th CENTURY ENGLISH INN

Menu For December Evenings. £10·70

Smoked scotch salmon filled with prawns and
served with caviar and cucumber salad.

Chilled ogen melon with fresh tangerines and
orange brandy.

Avocado pear filled with prawns and baked with
a cheese and mushroom sauce.

Cocktail of scampi, scallops, crab and prawns
served with marie rose sauce.

Terrine of chicken liver pâté.

Cream of leek and potato soup.

Smoked mackerel with french bean and mustard
salad.

The Cricketers' arbroath smokies.

Prime local venison with a black cherry and
port wine sauce.

Tournedos of beef with madeira sauce and pâté
de foie gras.

Roast duckling with apricots, red and green
capsicums with a brandy and cream sauce.

Poached lemon sole filled with crabmeat with a
mushroom and lobster sauce, glazed with
parmesan.

Parsley chop with a sauce of gherkins, mushr
herbs and ham.

Whole baby chicken with garlic, onions, olives,
tomatoes and thyme.

Sirloin steak with a red wine, shallot and
mushroom sauce.

Veal cutlet with calvados, mushrooms and apples
finished with fresh cream and almonds.

Selection of vegetables. Sweets from the trolley.

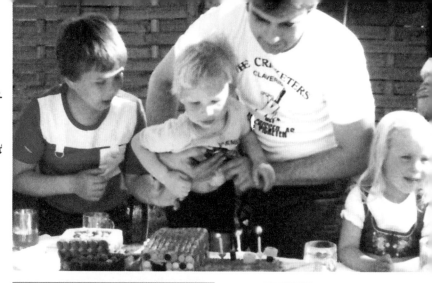

The Cricketers

This was the place where I grew up and spent all of my childhood. There were all sorts of customers from travellers to businessmen, there was lots of comfort food like pies, puddings, homemade bread, roast dinners and Mavis's mega Yorkshire puddings, and exciting things on the menu like fish days with scallops and lobster. We also had local beers, pale ale and stout, as well as that cutting-edge new drink called Appletiser. This is where my dad drilled me to work every single department of the business, and even though I was bad at school, this set me up for life. So thanks, Mum and Dad, good times. And I must say: it was a real pleasure to serve such nice customers and locals.
www.thecricketers.co.uk

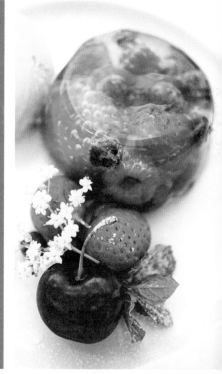

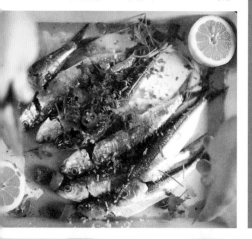

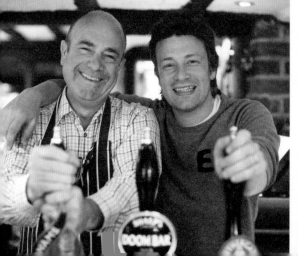

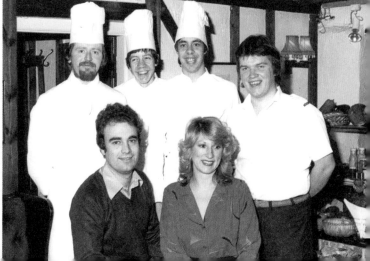

HAPPY FISH PIE

Fish pie is one of the cornerstones of great British comfort food, not really surprising when you consider that even when you're furthest inland in Britain you're still no more than seventy miles from the sea. I've called this version 'happy fish pie' because it's simple, delicious, and makes use of more underused varieties of fish. I stuck a fish tail in it right before baking and everyone seemed to like it so I just keep doing it now. These days it's so important to buy delicious but less famous fish like gurnard, coley and pouting, which are just as wonderful as cod but much more plentiful. If you are going to use cod or haddock, the best advice I can give you is to make sure it's MSC approved. Enjoy.

SERVES 6 TO 8

- 2 large leeks
- 2 large carrots
- 2 sticks of celery
- 2 knobs of butter
- 2 rashers of quality smoked streaky bacon, roughly chopped
- sea salt and white pepper

- 2 sprigs of fresh rosemary, leaves picked and finely chopped
- 2 fresh bay leaves
- 1kg Maris Piper potatoes
- olive oil
- 1 whole nutmeg, for grating
- 1 x 300ml tub of single cream

- 2 teaspoons English mustard
- 2 handfuls of grated mild Cheddar cheese
- 1 lemon
- 1kg fish fillets, skinned and pin-boned (gurnard, coley, pouting, trout would be a lovely mixture)

Strip the tough outer leaves of the leeks back, then halve, wash well and finely slice the rest. Roughly chop the carrots and celery. Get a nice casserole-type pan that's not too high-sided (roughly 20 x 30cm) and add a knob of butter and the chopped bacon. When it starts looking crisp and golden, add all the herbs and prepared vegetables to the pan. Season, then put the lid on, turn the heat down a touch and cook for around 15 minutes, stirring every now and again until sweet and tender.

Preheat the oven to 220°C/425°F/gas 7. While the vegetables cook, peel the potatoes (or leave the skins on if you like), cut into 2cm chunks and boil in salted water for around 12 to 15 minutes, or until just cooked. Drain, then leave them to steam dry for a few minutes before returning them to the empty pan. Mash with a drizzle of olive oil and a generous knob of butter. I don't like to mash too much because it can make the potato gluey rather than light and insanely crisp. Season with care and add a nice grating of nutmeg.

When the leeks are sweet, add the cream and mustard, simmer for a few seconds, then turn the heat off and sprinkle in half the grated Cheddar. Stir and season to taste, then grate in a good few swipes of lemon zest, squeeze in the juice and stir again. Cut the fish into 2cm chunks and dot them evenly around the sauce. Jiggle the dish gently so the fish gets slightly submerged in the beautiful thick sauce. Sprinkle the rest of the Cheddar on top. Put forkfuls of mash all over until the surface of the pie is evenly covered. Use a fork to pat, poof and rough it up, leaving a few little gaps for the sauce to bubble through. Put the dish at the top of the oven for 30 minutes, or until golden, crisp, bubbling and delicious. Serve with fresh lovely things like peas, beans or spinach.

PS: Here the pie is baked straight away, but if you want to make it in advance, allow everything to cool before assembling, then bake for about 45 minutes at 180°C/350°F/gas 4.

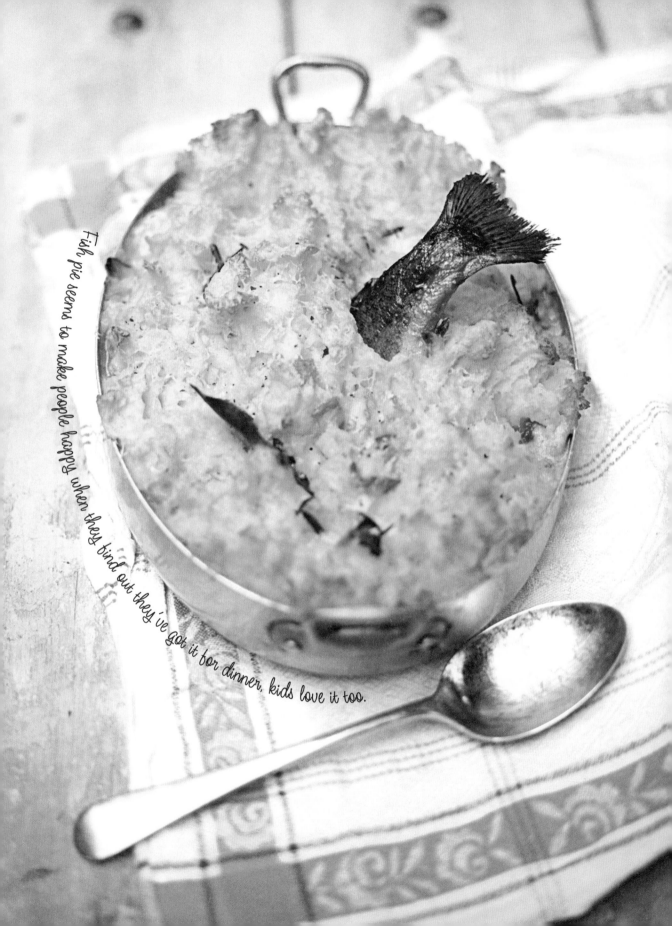

Fish pie seems to make people happy when they find out they've got it for dinner, kids love it too.

PALE ALE FONDUE
ARTISAN CHEESES • SWEET ONIONS

I've enjoyed many a fondue on skiing holidays in Switzerland and France, but making this great mountain classic with wonderful artisan British cheeses is a total joy. Choose your cheeses wisely and use a nice pale ale or cider in place of wine, and you'll have the most delicious dip. The most important thing is to blend great cheeses that melt nicely and give incredible flavours. Depending on which cheeses you use, your fondue might be a little more rustic than silky smooth, but that's fine. If you have loads of good buddies coming around, it's quite nice to make two separate batches of this, swapping in different cheeses, spices or alcohol for the second batch. Put both versions on the table and dip between the two. Your mates will love it.

SERVES 8

- ½ a white onion, peeled
- olive oil
- 1 tablespoon thyme tips
- 100ml quality smooth pale ale
- 200g quality Cheddar cheese, grated
- 200g quality Cheshire or Red Leicester cheese, grated
- 2 tablespoons single cream

Put a large saucepan on a medium heat and fill it one-third of the way up with boiling water. Find a bowl that fits on the top of your pan without touching the water and put it to one side. Carefully grate the onion on a box grater. Put a small pan on a medium heat and add a good lug of olive oil, the thyme leaves and the grated onion. Turn the heat down to low and cook for around 15 minutes, stirring occasionally, or until the onion has softened but not coloured.

Pour the beer into the onions and simmer for another 5 minutes, then tip into a heatproof bowl and place it over the pan of gently simmering water (the slower you can melt the cheese, the silkier it will be). Add all the grated cheese, then gently stir and mix everything together. Add the cream to loosen it slightly, and stir occasionally as the cheese melts down.

While your cheese melts, prepare, wash and cut any of the dipping bits you fancy (have a look at the list below, but really the sky's the limit, so use your imagination). At this point, it's all about fun and being dramatic, so pile it all in the middle of the table and people will go crazy for it. I like to take the fondue to the table still resting over the pan it cooked in, so that it holds its temperature and texture for longer; just make sure you remember to put the pan on a board so you don't burn your table.

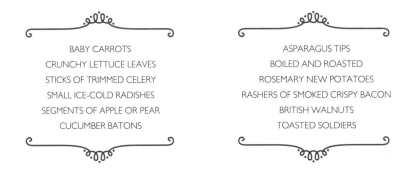

BABY CARROTS
CRUNCHY LETTUCE LEAVES
STICKS OF TRIMMED CELERY
SMALL ICE-COLD RADISHES
SEGMENTS OF APPLE OR PEAR
CUCUMBER BATONS

ASPARAGUS TIPS
BOILED AND ROASTED
ROSEMARY NEW POTATOES
RASHERS OF SMOKED CRISPY BACON
BRITISH WALNUTS
TOASTED SOLDIERS

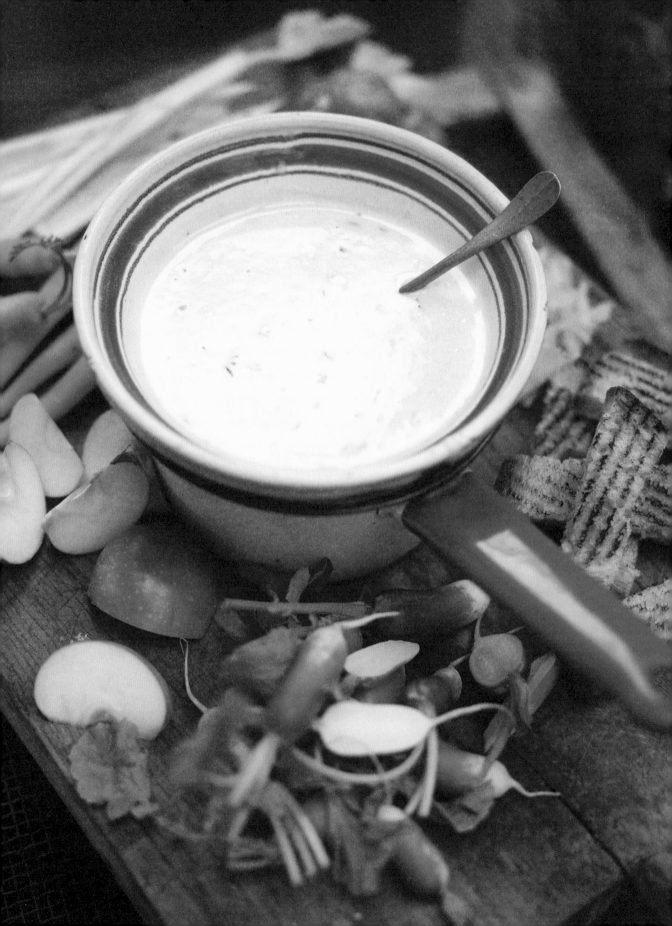

EASY PORK SCRATCHINGS
APPLE & PEAR SAUCE • TANKARD OF ALE

I don't know how it is that something this cheap and easy to make has come to be revered along with some of the finest foods, but it certainly has, and there's no denying that the British love these. As a child growing up in a pub restaurant it was clear to see that anyone with a small bowl of puffy golden scratchings and a pint of local ale in front of them was content – throw in some half-decent conversation and they'd be in seventh heaven. You should be able to get pork skin from your butcher without any trouble; if you ask nicely he might even slice it up for you. These are really good for nibbles at parties. I like to cook the apple and pear sauce a little less in the summer, then take it further in the pan during the winter months so it gets khaki and dark and feels more like comfort food.

MAKES 20 TO 25 PIECES

For the pork scratchings
- 1kg free-range pork skin
- olive oil
- 1 teaspoon ground white pepper
- 1 handful of fennel seeds
- sea salt

For the sauce
- 500g apples and pears
- a knob of butter
- 3 tablespoons white sugar
- 4 sprigs of fresh rosemary
- zest of ½ a lemon
- a splash of cider

Preheat the oven to full whack (about 240°C/475°F/gas 9). Using a very sharp knife or a Stanley knife with a clean blade, cut the pork skin into 1.5cm slices. Drizzle it with a little olive oil, then dust with the white pepper, fennel seeds and a few pinches of sea salt and rub these in. Put the skin into your largest roasting tray in a single layer, then whack into the oven for 30 to 35 minutes, until golden and puffy. All scratchings differ depending on how moist the skin is, so use your instincts and give them more time if needed.

While your crackling is crisping up, peel and quarter your apples and pears. Carefully remove and discard the cores, then roughly chop into 2cm chunks. Put into a medium pan with a knob of butter, the sugar, rosemary, lemon zest and a splash of cider. Place on a medium to high heat with a lid on until thick and gorgeous, checking and stirring occasionally. Have a taste – you may need more sugar. But keep in mind that it shouldn't be as sweet as a crumble filling – it needs to have some acidity to cut through the richness of the pork.

After about 20 minutes the fruit should be really nice and soft, so pull out the rosemary sprigs, then mash it up so you get a mix of smooth and chunky. Mix well, spoon into a bowl and serve next to the crackling and a tankard of ale. Put any leftover sauce into a clean jam jar and use up over the week with cold ham or a cheeseboard.

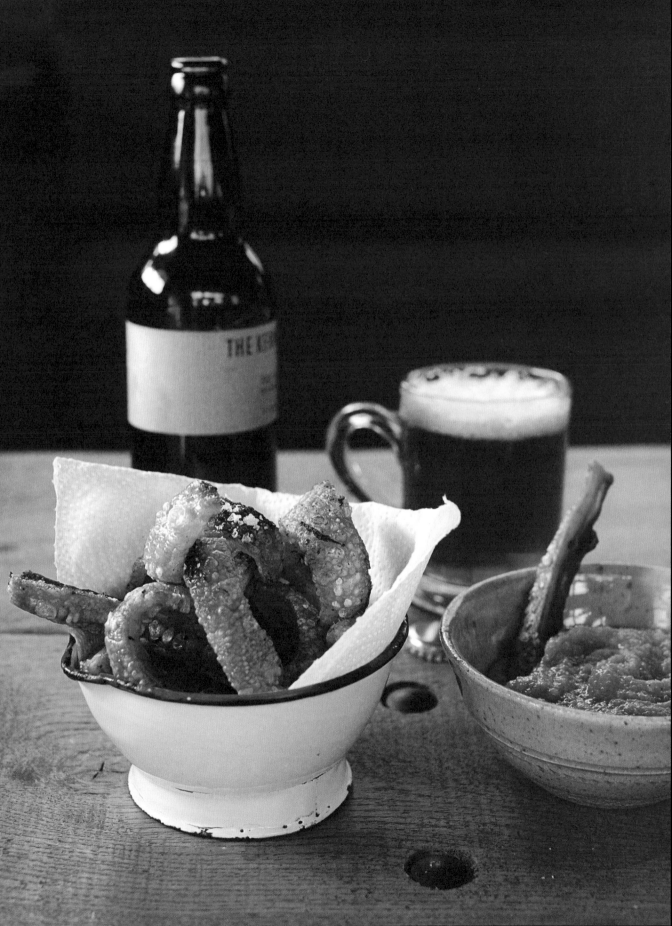

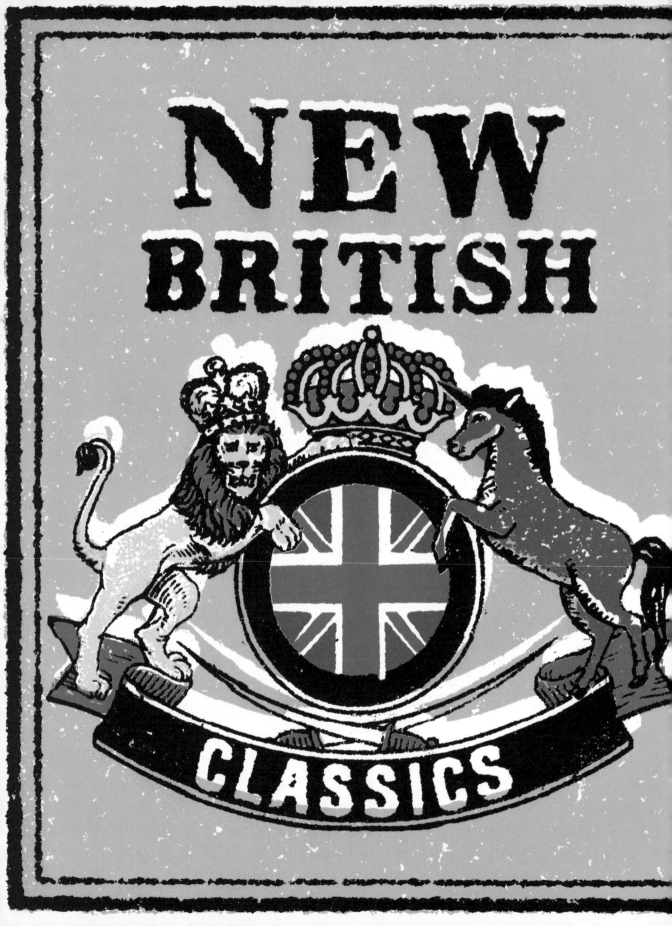

Britich food today is blessed with flavours, influences and ingredients from all corners of the world. Over our long history, foreign armies, visitors and immigrants have brought ingredients, cooking methods and radical new flavours to our tables. And like magpies, the British Empire of old explored and traded its way around the globe, bringing home the most exciting spices and glittering dishes. Over time, these things have become loved and revered. So much so, we now think of them as our own. **The food in this chapter is really a nod to this diversity. I hope it gets you going and acts as a celebration of modern British food. There's a great update on a classic Scottish haggis, as well as one of my favourite recipes in this book, Empire roast chicken - a cross between a roast chicken dinner and an Indian feast. It's quickly becoming one of my new family classics.**

EMPIRE ROAST CHICKEN

BOMBAY ROASTIES • AMAZING INDIAN GRAVY

SERVES 4 TO 6

For the chicken and marinade
- 1.4kg free-range chicken
- 1 heaped tablespoon each finely grated garlic, fresh ginger and fresh red chilli
- 1 heaped tablespoon tomato purée
- 1 heaped teaspoon each of ground coriander, turmeric, garam masala and ground cumin
- 2 heaped teaspoons natural yoghurt
- 2 lemons
- 2 level teaspoons sea salt

For the gravy
- 1 stick of cinnamon
- 3 small red onions, peeled
- 10 cloves
- 3 tablespoons each of white wine vinegar and Worcestershire sauce
- 3 level tablespoons plain flour
- 500ml organic chicken stock
- *optional:* natural yoghurt, to serve

For the Bombay-style potatoes
- 800g new potatoes
- sea salt and ground pepper
- 1 lemon
- 2 or 3 tablespoons olive oil
- a knob of butter
- 1 heaped teaspoon each of black mustard seeds, cumin seeds, garam masala and turmeric
- 1 bulb of garlic
- 1 fresh red chilli, deseeded and finely sliced
- 2 tomatoes, roughly chopped
- 1 small bunch of fresh coriander

Ask any British person what their two favourite meals are and I reckon most people would say their mum's roast chicken, and a curry. Well, welcome to Empire roast chicken, a combination of both of those things. Your friends and family are going to love it. I love it. You will love it.

Slash the chicken's legs a few times right down to the bone. Get a roasting tray slightly bigger than the chicken, then add all of the marinade ingredients and mix together well. Put on a pair of clean rubber gloves, then really massage those flavours over and inside the chicken so it's smeared everywhere. Don't be shy! Ideally marinate overnight in the fridge.

Preheat the oven to 200°C/400°F/gas 6 and organize your shelves so the roasting tray can sit right at the bottom, the chicken can sit directly above it, right on the bars of the shelf, and the potatoes can go at the top. Halve any larger potatoes, then parboil them in a large pan of salted boiling water with a whole lemon for about 15 to 20 minutes, or until the potatoes are cooked through. Drain the potatoes then let them steam dry. Stab the lemon a few times with a sharp knife and put it right into the chicken's cavity. Move the chicken to a plate.

Roughly chop the onions and add to the roasting tray along with the cinnamon stick, cloves, vinegar and Worcestershire sauce, then whisk in the flour. Pour in the stock or water, then place this right at the bottom of the oven. Place the chicken straight on to the bars of the middle shelf, above the roasting tray. Cook for 1 hour 20 minutes.

Put another sturdy roasting tray over a medium heat and add the olive oil, a knob of butter, the mustard and cumin seeds, garam masala and turmeric – work quickly because if the fat gets too hot the mustard seeds will pop everywhere. Halve a bulb of garlic and add it straight to the pan, with the sliced chilli and chopped tomatoes. Add your drained potatoes to the tray, mix everything together, then season well. Finely slice and scatter in the coriander stalks, and keep the leaves in a bowl of water for later. After the chicken has been in for 40 minutes, put the potatoes in.

Once the chicken is cooked, move it to a board and carefully peel off the dark charred bits to reveal perfect chicken underneath. Pass the gravy through a coarse sieve into a pan, whisking any sticky goodness from the pan as you go. Bring to the boil and either cook and thicken or thin down with water to your preference. Put it into a serving bowl and drizzle over a little yoghurt. Get your potatoes out of the oven and put them into a serving bowl, then serve the chicken on a board next to the sizzling roasties and hot gravy. Sprinkle the reserved coriander leaves over everything and serve with any condiments you like. Life doesn't get much better.

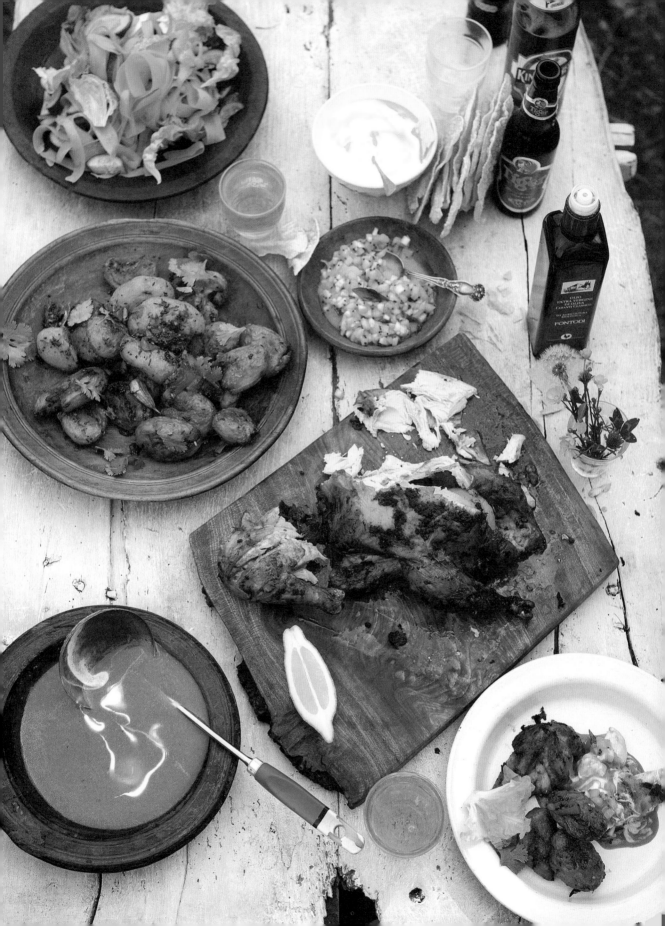

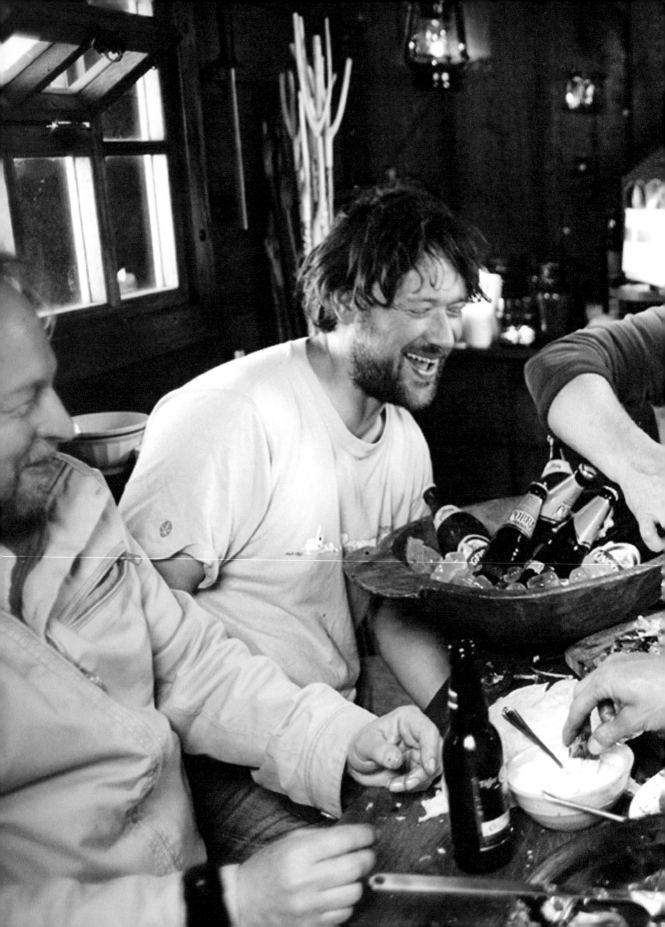

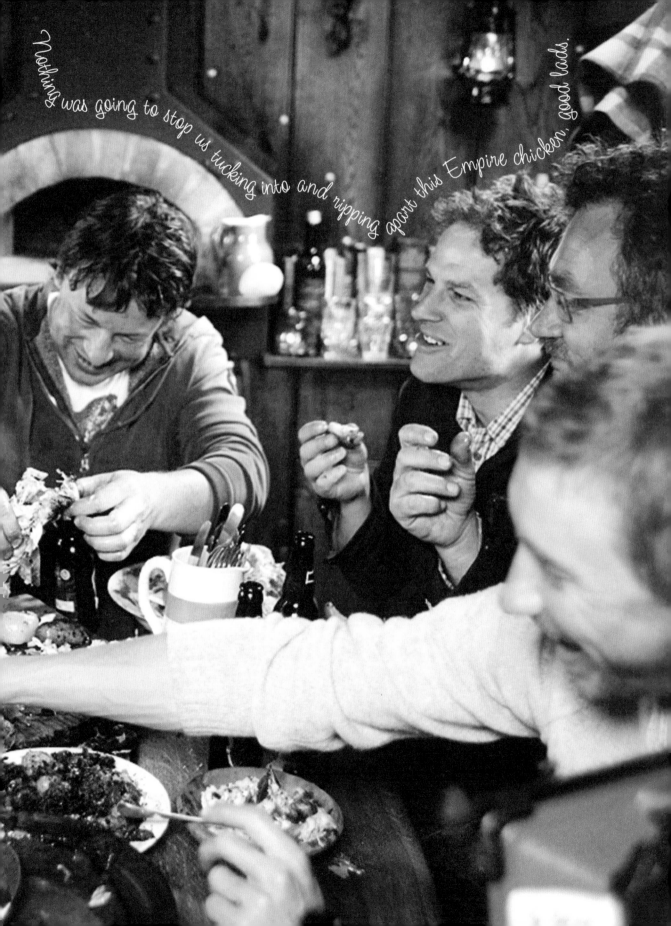

Nothing was going to stop us tucking into and ripping apart this Empire chicken, good lads.

ROASTED VEG VINDALOO
GOLDEN GNARLY CHICKEN SKEWERS

SERVES 6 TO 8

For the paste
- 1 whole bulb of garlic, cloves separated and peeled
- 1 heaped tablespoon each of turmeric and garam masala
- 2 heaped tablespoons raisins
- 1 level teaspoon each of sea salt and ground cumin
- 1 heaped teaspoon fennel seeds
- 2 dried red chillies
- a bunch of fresh coriander, leaves picked and stalks chopped
- 1 red onion, peeled and roughly chopped
- 200ml white wine vinegar
- 2 tablespoons each of Worcestershire sauce and rapeseed or olive oil

For the chicken skewers
- 4 x 150g skinless free-range chicken breasts
- rapeseed or olive oil
- 1 lemon

For the curry
- 1kg large ripe tomatoes
- sea salt and ground pepper
- 1 cauliflower, broken into florets, stalk sliced, leaves removed
- 3 red onions, peeled and roughly sliced
- 1 x 400g tin of chickpeas
- 500ml organic chicken or vegetable stock
- 500g mixed peas, broad beans and sweetcorn
- 1 x 200g bag of baby spinach
- natural yoghurt, to serve
- 1 fresh red chilli, deseeded and finely chopped

I was cooking with some of the Goan community in Leeds and was interested to learn that vindaloo, a curry famous all over the UK, is actually from Goa but has European roots. That part of India was, for many hundreds of years, actually under Portuguese control. It was the Portuguese who introduced vinegar to Goa and put the 'vin' (vinegar) in vindaloo ('loo' was the garlic). With this recipe, you're creating a wonderful standout vegetable curry but then adding a meat kicker for any non-veggies at the table. It's a great one for a mixed dinner party – everyone's happy.

Preheat your oven to 200°C/400°F/gas 6. Put all the paste ingredients except the coriander leaves into a liquidizer and whiz until smooth, then scrape the paste out into a bowl. Roughly chop the tomatoes and add to the liquidizer, season well, then blitz until smooth and put aside for later. In a large casserole-type pan, toss the cauliflower florets and red onions with half the curry paste. Add 600ml of water, and roast in the hot oven for 40 minutes, stirring halfway through. Meanwhile, cut the chicken into finger-sized strips, toss them in the bowl with the remaining curry paste, cover and pop into the fridge.

After 40 minutes, carefully move the hot pan from the oven to the hob. Drain and add the chickpeas, along with the stock and blitzed tomatoes and simmer on a medium heat for about 30 minutes, or until the consistency you like. Meanwhile, preheat a large griddle pan over a high heat. Thread the chicken pieces on to 6 or 8 metal or wooden skewers. Drizzle with a little oil, season from a height, and cook on the screaming hot griddle for around 10 to 12 minutes, turning each one every now and again, until gnarly, sizzly and cooked through. Squeeze over some lemon juice and give the pan a good shake, scraping the bottom of the pan for around 30 seconds to get all the intense flavour. Transfer everything to a plate and set aside.

Go back to your curry and mash a few times to thicken up the sauce. Add the delicate veggies (corn, peas, beans and spinach) for the last 3 minutes of cooking, then have a taste and correct the seasoning. Marble through a few dollops of yoghurt, scatter over the reserved coriander leaves and chopped fresh chilli (leave the seeds in for extra heat), then take straight to the table. Serve with fluffy rice, the chicken skewers and anything else you fancy.

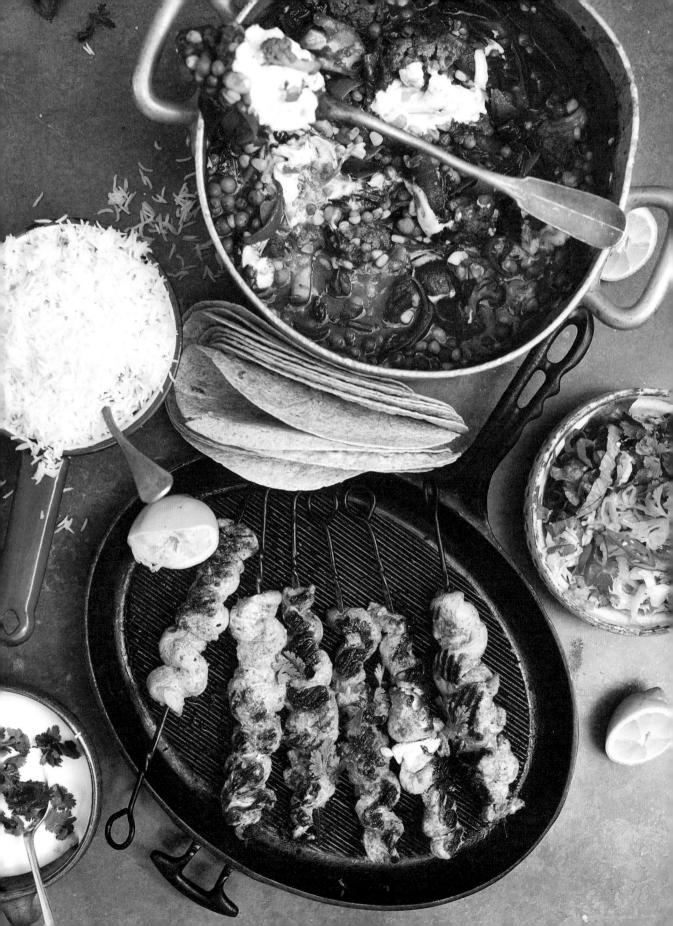

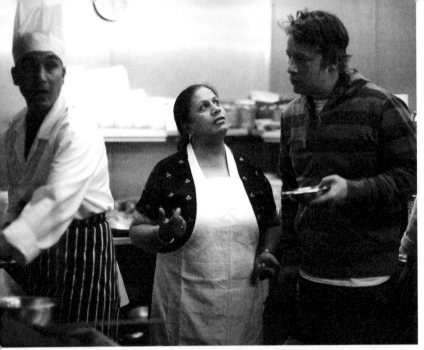

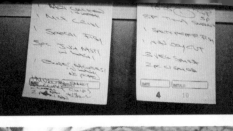

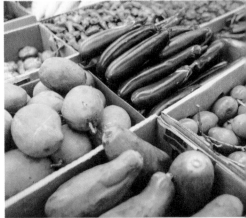

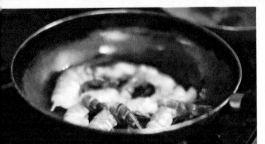

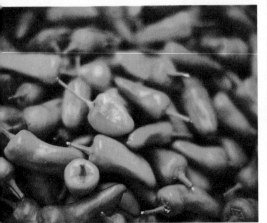

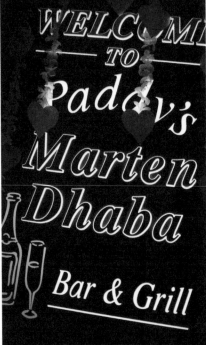

WELCOME TO Paddy's Marten Dhaba

Bar & Grill

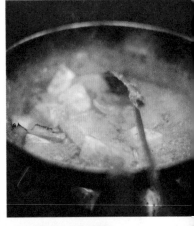

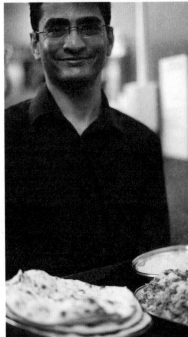

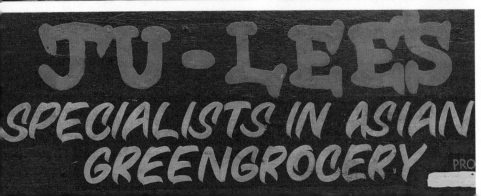

JU-LEES

SPECIALISTS IN ASIAN GREENGROCERY

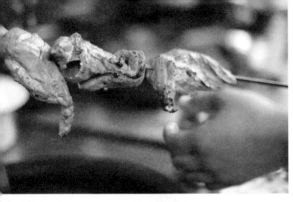
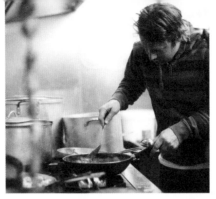
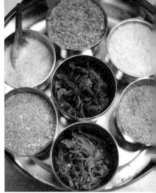
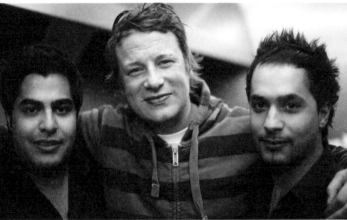
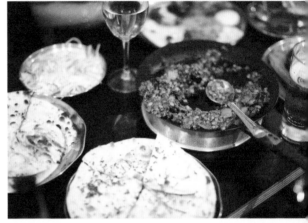

Paddy's Marten Dhaba Bar and Grill

Paddy's Bar and Grill is a brilliant Indian restaurant in a lovely old pub. What I love about these guys is that the menu represents many different and specific areas of Indian cooking, like Gujarati, Punjabi and Keralan. These regions are represented by their chefs, which makes it incredibly authentic, and also a testament to the fact that our great British Indian communities have been in Britain for so long that we're now going beyond the food being just Indian, and getting into specific regions. The pub is in Leicester, which is predicted to be one of the first minority majority cities. I loved everything I tried. It's called Paddy's because when it opened the locals couldn't pronounce Pradip, the dad's real name, so they just called him Paddy. Now the sons Rajiv and Ravi are both working the floor as well, with their mighty mum Amita in the kitchen cracking the whip – she's brilliant. What a lovely place.

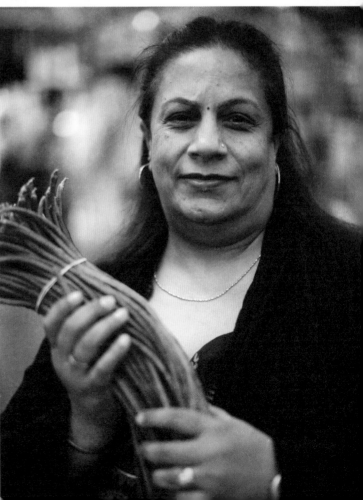
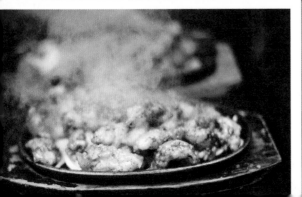

ER'S DIAMOND JUBILEE CHICKEN

SERVES 4 TO 6

- 8 large free-range chicken thighs, bone in and skin on
- 1 heaped tablespoon garam masala
- 1 level teaspoon cumin seeds
- 1 level teaspoon turmeric
- ½ teaspoon chilli powder
- olive oil
- sea salt and ground pepper
- a thumb-sized piece of fresh ginger, peeled
- 4 cloves of garlic, peeled
- 1 lemon
- a handful of cashews or almonds
- 2 heaped tablespoons sesame seeds
- ½ a ripe pineapple, peeled and cored
- ½ a cucumber, seeds scraped out
- 6 spring onions, trimmed
- 1 fresh red chilli
- 250g natural yoghurt
- 2 limes
- a small bunch of fresh coriander

June 2012 is Queen Elizabeth II's sixtieth year on the throne, and her official eighty-sixth birthday. The dish we know as Coronation chicken was created in honour of her 1953 coronation, and I'm sure it was probably an update on Jubilee chicken, which was created for King George V's Silver Jubilee in 1935. Coronation chicken is served with salad and in sandwiches in restaurants, cafés and supermarkets all over Britain, and unfortunately it's become one of those things that's often done very badly. So let me introduce you to Diamond Jubilee chicken! I'm amplifying the crispy-skinned tender chicken, using lovely spices, sweet ripe fruit, fresh herbs and citrus to make it worthy of the occasion. I'll be offering to make it for her when the Jubilee rolls around (though I might calm the chillies down a bit!).

Preheat the oven to 190°C/375°F/gas 5. Put the chicken thighs into a bowl with all the spices, a drizzle of olive oil and a pinch of salt and pepper. Grate in the ginger and garlic, and squeeze in the juice of the lemon. Feel free to put some rubber gloves on, then mix and rub those flavours all over the chicken. Arrange the thighs in a snug-fitting roasting tray in a single layer, skin side up, and cook at the top of the oven for around 50 minutes, or until the meat pulls away easily from the bone.

Once cooked, remove the chicken skin and place it upside down on a separate roasting tray. Scatter the nuts and seeds over the skin, then put it back into the oven for around 10 minutes, or until the skin is really crispy and the nuts are toasted (don't burn them, set the alarm!). Remove from the oven and leave to cool. Meanwhile, chop the pineapple and cucumber into 1cm cubes and sprinkle them on to a beautiful serving platter, then finely slice the spring onions and chilli and add those to the platter too, saving a little fresh chilli for garnishing.

Spoon away any fat from the roasting tray, leaving the juices behind, then use two forks to pull the chicken meat apart in the tray, discarding the bones and any wobbly bits. Move all the delicious meat to the serving platter then, in the tray mix three quarters of the yoghurt, the juice of 2 limes, and the chopped coriander stalks, keeping the leaves aside. Mix everything up nicely, scraping all the goodness from the bottom of the tray, then taste and season to perfection.

Pour the sauce all over the platter, then toss and mix everything together using two forks. Clean around the edges of the platter if it's messy, then sprinkle over the crispy skin, toasted nuts and seeds, the coriander leaves and red chilli. Drizzle over the rest of the yoghurt and serve.

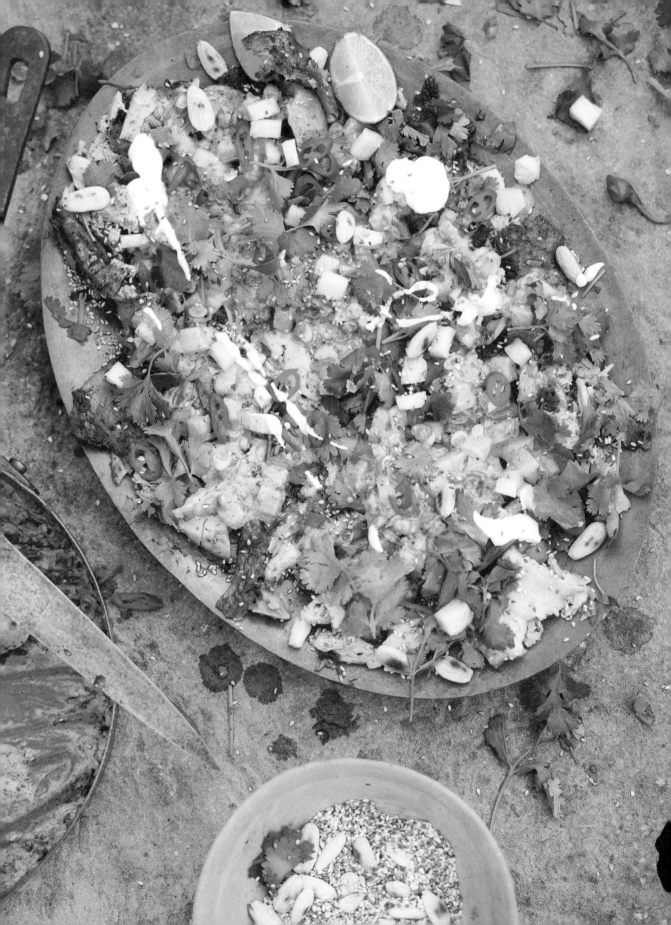

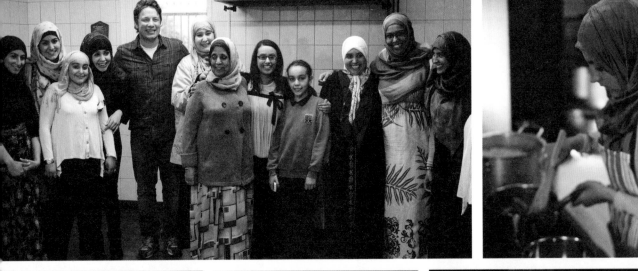

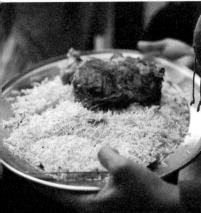

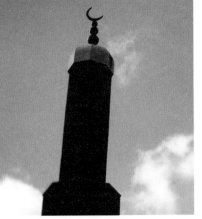

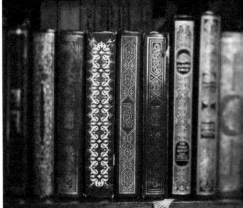

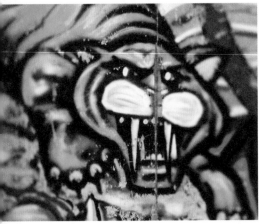

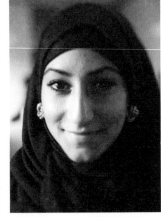

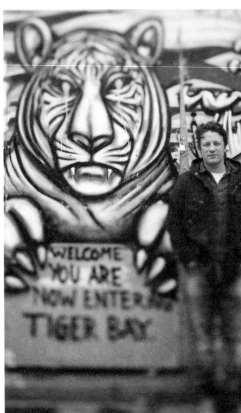

WELCOME
YOU ARE
NOW ENTERING
TIGER BAY

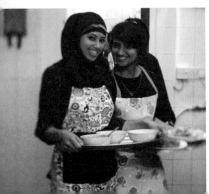

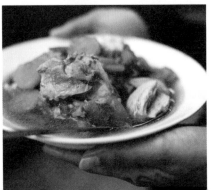

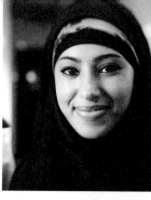

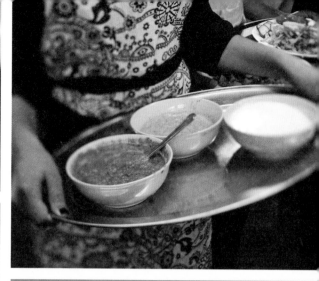

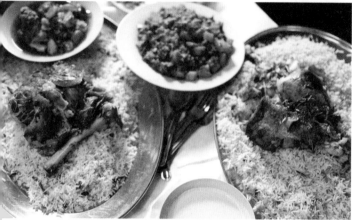

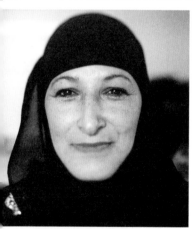

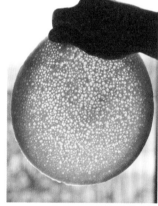

Welsh Yemeni Community

Some of the most delicious food I've had in ages was cooked by the Yemeni ladies in a community centre in Bute Town in Cardiff, historically known as Tiger Bay. Back in the industrial revolution, British steam ships were sailing across the world, stopping at ports like Aden in Yemen. The Yemeni men were strapping, strong lads who got work stoking the coal on the ships that travelled back to Cardiff, and many of them stayed in Wales, which is how the Yemeni community first began. The ladies' cooking was intelligent and comforting, and its genius was the biggest culinary secret I'd uncovered in a long time. Mainly because, in Yemeni culture, they don't really have restaurants - it's all about the home. So you're not going to nip down the road and get a Yemeni, like we do with an Indian or a Chinese. The fun and happiness I had with these lovely, friendly ladies, as you can see from all their faces, was inspiring. I think it's important that we realize we have our own Yemeni communities here in Britain that can let us know what Yemen is really all about, instead of just the soundbites we hear on the news.

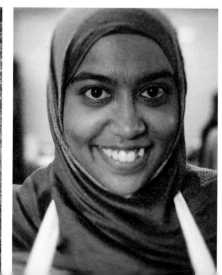

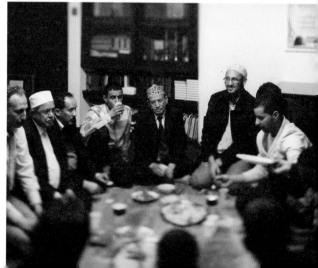

SERVES 4

For the lamb and marinade
- 1 heaped teaspoon coriander seeds
- 1 level teaspoon cumin seeds
- a generous pinch of turmeric
- 2 bird's-eye chillies, stalks removed, finely sliced
- 2 cloves of garlic, peeled and finely sliced
- sea salt and ground pepper
- olive oil
- 8 long lamb cutlets, not trimmed, fatty side scored

For the spiced nuts
- 50g blanched almonds
- 50g shelled pistachios
- 1 tablespoon sesame seeds
- a pinch of ground cumin

For the cucumber dip
- ½ a cucumber
- a handful of fresh mint leaves
- 100g natural yoghurt
- ½ a lemon

For the spicy tomato dip
- 2 large ripe tomatoes
- 1 fresh red chilli
- a few sprigs of fresh coriander
- a little feta cheese, for crumbling over
- ½ a lemon

I came up with this recipe when I was in Wales, which produces some of the best lamb in the world. Ask your butcher for extra long lamb cutlets, untrimmed, so you have big Captain Caveman style chops to gnaw on. Marinate the lamb overnight if you can, to really intensify the flavours, which are inspired by the amazing Yemeni cooks I met in the old Tiger Bay community near the docks in Cardiff. Their community has been there for over 200 years, ever since the coal boom of the industrial revolution brought their ancestors to Wales. Their food hasn't become famous in the same way other cuisines have. But it should have. It's some of the most exciting food I've seen in a long time.

Pound the marinade spices, chillies and garlic to a paste using a pestle and mortar add a good pinch of salt and pepper, then muddle in just enough olive oil to make the mixture nice and loose. Get a roasting tray, put in the cutlets and rub the marinade all over them. Cover with clingfilm and put into the fridge, or to one side if you're cooking right away.

Now get all your little dips ready. Put the nuts, sesame seeds, cumin and a pinch of salt into a dry frying pan and toast for a few minutes, tossing occasionally. Once golden, tip them into the mortar and pound up a few times until fine and crunchy, then pour them into a little bowl. Coarsely grate the cucumber on a box grater, then transfer it to a bowl, squeezing out any excess liquid. Finely chop the mint and add it to the bowl with the yoghurt, a good pinch of salt and pepper, and a good squeeze of lemon juice. Stir, then put into a little bowl next to the toasted nuts.

Halve the tomatoes and rub each half, cut side down, on the finer side of the grater so you end up with a fresh tomato slurry. Discard the skins, then finely grate in half the chilli. Season with salt and pepper, stir in a squeeze of lemon juice, sprinkle over some coriander leaves, and crumble over a little feta. Have a taste, adjust if you want it a bit spicier, or saltier, then put it into a little bowl next to the other dips.

Heat a griddle pan on a high heat and cook the lamb cutlets for around 4 minutes on each side, standing them on their fatty sides for a minute or two extra to crisp up. Once they are sizzling and golden, they're done. Pile them on a board, then get stuck in and encourage everyone to dunk the chops in the dips and some of the bashed-up nuts. Lovely with flatbreads or rice.

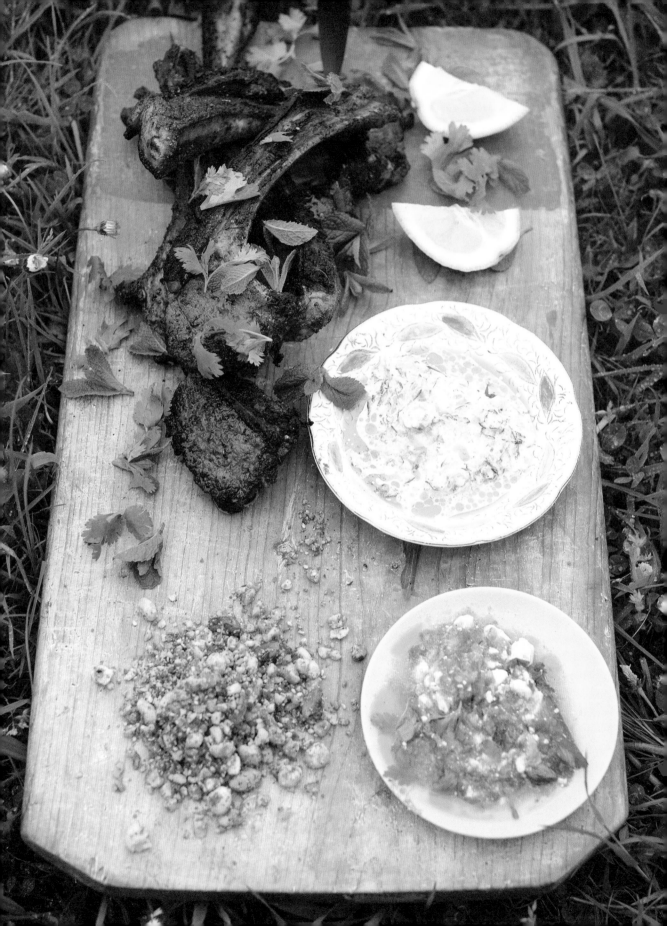

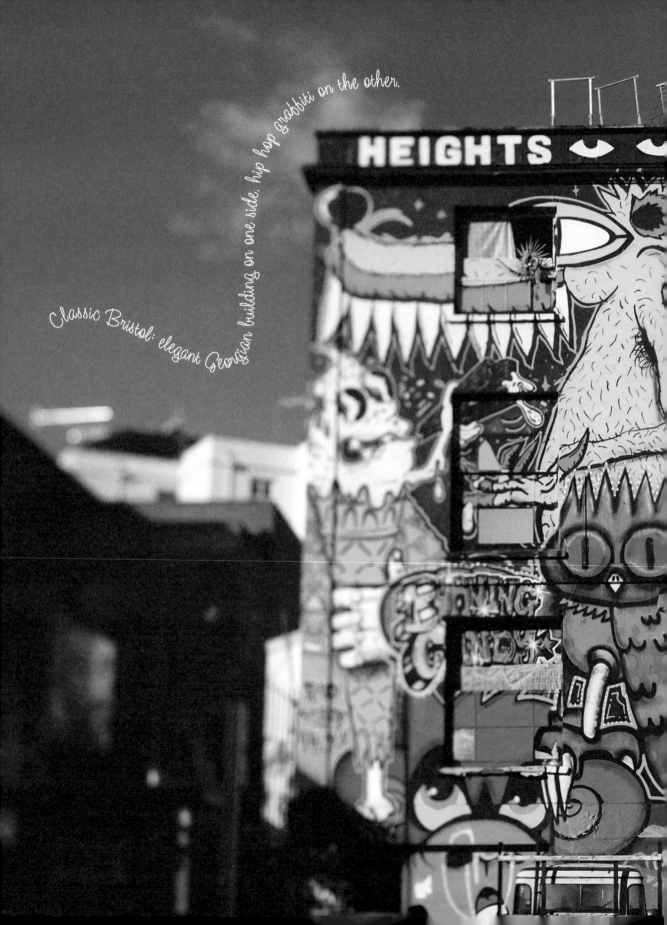

Classic Bristol: elegant Georgian building on one side, hip hop graffiti on the other.

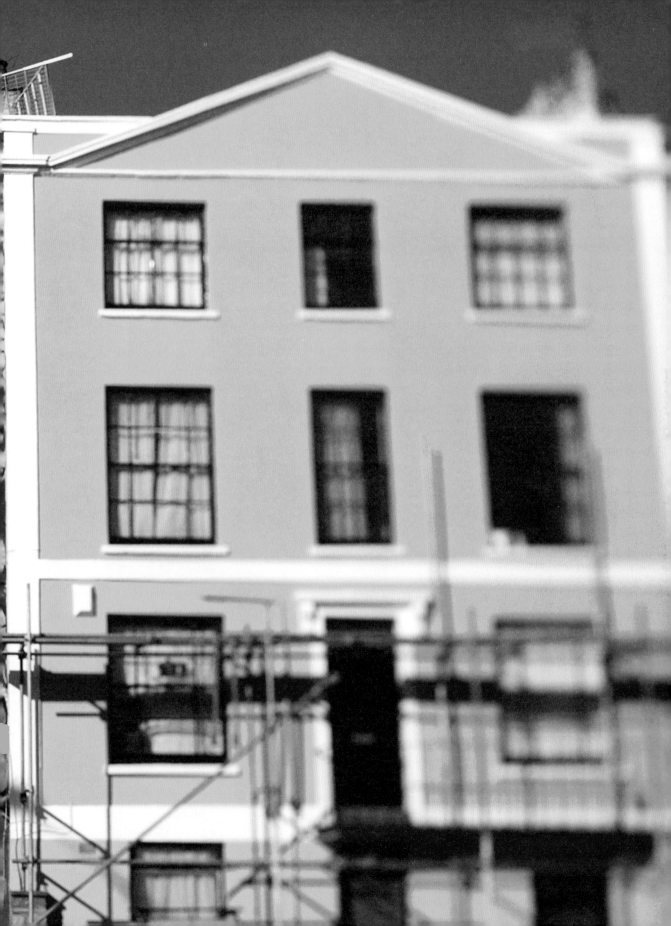

EASY ESSEX HAGGIS
NEEPS & TATTIES SHEPHERD'S PIE STYLIE

SERVES 16

- 3 medium onions, peeled and quartered
- 3 sticks of celery, trimmed and roughly chopped
- 3 rashers of quality smoked streaky bacon
- 8 sprigs of fresh thyme, leaves picked
- olive oil
- 3 heaped teaspoons allspice
- 3 heaped teaspoons finely ground pepper
- 1 level teaspoon ground cloves
- sea salt
- 1 whole nutmeg
- olive oil
- 500g chuck steak
- 500g shoulder of lamb or mutton
- 1 pig's or lamb's heart
- 250g lamb's kidneys
- 250g chicken livers
- 10 fresh bay leaves
- 1.5 litres beef stock, preferably organic
- 500g pinhead oats (coarse ground oatmeal)
- 50ml whisky
- 1 lemon
- 1 orange
- 2 tablespoons Worcestershire sauce

This recipe is inspired by a particularly delicious version I tried at the Ubiquitous Chip restaurant in Glasgow. They serve their haggis on large spoons instead of in the sheep's stomach (which is the traditional way). So I've decided to write a recipe that anyone, anywhere in the world, can make as long as they have access to a fairly decent butcher. I think it still preserves the beautiful soul and attitude of haggis, and my mate Peter Begg, who is 110% Scottish, says it's the nicest haggis he's ever had. That made my year, so what are you waiting for? Crack on!

Put the onions and celery into a food processor with the bacon and thyme leaves and pulse until finely chopped. Put a very large casserole-type pan (roughly 25cm in diameter) on a medium heat, add a good lug of olive oil, then add the allspice, pepper, ground cloves, a good pinch of salt, and grate in the nutmeg. Stir for a few minutes, until it's smelling fantastic, then tip in everything from the food processor and cook for a few minutes, stirring occasionally until the veg are starting to soften.

Cut the steak into roughly 2cm pieces and pulse in a food processor until it looks like mince. Add to the pan of veg, then do the same with the lamb or mutton and the heart. Get rid of any sinewy bits. Halve the kidneys, and quickly rinse them and the livers in a bowl of water. Drain, then pulse in the processor once or twice – don't purée them! Add to the pan, then cook and stir everything for about 15 minutes, or until the meat starts to colour. At this point, add the bay leaves and 500ml of stock or water, then cover with a lid and leave to blip away on a low heat for around 2 hours, stirring now and then to make sure it doesn't catch and adding a splash of water if needed.

Preheat the oven to 180°C/350°F/gas 4. After 2 hours, spoon a few ladles of the haggis mixture (avoiding the bay leaves) into the clean food processor and blitz to a fairly smooth consistency. Stir this back in to add a lovely creaminess. Spread the pinhead oats on a baking tray and toast in the oven for about 25 minutes, or until golden. Stir into the haggis mixture, then add the remaining stock. Simmer with the lid off for about another 30 to 35 minutes. This is a great time to cook your neeps and tatties (see page 334).

Once the time is up, fish out the bay leaves and continue cooking until you've got a nice thick consistency. Turn the heat off, then correct the seasoning to push it to the point of perfection. Stir in the whisky, a few gratings of lemon and orange zest and the Worcestershire sauce. Taste and correct the flavours if needed, then put the lid on and leave until you're ready to serve – preferably with plenty of good friends and a dram or two of fine Scottish whisky.

PS: Put the leftover haggis into an earthenware-type dish and top it off with neeps and tatties. It makes the most exciting sorta-shepherd's pie.

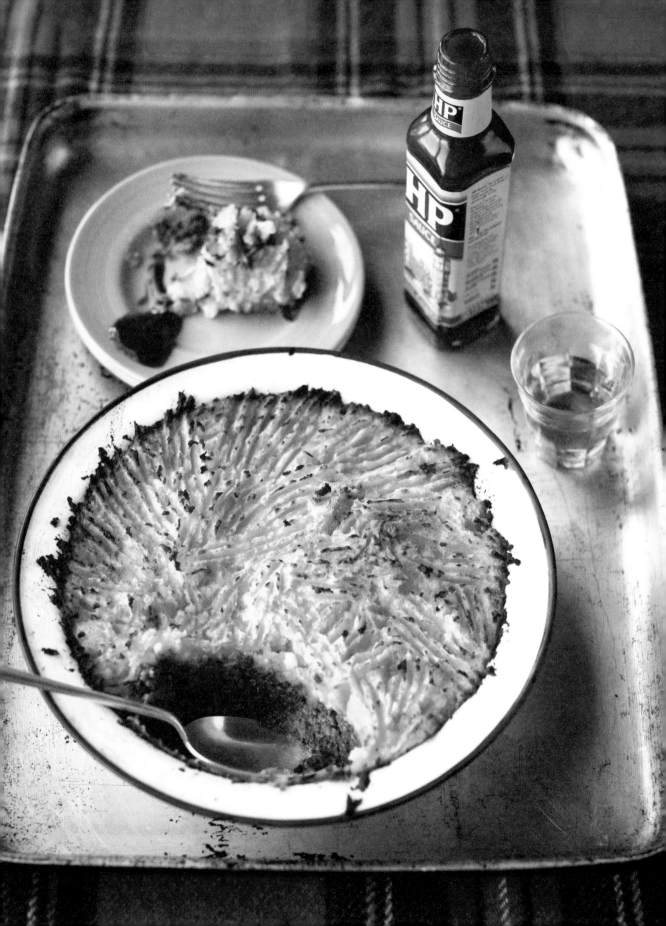

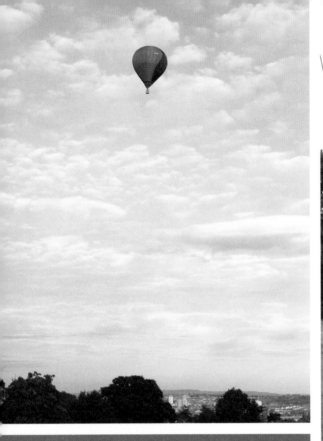

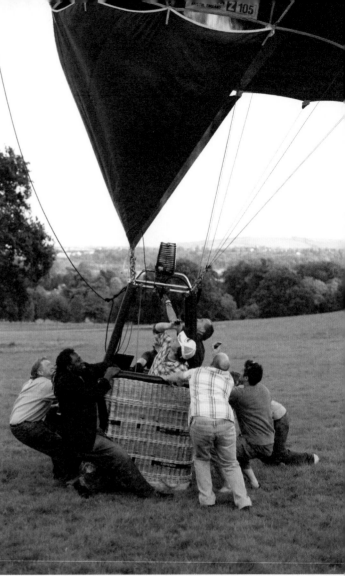

Beautiful Bristol

Bristol is a really exciting, multicultural city in the heart of some really beautiful countryside, and, as you can see, with me hanging in a basket God knows how high in the air, it's one of the busiest ballooning areas in the world. The communities represent a wonderfully diverse ethnic mix. Bristol ports used to be some of the busiest in Europe and were specifically linked with the slave triangle between Britain, the West Indies and Africa. As a result of that dark time, ingredients from these places became part of our cooking, and made it much nicer and more exciting along the way.

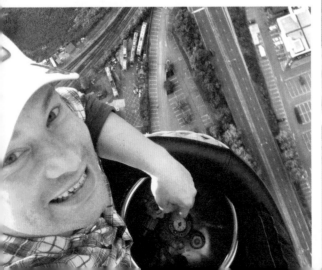

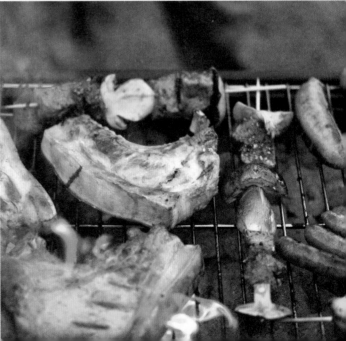

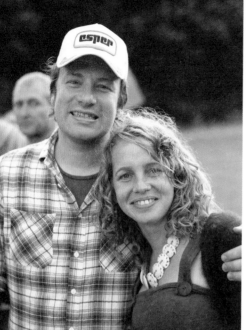
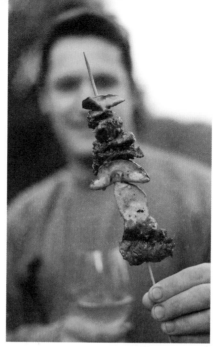
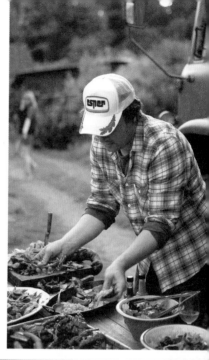
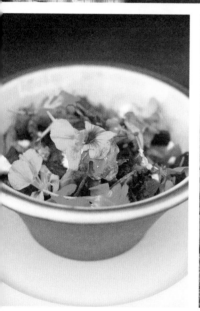
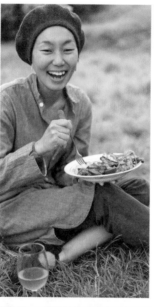
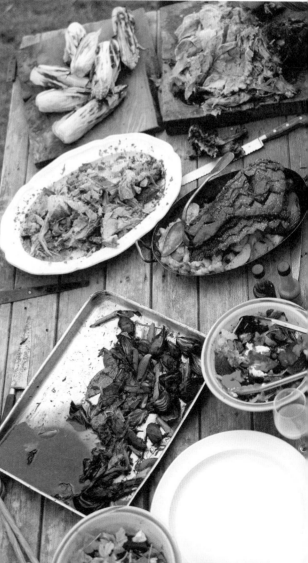
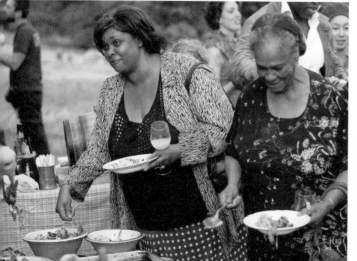

JERK-DRESSED BRISTOL PORK
CRUNCHY CRACKLING • ORCHARD APPLE SAUCE

Just about everyone gets excited when they see roast pork on the table. But even though a whole roasted shoulder is really impressive, it's actually a 'slam and go' recipe. Of course it's lovely served with roast potatoes and the orchard sauce on page 380, but lately, I've been pulling all the meat apart and tossing it through this great jerk salsa – hell, yeah! The flavours of Jamaica and Britain really work well together – and actually many of the same spices found in jerk can also be found in some of the most quintessentially British puddings, syrups and even our beloved mulled wine. This is my version of jerk-dressed pork, and I love it.

SERVES 12 WITH LEFTOVERS

- 5kg free-range shoulder of pork, bone in, skin on
- sea salt and ground pepper
- a generous pinch each of dried rosemary and thyme
- 1 whole nutmeg, for grating
- olive oil
- 2 x 500ml bottles of quality cider

For the jerk salsa
- 1-2 fresh Scotch bonnet chillies (to taste)
- 2 bunches of spring onions, trimmed
- 1 level teaspoon ground cinnamon
- 1 level teaspoon ground cloves
- 2 level teaspoons ground allspice

- 3 limes
- a thumb-sized piece of fresh ginger, peeled
- a few fresh bay leaves
- 2 cloves of garlic, peeled
- 1-2 tablespoons honey
- extra virgin olive oil
- a large bunch of fresh coriander

Preheat the oven to full whack (about 240°C/475°F/gas 9). Carefully score the skin and fat on the shoulder into zigzags about 1cm deep, using a very sharp knife or a clean Stanley knife. Sprinkle and rub in a good pinch of salt, pepper, dried rosemary, thyme, and a few good gratings of nutmeg. Add a lug of olive oil, then rub those flavours all over the meat and into the scores. Place the pork, skin side up, in your largest roasting pan. Pour one of the bottles of cider into the bottom of the tray, put into the hot oven for 30 minutes so the crackling gets going, then turn the heat down to 130°C/250°F/gas ½.

After the pork has been in for an hour, add the rest of the cider and cook for a further 6 to 7 hours, or until the meat pulls apart easily. Halfway through the cooking time cover with a double layer of tin foil.

Once the pork is perfectly cooked, move it to a large serving board or platter. Carefully pour any fat from the roasting tray into a Kilner jar for some lucky roast potato some day, but leave the wonderful flavourful cooking juices in the pan. Then add the Scotch bonnets to a liquidizer with the spring onions, spices, the juice from the limes, ginger, bay leaves, garlic, a squeeze of honey and 2 lugs of extra virgin olive oil. Pulse together until you get a salsa consistency, then mix the salsa into the juices in the roasting tray, have a taste and balance out the salt and acid if needed. It should have attitude and loads of personality. Pour that salsa on to a platter, then pull the crispy crackling off the shoulder, get rid of any flobbery fat underneath, and use two forks to roughly pull the meat apart. Pile the meat on top of the salsa and toss together quickly. Tear over any coriander leaves and snap those wonderful zigzags of crackling on top of the meat and serve next to your orchard sauce. Rock 'n' roll!

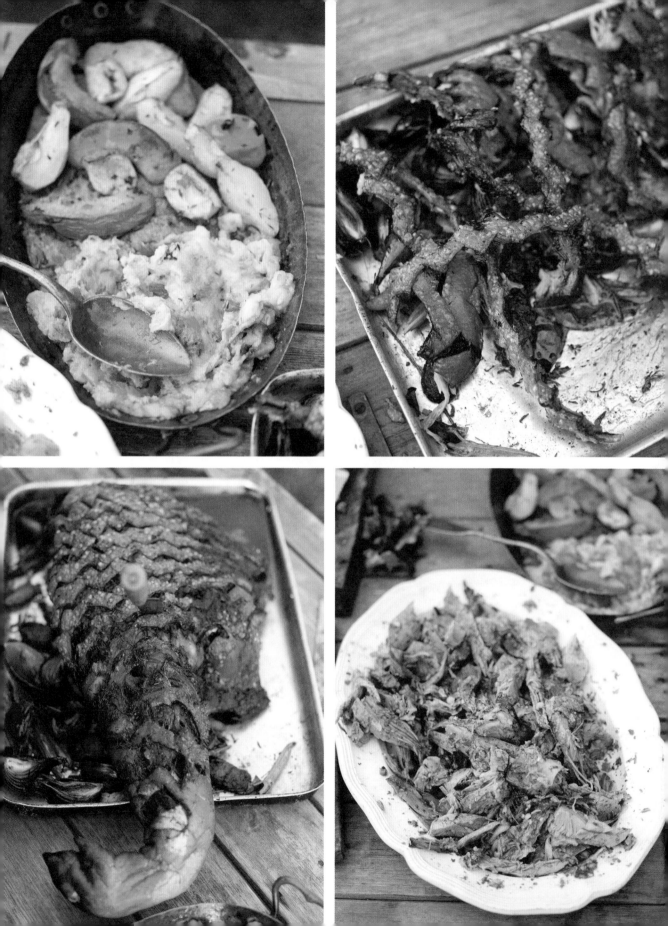

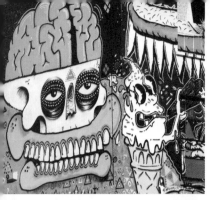

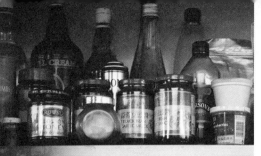

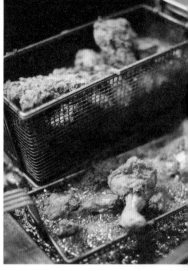

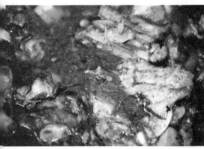

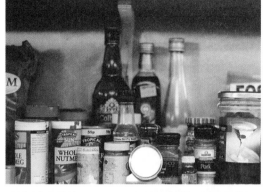

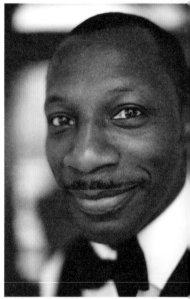

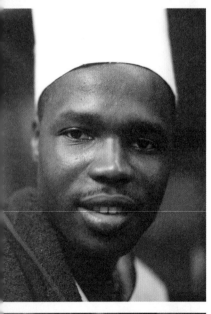

Rice & Things

Rice & Things in Bristol is run by a very cool dude, Chef Neufville. His food is excellent, his seasoning is sublime, and he built up his business, bought the building, and a beautiful pad in his homeland of Jamaica, starting as a hardworking immigrant who came to England with nothing. That's the kind of man I admire. He was passionate that I taste the flavours and feel the positive energy of the Caribbean instead of the stereotypes; this dude was a very special guy.

www.riceandthings.co.uk

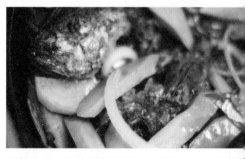

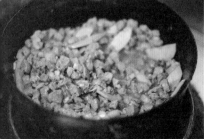

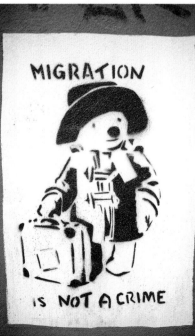

MIGRATION

IS NOT A CRIME

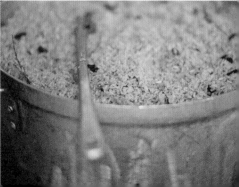

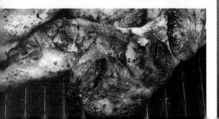

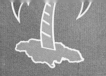

Exclusive Jamaican Restaurant

Tel: 07890 627749   Tel: 924 4

Me and all the gang at Rice & Things; this restaurant is amazing.

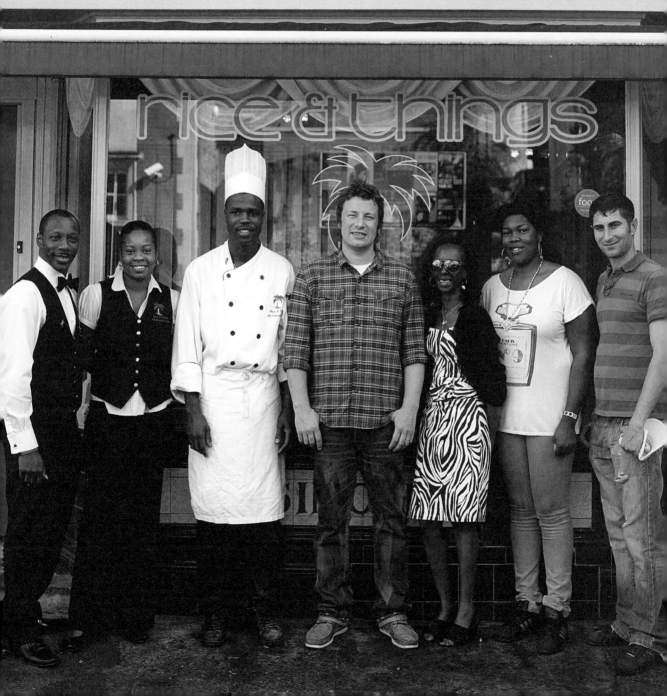

Afternoon TEA

Snacking is nothing new; we humans are all born to snack, but it took a lady-in-waiting to turn it into a British institution. The Duchess of Bedford was Queen Victoria's friend and lady-in-waiting in the 1840s. In those days, dinner was served fashionably late, at about 8 pm, but understandably, people got really hungry between lunch and dinner. So the Duchess started requesting tea and bread and butter in the afternoons, and would invite a few of her friends along. It caught on really quickly, and along the way delicate little sandwiches, cakes and scones were added, until eventually we ended up with something really special. **The things in this chapter are some of my favourite afternoon tea treats. Admittedly, there's a fine line between desserts and afternoon tea, but it's hardly a daily occurrence these days, and if you can sit down with a nice slice of delicate sponge and a cup of tea why wouldn't you? I don't know anyone that doesn't love it, regardless of where they're from.**

MY NAN'S ST CLEMENT'S CAKE

This cake reminds me of my nan, and also of some of the older customers who used to come into my parents' pub. The old dears would come up to the bar and ask for a half pint of Guinness for themselves and a St Clement's for the wife, which is a simple orange juice and lemonade combo. It's named after that nursery rhyme we all grew up singing, which I've realized is actually quite a sinister song about owing people money and chopping off heads! But putting that aside, this cake is as sweet and lovely as you'd want it to be. The icing that seeps into the sponge adds flavour, and once the top layer firms up it becomes a sherbety, citrusy delight. If you really smother the cake well, it will help to keep it nice and moist for quite some time. This recipe also makes the sweetest little cupcakes.

SERVES 12

- 125g unsalted butter, softened, plus extra for greasing
- 225g golden caster sugar
- 4 large free-range eggs
- 1 large orange
- 200g ground almonds
- 100g self-raising flour

For the lemon icing
- 225g icing sugar
- 1 lemon

Preheat your oven to 180°C/350°F/gas 4. Grease a 20cm loose-bottomed springform cake tin with a knob of butter, then line the base with greaseproof paper.

Beat the softened butter with 125g of the caster sugar until it's light and creamy, then crack in the eggs, one at a time, beating each one in well before adding the next. Finely grate in most of the orange zest, keeping back a few scrapings of the zest in a clingfilm-covered bowl. Fold in the ground almonds and sift in the flour. Mix and gently combine everything, then spoon the cake batter into your prepared tin and bake in the oven for about 30 minutes, or until risen and lightly golden. To check that the cake is cooked through, poke a skewer or cocktail stick into the centre of the sponge. If it comes out clean, it's done; if not, cook it for a few more minutes. Leave to cool for a few minutes in the tin while you make the orange syrup.

Put the remaining 100g of caster sugar into a pan and add the juice of the zested orange. Place the pan on a medium heat for a few minutes, or until the sugar has dissolved. While the cake is still hot, poke lots of little holes in the top with a cocktail stick and pour the syrup all over it. Once all the syrup has been absorbed, move the cake to a wire rack to cool completely.

To make the icing, sift the icing sugar into a bowl and grate in most of the lemon zest. Keep back a few gratings, add them to the bowl of reserved orange zest, and cover again with clingfilm. Squeeze the lemon juice over the icing sugar and mix, adding more juice if needed until you get a good drizzling consistency. Keep aside until the cake has completely cooled, then transfer it to a serving plate and pour that lemony icing all over the top, letting it drizzle down the sides. Sprinkle over the reserved orange and lemon zest, and serve.

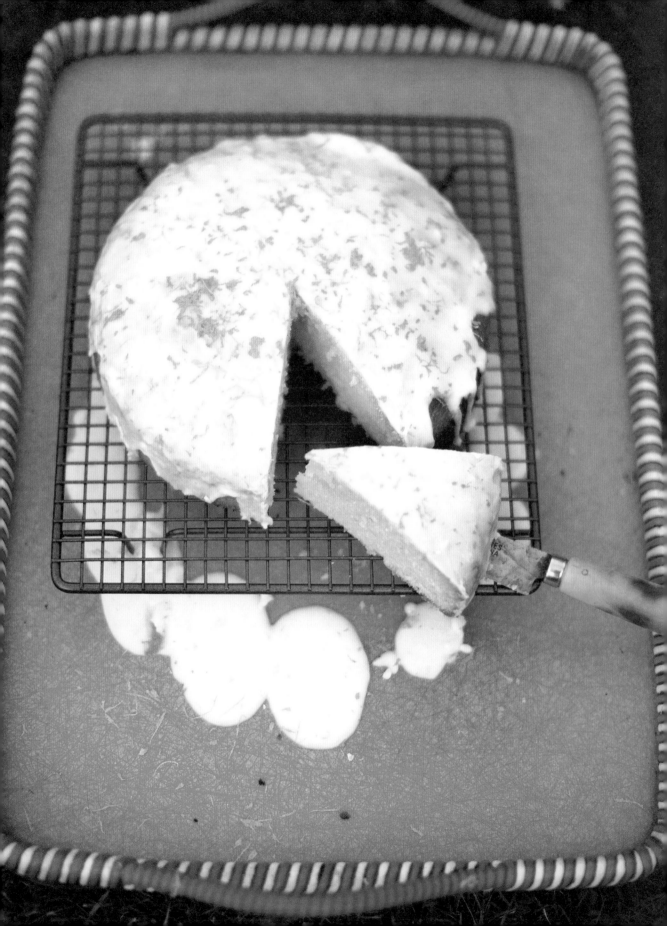

EARL GREY TEA LOAF

When I put this old-fashioned, humble fruit loaf through the rigorous recipe-testing process I always use for these books, the feedback on it was remarkable. Yes, the dried fruit in it is exciting and lovely, but I think it's the Earl Grey tea-infused syrup that makes people do a complete double take. I guess it's not surprising – everyone knows we Brits love our tea! If you make this, I hope you get the same great response I've had.

SERVES 12

- 6 Earl Grey teabags
- 400g dried fruit, such as raisins, sultanas, cherries, cranberries
- 1 orange
- 1 large free-range egg
- 300g golden caster sugar
- 400g self-raising flour
- 1 level teaspoon mixed spice
- 1 whole nutmeg, for grating
- 1 lemon
- Wensleydale cheese, to serve

Put 4 of the teabags into a measuring jug and add 300ml of boiling water. Leave to brew for a few minutes, then remove the teabags. Put the dried fruit into a large mixing bowl, grate over the zest of the orange and pour over the hot tea. Give it a good stir, then cover and leave to one side for a few hours, ideally overnight – so the fruit swells and soaks up all the tea.

When the fruit is completely rehydrated, preheat your oven to 180°C/350°F/gas 4. Line a 1 litre loaf tin with greaseproof paper – the easiest way to do this is to use one piece to line the sides and bottom, then a long strip to cover the ends of the tin.

Whisk the egg and add to the bowl of fruit along with 200g of the caster sugar. Add the flour, mixed spice and a few good gratings of nutmeg, and squeeze in the juice of the orange. Mix until you have a dough-like consistency (it might seem a little bit dry, but it'll be fine). Spoon the mixture into your lined tin and bake in the oven for around 1 hour 10 minutes, or until cooked through. To test it, poke a skewer or a cocktail stick into the middle of the cake. If it comes out clean, it's cooked; if not, give it a few more minutes.

Meanwhile make your syrup. Put the 2 remaining teabags into a pan with 200ml of water and the zest and juice of the lemon. Gently bring to the boil, removing the teabags after a couple of minutes. Add the remaining 100g of caster sugar and bring back to the boil without stirring – keep it on a medium heat so that you have a steady boil for around 5 to 10 minutes, or until the mixture has reduced by half and you have a lovely golden syrup. Pour this into a jug.

As soon as the loaf comes out of the oven, use a cocktail stick or a skewer to make lots of little holes in the top, then pour the syrup all over it. Once the syrup has been absorbed, transfer the loaf to a wire rack and leave to cool completely. Serve with a cup of tea and some butter, or with a few glasses of sherry and a nice Wensleydale cheese as an after-dinner treat.

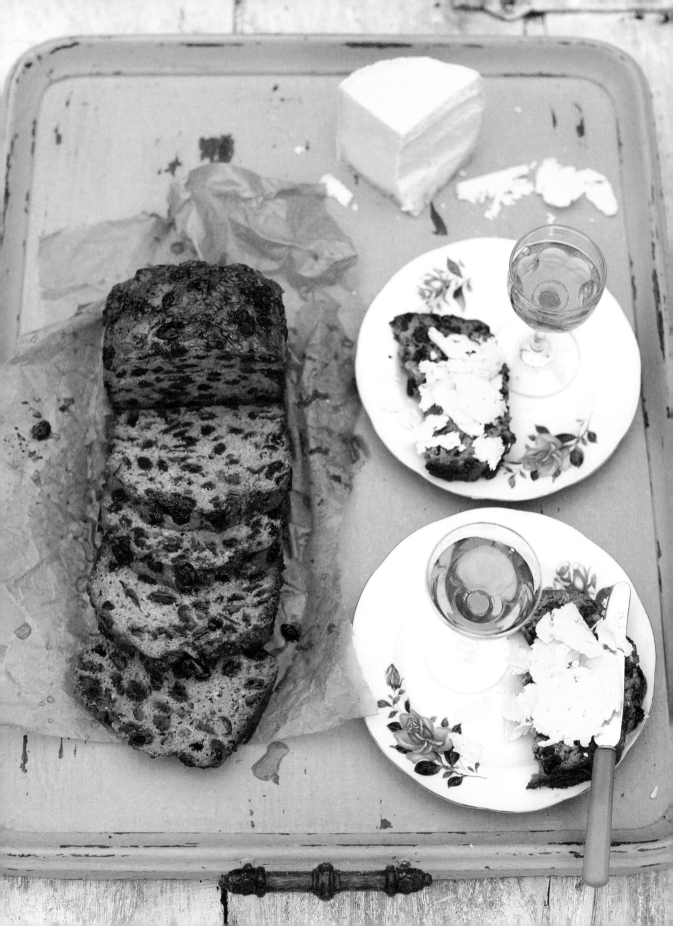

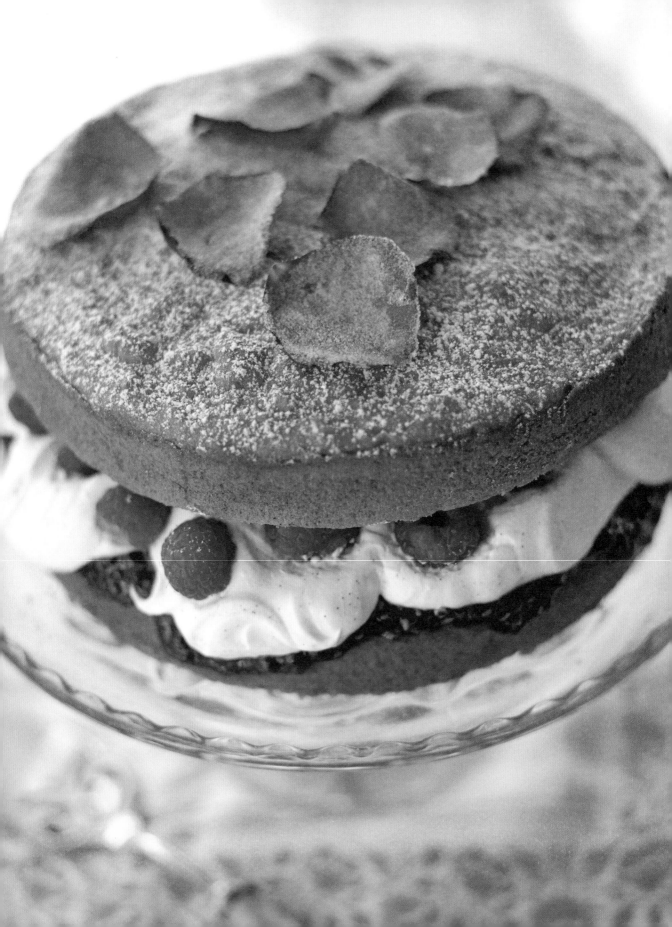

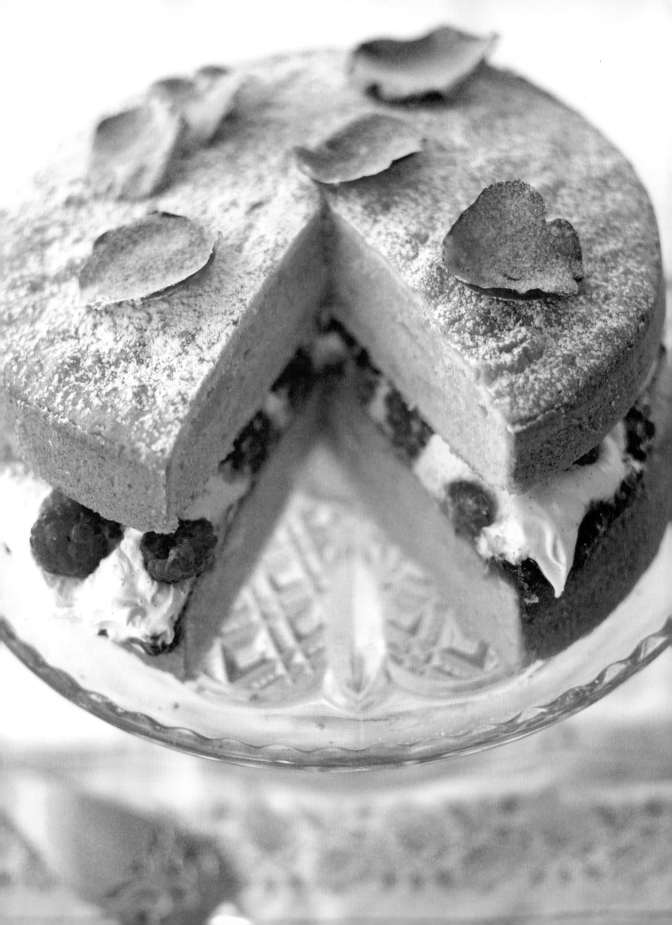

QUEEN VICTORIA SPONGE

Sponge cakes are something Britain does so well. For some reason, when you see a good Victoria sponge, regardless of what's happening at that moment, you just somehow feel everything's going to be all right. For sure, this cake would originally have been just straight sponge and jam, but then it evolved and promoted itself to another level, so that now it often has sweet cream in between the layers and all sorts of summer berries on top. I've added crystallized rose petals to my version, for extra prettiness. For me, this beautiful afternoon tea is really about precision sponge making, wonderful jam and gorgeous Jersey cream. If you can pull that off, you'll have perfection and smiling faces at the table.

SERVES 10

- 250g softened unsalted butter, plus extra for greasing
- 250g self-raising flour, plus extra for dusting
- 250g golden caster sugar
- 4 large free-range eggs
- zest of 1 orange
- a few drops of rosewater, to taste

- 4 tablespoons good-quality raspberry jam
- 150g fresh raspberries
- icing sugar, for dusting

For the crystallized rose petals
- 1 large free-range egg white
- a handful of rose petals
- white caster sugar

For the vanilla cream
- 150ml Jersey double cream
- ½ a vanilla pod, split lengthways and seeds scraped out
- 2 teaspoons caster sugar

Preheat your oven to 190°C/375°F/gas 5. Grease two 20cm sandwich tins all over with a few knobs of butter, line the bases with greaseproof paper, then dust lightly with flour.

Beat the butter and sugar together until very light and fluffy. Add the eggs one by one, making sure you beat each one in well before you add the next, then fold in the orange zest and the flour. Divide the cake mix between the prepared tins. Spread it out well with a spatula and bake for 20 to 25 minutes, or until golden brown and risen and a skewer comes out clean. Allow to cool slightly, then carefully turn out on to a baking rack to cool completely.

Mix a few drops of rosewater into your jam, but don't go crazy with it – it's very strong!

For the crystallized petals, turn the oven right down to 110°C/225°F/gas ¼ and whisk the egg white to stiff peaks. Use a pastry brush to coat the rose petals on both sides with a very thin layer of the egg white, then sprinkle over some caster sugar. Shake off the excess sugar and lay the petals on a baking tray lined with greaseproof paper. Bake for 3 to 4 minutes in the oven, until the petals are firm to the touch.

Whip the cream with the vanilla seeds and sugar until you get soft peaks. Spread the jam and then the vanilla cream over one of the cakes and scatter the raspberries on top. Place the second cake on top, dust with icing sugar and decorate with the crystallized rose petals. Serve on a beautiful cake stand to really show off your creation, and enjoy.

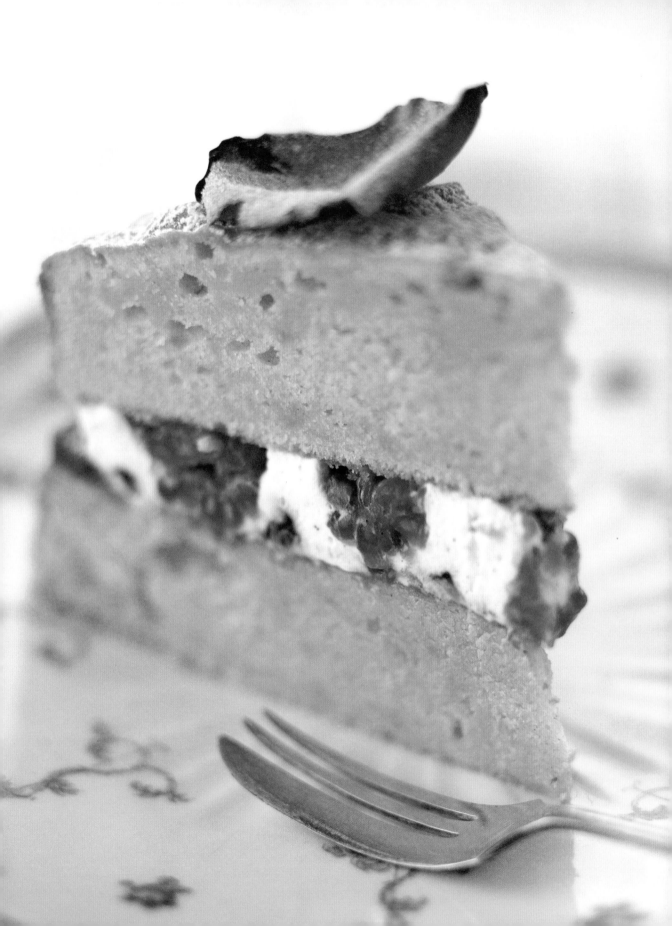

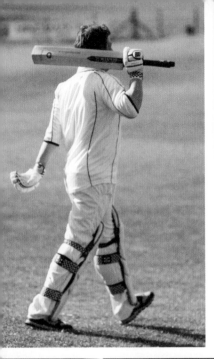

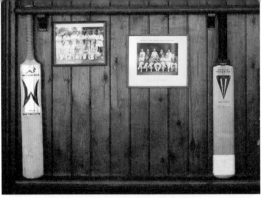

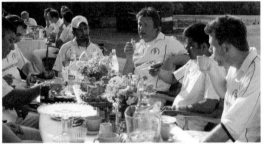

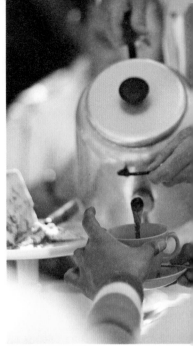

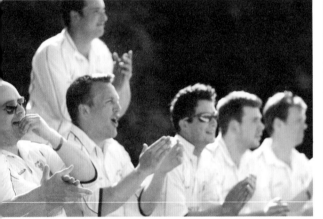

Cricket Tea

Growing up in a pub called The Cricketers I was very used to pulling pints and feeding the players after their matches. After twenty-five years of not playing cricket, it was a pleasure to get back on the pitch. Unbelievably, I managed to bowl someone out first time, so I reckon with a bit of practice I could become a dangerous force once again. It was a great day, and reminded me how brilliant the rituals around cricket are, especially the breaks for lunch and afternoon tea, which are taken very seriously. How civilized! Through the British Empire of old, the game became much loved around the world, and as these guys I played against reminded me, Indian cricketers now teach the English team a thing or two on the international stage!

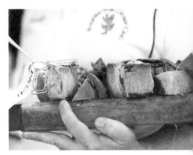

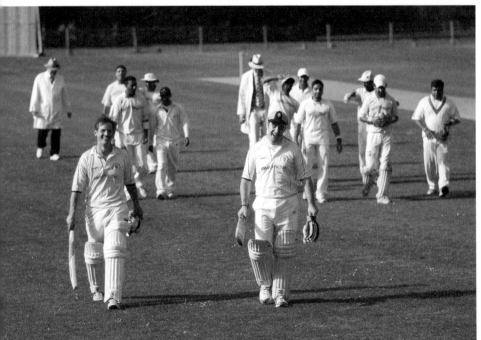

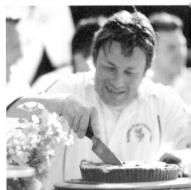

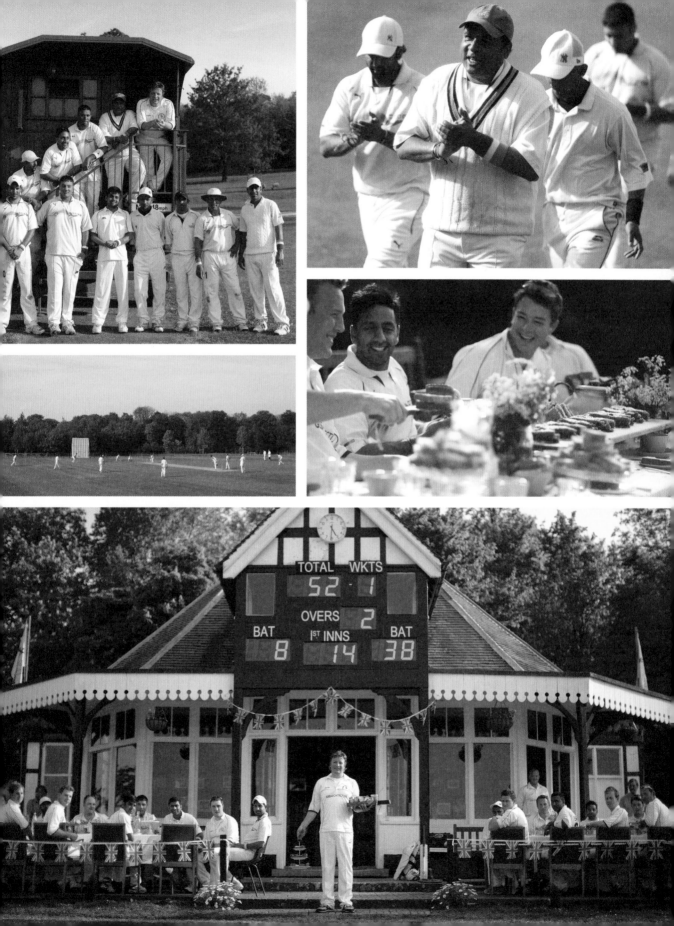

SOUR CRANBERRY BAKEWELL
ORANGE & LEMON SHERBET DRIZZLE SAUCE

SERVES 12 TO 16

For the pastry
- 250g plain flour,
  plus extra for dusting
- 100g icing sugar, sifted
- 125g cold unsalted butter,
  cut into cubes
- 1 orange
- 1 large free-range egg,
  beaten
- a splash of milk

For the cranberry jam
- 500g fresh or frozen
  cranberries
- 150g golden caster sugar
- 2 oranges

For the frangipane
- 100g blanched hazelnuts
- 100g shelled walnuts
- 250g cold unsalted butter,
  cut into cubes
- 250g golden caster sugar
- 1 lemon
- 1 orange
- 3 large free-range eggs
- 60g plain flour

I'm really excited about this tart. It's my contribution to the evolutionary journey of the great British Bakewell tart, which was born when somebody in a pub kitchen made a mistake while making a Bakewell pudding. I'm using hazelnuts and walnuts in place of almonds to give the filling a wicked sort of praline flavour.

Sift the flour and half the icing sugar into a large bowl, then rub in the butter until the mixture resembles breadcrumbs. Mix in the zest of the orange, then add the beaten egg and a small splash of milk and mix together until you have a ball of dough. Don't work it too much. Lightly flour the dough, wrap it in clingfilm, then chill in the fridge for 30 minutes. After that time, roll the pastry out on a clean floured surface until it's about 0.5cm thick. Loosely roll it around the rolling pin, then unroll it over a 25cm loose-bottomed tart tin. Ease the pastry into the tin, pushing it into the corners. Trim off any excess overhanging pastry, wrap that in clingfilm and use it for jam tarts (see page 178) if you like. Prick the base of the tart all over with a fork. Cover with clingfilm and chill in the fridge for another 30 minutes.

Preheat the oven to 180°C/350°F/gas 4. Remove the clingfilm from the chilled base, then line it with scrunched-up greaseproof paper and dried rice. Blind bake for 12 minutes, then remove the paper and rice and bake for a further 5 minutes. Meanwhile, put a large pan on a medium heat and add the cranberries, sugar and the zest and juice from 1½ oranges. Bring to the boil, then reduce to a simmer over a medium to low heat and cook for 15 minutes, stirring occasionally, until lovely and jammy. At this point, take the pan off the heat and leave to cool.

Blitz the nuts for the filling in a food processor until really fine. Tip into a clean bowl, then put the butter and sugar into the food processor and whiz until pale, creamy and fluffy. Grate the zest of the lemon and orange into the food processor, then crack in the eggs, one at a time, keeping the food processor running until well mixed. Tip the blitzed nuts back into the food processor along with the flour, and blitz again to mix. Set aside.

Spread a third of your cooled cranberry jam mixture over the base of your pastry case, then spoon over the frangipane and gently spread it out. Dot a few more blobs of cranberry jam on top, and put the rest of it aside (it will be delicious on toast and makes the perfect filling for jam tarts – see page 178). Cook the tart in the hot oven for 45 to 50 minutes, or until golden and set. Once cooked, leave to cool for 20 minutes, then transfer to a wire rack while you make your icing.

Put the remaining icing sugar into a bowl, then squeeze in drops of juice from the zested orange and lemon until you have a nice thick drizzly mixture. Serve the tart drizzled with that zesty icing, and with a little dollop of cream, if you like.

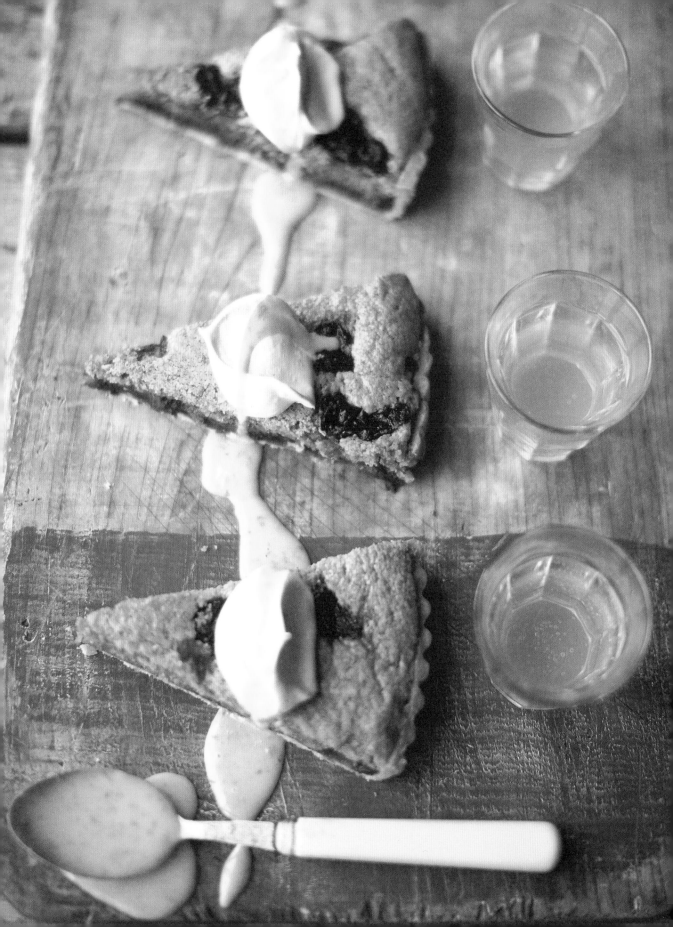

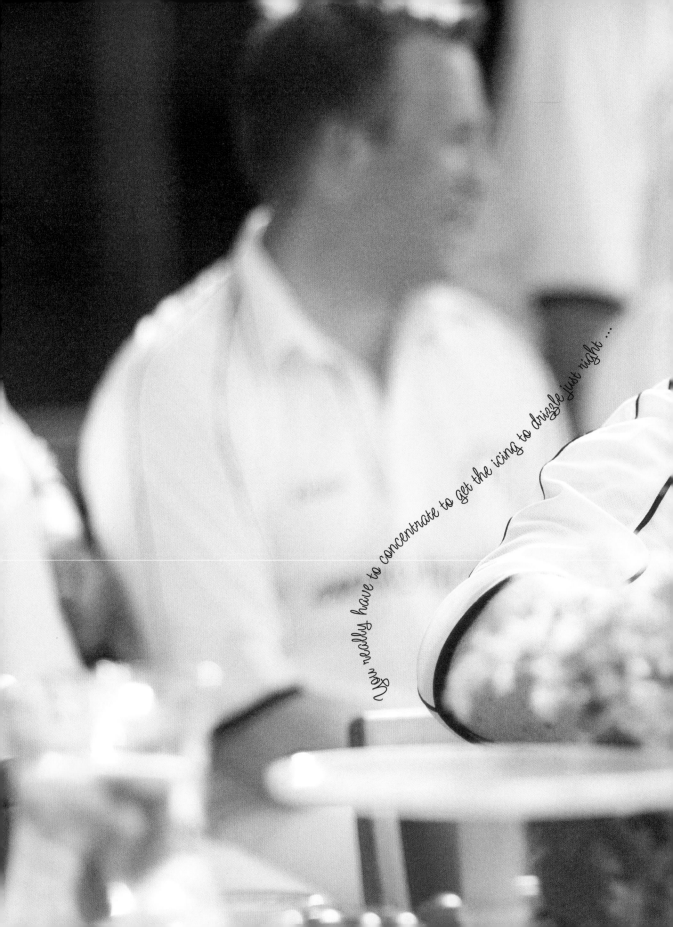

You really have to concentrate to get the icing to drizzle just right ...

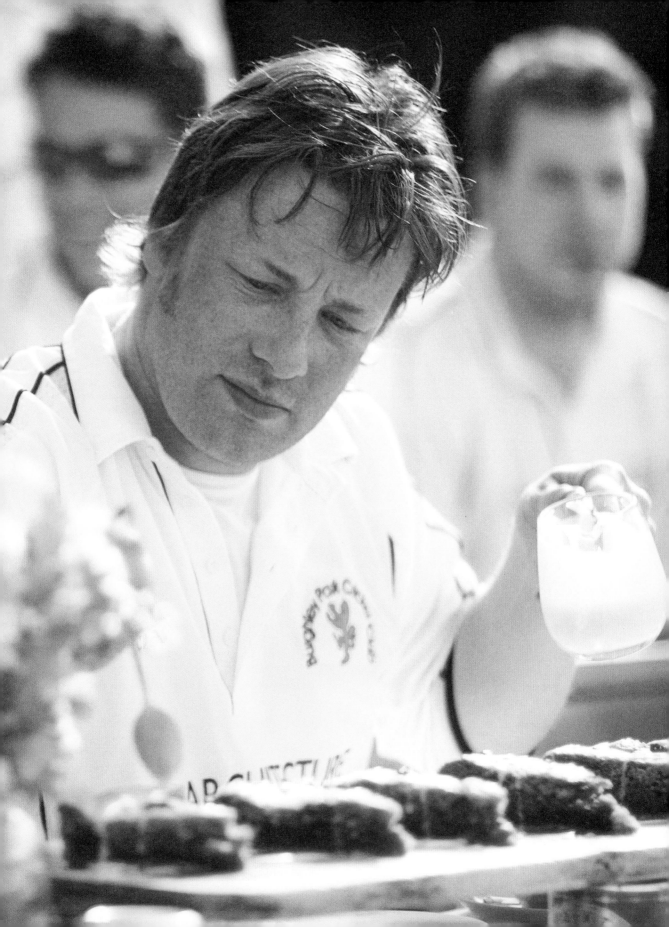

RAINBOW JAM TARTS

Jam tarts are definitely a part of my childhood. They are humble, cheap to make and such a pretty little treat. It's funny how simple pastry with a blob of jam can turn into something so exciting, with chewy bits, bubbling bits, crunchy bits and jammy jelly bits. Even if you cheat a little, and buy ready-made pastry, just the ritual of filling these tarts with your favourite jams and then baking them can be really relaxing. The beauty of these for me is playing with the different jam or jelly flavours so you get a rainbow of colours. Just about every supermarket in Britain stocks a great selection of posh jams: strawberry, blackberry, blueberry, gooseberry, apricot, cranberry … the sheer number of fillings available now makes these even more exciting than the ones I had as a kid.

MAKES ROUGHLY 30 LITTLE TARTS

For the sweet pastry
- 250g plain flour, plus extra for dusting
- 250g icing sugar
- 125g unsalted butter, softened
- a pinch of sea salt
- 1 large free-range egg
- 1 orange or lemon
- a splash of milk

For the fillings
- 30 heaped teaspoons of your favourite jams, curds, marmalades and jellies

Put the flour, sugar and butter into a food processor with a pinch of salt and pulse until you have a mixture that looks like breadcrumbs. Crack in the egg, grate in the zest from your orange or lemon and pulse again, adding a little splash of milk to bring everything together, if needed. Wrap the dough in clingfilm and pop it into the fridge to rest for 30 minutes.

Preheat the oven to 180°C/350°F/gas 4. Dust a clean surface and a rolling pin with flour and roll out the pastry so it's 0.5cm thick. Get yourself a few 12-hole jam tart trays (or cook the tarts in batches) and a fluted pastry cutter just a little bigger than the holes of the tray (normally around 6cm). Cut out rounds of pastry and gently push them into the wells so they come up the sides. Any leftover pastry can be gently pushed back into a ball and rolled out to make a few more tarts. Put 1 heaped teaspoon of filling into each jam tart, interspersing and alternating the flavours of jams, curds or jellies.

Pop the trays on the middle shelf of the oven and cook for around 12 to 15 minutes, or until the pastry is golden and the filling is thick and bubbling. Remove from the oven, leave in the tray to firm slightly, then transfer to a wire rack and leave to cool for a few minutes before serving.

PS: I know this might sound a bit girly, but if you can track down a lovely old tart tin from an antique shop, then serve these straight out of the tin - it looks really good, as the old tins are really cute. See, I told you it was girly!

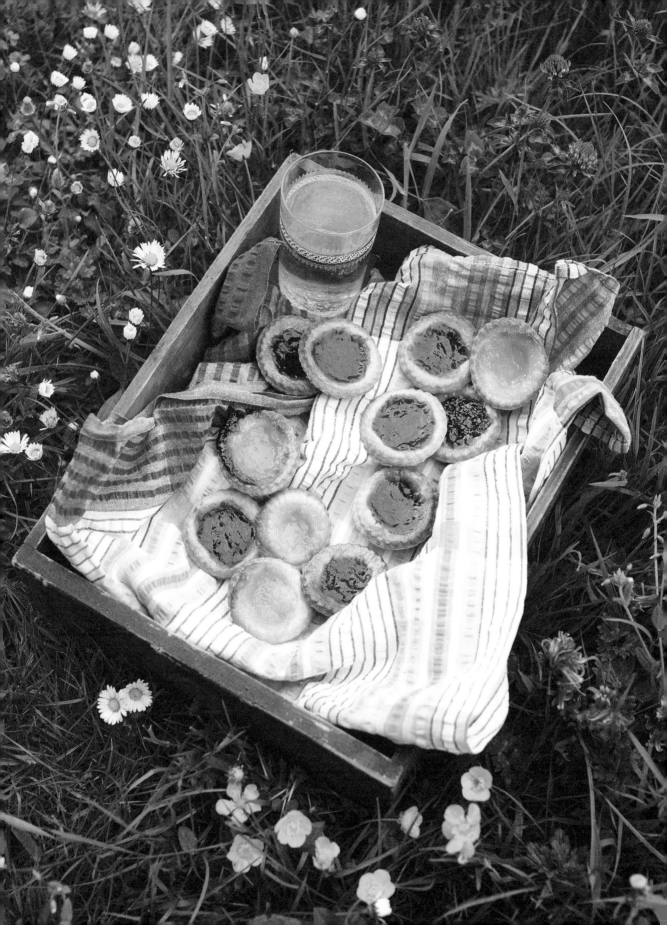

SCOTTISH SHORTBREAD

I know you can buy shortbreads everywhere these days, but great as some of those biscuits can be, nothing comes close to a batch cooked that day, or even that week. It's having the real version of something, rather than the 'buy one get one free' version, that makes us appreciate it. The simplicity of these biscuits makes them a wonderful base for desserts with cream and fruit, or a crumbly topping for trifles and stewed fruits. But for me the very best way to celebrate this humble biscuit is with a cup of tea.

You can have these biscuits plain, or scent them with everything from lemon or tangerine, to lavender, lemon thyme or caraway seeds. Just don't go mad with these flavours, because a little goes a long way and these are nicest when the flavours are subtle.

MAKES 12 PIECES OF SHORTBREAD

- 200g plain flour, plus extra for dusting
- 50g caster sugar, plus extra for sprinkling over
- 125g unsalted butter

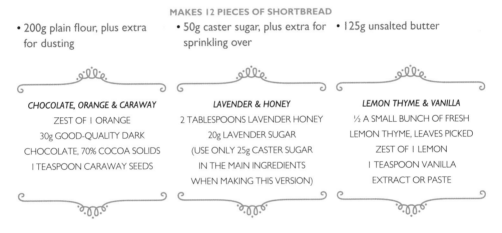

CHOCOLATE, ORANGE & CARAWAY
ZEST OF 1 ORANGE
30g GOOD-QUALITY DARK
CHOCOLATE, 70% COCOA SOLIDS
1 TEASPOON CARAWAY SEEDS

LAVENDER & HONEY
2 TABLESPOONS LAVENDER HONEY
20g LAVENDER SUGAR
(USE ONLY 25g CASTER SUGAR
IN THE MAIN INGREDIENTS
WHEN MAKING THIS VERSION)

LEMON THYME & VANILLA
½ A SMALL BUNCH OF FRESH
LEMON THYME, LEAVES PICKED
ZEST OF 1 LEMON
1 TEASPOON VANILLA
EXTRACT OR PASTE

Preheat the oven to 170°C/325°F/gas 3. Mix the flour and sugar together in a mixing bowl. Rub in the butter with your thumb and forefinger, then add your chosen flavourings (if you're using chocolate or seeds you might want to push these into the dough at the end, after you've rolled it out) and squash, pat and push it into a dough. Don't knead it, you just want to pat it down flat. Push or roll it out until it's 1cm thick - do this directly on to a baking sheet lined with greaseproof paper so you don't have to move it. Once it's in the shape you like - which could be square, round, or a few small finger-shapes - feel free to thumb or pinch the edges. If it splits or tears, just press it back together - but remember, the less you work the dough, the shorter and better these biscuits will be.

If you want to score lines on the shortbread so that you can click the biscuits off into pieces later, you can. Sprinkle over some caster sugar, then pop the baking sheet into the oven and cook for 20 to 30 minutes. Keep an eye on it - you want a lovely light golden colour (unless you're making the lavender honey version, which will be darker). Leave to cool, then put away in a tin or serve. These will be delicious for two or three days and make a lovely present for someone special.

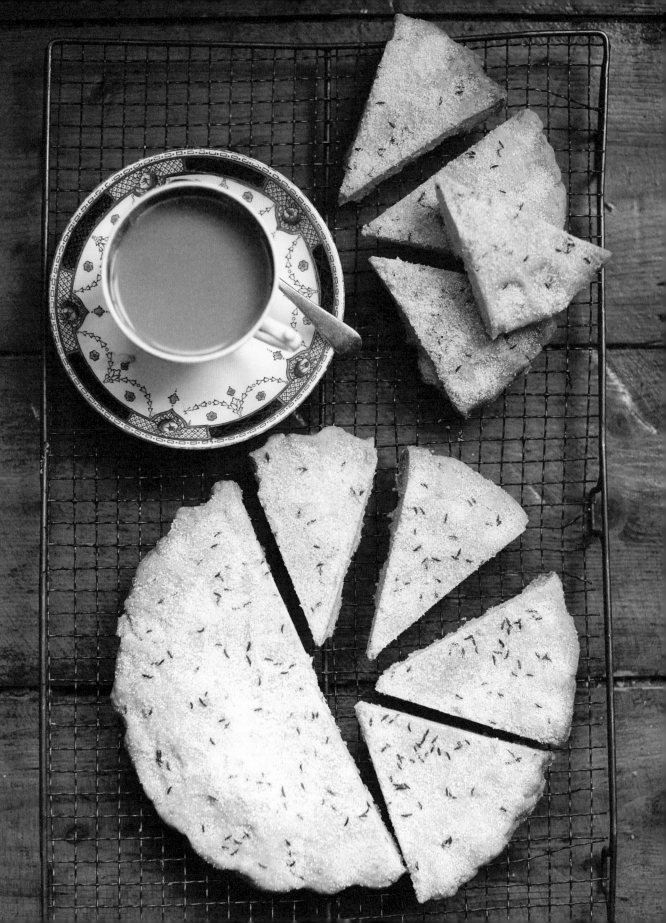

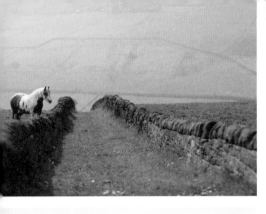

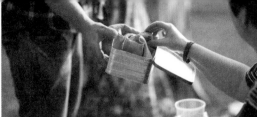

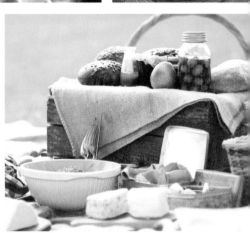

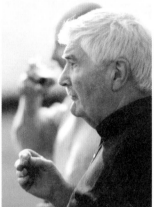

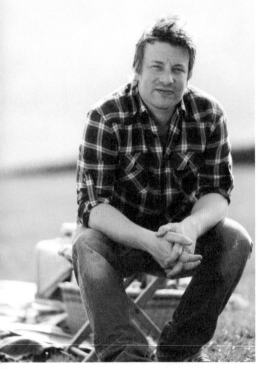

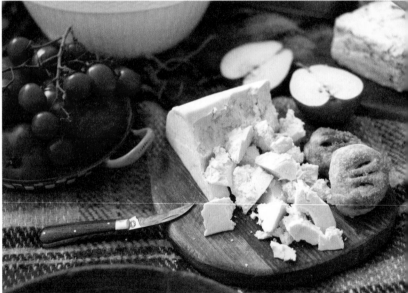

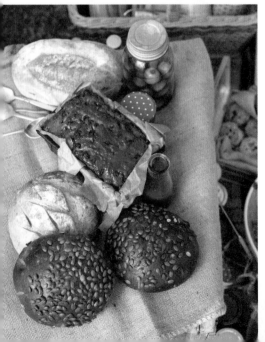

The Great British Picnic

We've been enjoying picnics since the days of the Industrial Revolution, when exhausted factory workers demanded a day off a week, and the weekend was born. They'd venture out of the cities on brand new steam trains for the day, and take portable lunches with them. What a beautiful tradition.

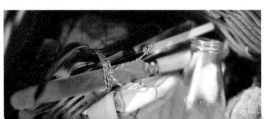

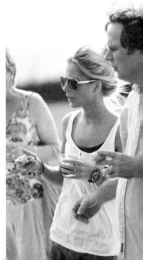

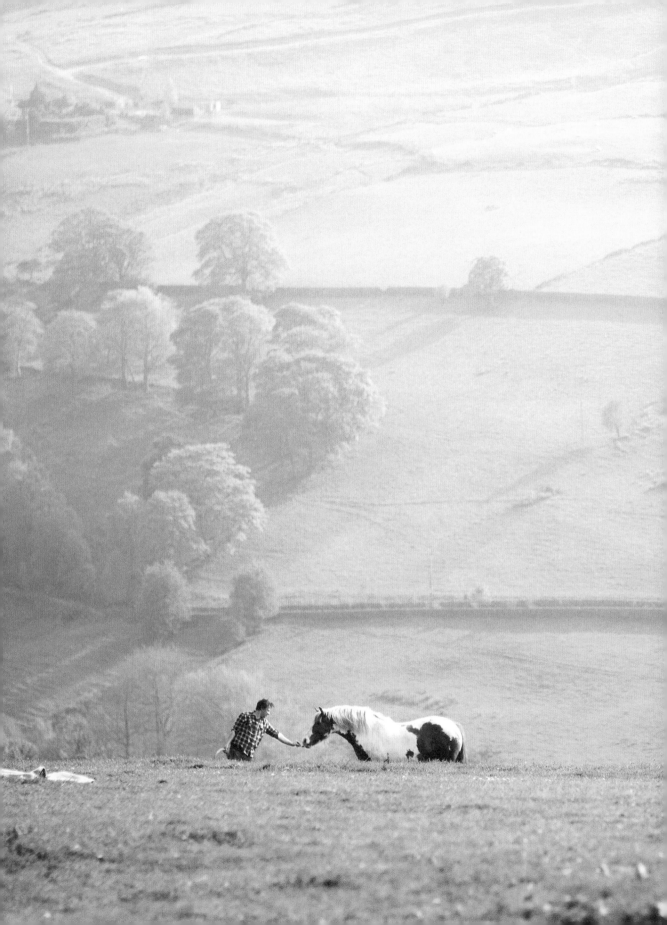

CHARMING ECCLES CAKES

My Eccles cakes are smaller and a little cuter than the traditional ones, but I think that makes them perfect little treats for teas, parties and any other sort of sharing occasion. I've added some really exciting sour fruits to the traditional currant and raisin filling, and also added a fresh bay leaf, for a tutti-frutti vibe. These really are exceptionally good served with a brilliant cheese and a little glass of port for dessert, or as a treat at a picnic. Hope you enjoy.

SERVES 16

For the filling
- 1 large fresh bay leaf
- 1 lemon
- 1 orange
- 1 whole nutmeg, for grating
- 1 level teaspoon mixed spice
- 100g demerara sugar, plus extra for sprinkling

- 150g mixed dried fruits, such as golden sultanas, sour bilberries, raisins, cranberries, apricots
- 2 balls of stem ginger, finely chopped, plus 1 teaspoon syrup
- 75g apple (just over half an apple), core removed

For the pastry
- plain flour, for dusting
- 1 x 500g all-butter puff pastry
- 1 large free-range egg, beaten
- icing sugar, for dusting

Preheat the oven to 200°C/400°F/gas 6. Strip the bay leaf off its thick stalk and bash it up with a pestle and mortar to break it down and release the oils. Finely grate in the fragrant yellow zest of the lemon and the zest of the orange as well as about half the nutmeg, and add the mixed spice and the demerara sugar. Muddle everything around a few times, then put aside. Pop your dried fruit into a bowl - finely chopping the apricots first, if using - along with the ginger and syrup, then tip in your flavoured sugar. Cut the apple into 1cm chunks and add to the bowl of dried fruit, then quickly mix to combine and put aside.

Dust a clean surface and a rolling pin with plain flour and roll the puff pastry out to about 3mm thick, dusting with more flour as you go. Cut out rounds with a 10cm cookie cutter - just pull any leftover pastry into a ball and roll that out too; it might rise slightly differently, but that's all right. You should end up with 16 rounds in total.

Line two baking trays with greaseproof paper. Put a tablespoon of fruit filling into the middle of each pastry circle, then stretch the pastry up and over the filling, bringing it together on top and sealing it in the middle. Arrange your Eccles cakes on the baking trays, with the sealed side facing down, then use a knife to make three little slits in the top. Some of the juices from the filling might spill out a bit as the cakes cook, but that's only going to create sticky golden caramelized bits later, so it's not a bad thing. Quickly egg wash each cake, then dust a little icing sugar over each one and sprinkle with a pinch of demerara sugar. Bake in the oven for 15 to 18 minutes, until they're golden, puffy and beautiful, then leave to cool and serve as part of a picnic spread, or with a nice cup of tea.

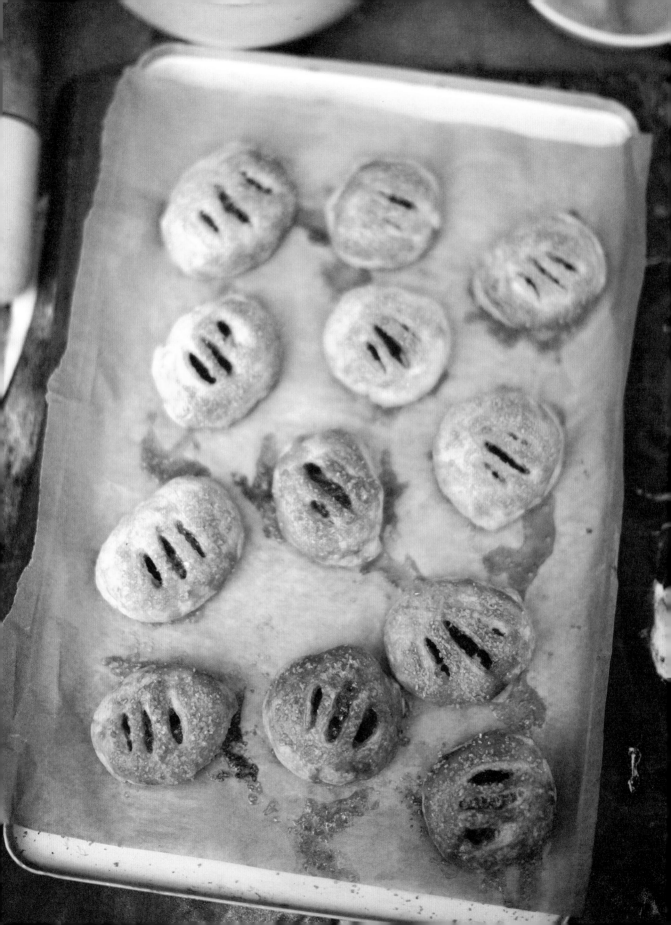

CRUMBLIEST SCONES

Scones are wonderfully British, delicious, and so simple even a five-year-old could make them. There's a magic hour just after they come out of the oven when they are so heavenly I just can't imagine why anyone would prefer store-bought scones. Just remember that the less you touch the dough, the shorter and crumblier your scones will be.

MAKES 16 TO 20 SCONES

- 150g dried fruit, such as sour cherries, raisins, sultanas, chopped sour apricots, blueberries, or a mixture
- orange juice, for soaking
- 150g cold unsalted butter
- 500g self-raising flour, plus a little extra for dusting
- 2 level teaspoons baking powder
- 2 heaped teaspoons golden caster sugar
- sea salt
- 2 large free-range eggs
- 4 tablespoons milk, plus a little extra for brushing
- *optional:* Jersey clotted cream, good-quality jam or lemon curd, to serve

Put the dried fruit into a bowl and pour over just enough orange juice to cover. Ideally, leave it for a couple of hours. Preheat the oven to 200°C/400°F/gas 6. First and foremost, brilliant scones are about having the confidence to do as little as possible, so do what I say and they'll be really great; and the second and third time you make them you'll get the dough into a solid mass even quicker, even better.

Put your butter, flour, baking powder, sugar and a good pinch of sea salt into a mixing bowl and use your thumbs and forefingers to break up the butter and rub it into the flour so you get little cornflake - sized pieces. Make a well in the middle of the dough, add the eggs and milk, and stir it up with a spatula. Drain your soaked fruit and add that to the mixture. Add a tiny splash of milk if needed, until you have a soft, dry dough. Move it around as little as possible to get it looking like a scruffy mass - at this point, you're done. Sprinkle over some flour, cover the bowl with clingfilm and pop it into the fridge for 15 minutes.

Roll the dough out on a lightly floured surface until it's about 2 to 3cm thick. With a 6cm round cutter or the rim of a glass, cut out circles from the dough and place them upside down on a baking sheet - they will rise better that way (so they say). Re-roll any offcuts to use up the dough. Brush the top of each scone with the extra milk or some melted butter and bake in the oven for 12 to 15 minutes, or until risen and golden. At that point, take them out of the oven and leave them to cool down a little. Serve with clotted cream and a little jam or lemon curd.

PS: A great little tip if you don't want to bake a whole batch is to freeze the scones after you've cut them out. That way, you can come home from work, pop the little rounds of frozen dough into the oven and cook them at 180°C/350°F/gas 4 for 25 minutes, or until golden and lovely.

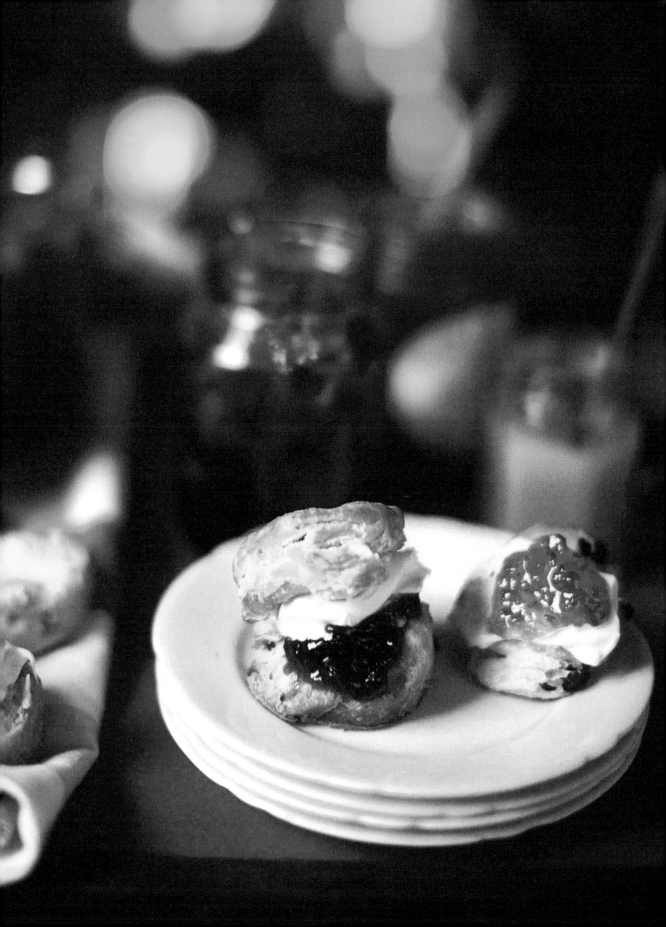

WALNUT & BANANA LOAF
NAUGHTY CHOCOLATE ORANGE BUTTER SPREAD

Not only is this one of the most scrumptious things to eat, it's also a total pleasure to make. The amount of smiles and oohs and aahs you're going to get when you serve it make it simply the best. If you can, try and use slightly overripe bananas as they'll give you a treacly, caramelly intensity that works so well. The chocolate butter is painfully enjoyable, but my nutritionist, Laura, has requested that I suggest just having a smidgen with a slice of the loaf, so I'm sure you'll all respect her wishes when tucking into this delight.

SERVES 16 WITH LOADS OF EXTRA BUTTER

- 100g shelled walnuts
- 500g (about 5 or 6) ripe bananas, peeled
- 125g unsalted butter, at room temperature
- 125g dark brown sugar
- 2 large free-range eggs
- 200g plain flour

- 2 level teaspoons baking powder
- 1 level teaspoon bicarbonate of soda
- 1 level teaspoon ground cinnamon
- a pinch of sea salt
- olive oil

For the chocolate butter
- 100g good-quality cooking chocolate (70% cocoa solids)
- zest of 2 oranges
- 150g unsalted butter, at room temperature
- 80g icing sugar

Preheat the oven to 170°C/325°F/gas 3. Spread the walnuts out on a baking sheet and pop them in the oven to gently toast for around 5 minutes, or until they smell fantastic. Meanwhile, quickly mash up the bananas with a fork or potato masher, so you've got a mixture of smooth and chunky, and put them aside.

Cream the butter and sugar together in a food processor, or by hand, until smooth and pale, and beat in the eggs one by one, scraping the sides as you go so everything gets mixed together, then spoon into a large bowl. Take the toasted walnuts out of the oven and put them on a chopping board. Quickly run a knife through them, leaving some halved and others fairly fine so you get a good range of textures. Add the mashed bananas and chopped up walnuts to the bowl of batter, then sift in the flour, baking powder, bicarbonate of soda, cinnamon and salt. Mix everything together until you have a nice smooth batter.

Tear off a metre of greaseproof paper, scrunch it and wet under a tap. Drizzle a little olive oil over both sides and rub that in, then push the scrunched greaseproof into a 1-litre loaf tin, getting it right down into the corners (it's ok if it's a bit scruffy). Transfer the batter to the tin and cook on the middle shelf in the oven for an hour. After this time, test the loaf by poking a skewer into the middle. If the skewer comes out clean the loaf is cooked, if not put the tin back in the oven for another few minutes.

While the loaf bakes, make your chocolate butter. Bash the chocolate up, pop it in a heatproof bowl and melt it slowly over a pan of gently simmering hot water. Once melted, carefully take the bowl off the pan, stir in the orange zest and put to one side to let the chocolate cool down a little.

Cream the butter and icing sugar together, then beat in the cooled chocolate until blended. Once you've got a nice even mixture, transfer it to a little pot or a cute butter dish and sprinkle on a tiny pinch of sea salt from a height to give it a little salty kick. Either put in the fridge to set for a few hours, or serve right away smeared on a slice of warm banana loaf. Keep any leftover chocolate butter in a jar in the fridge for another day, and just take it out of the fridge to soften before serving.

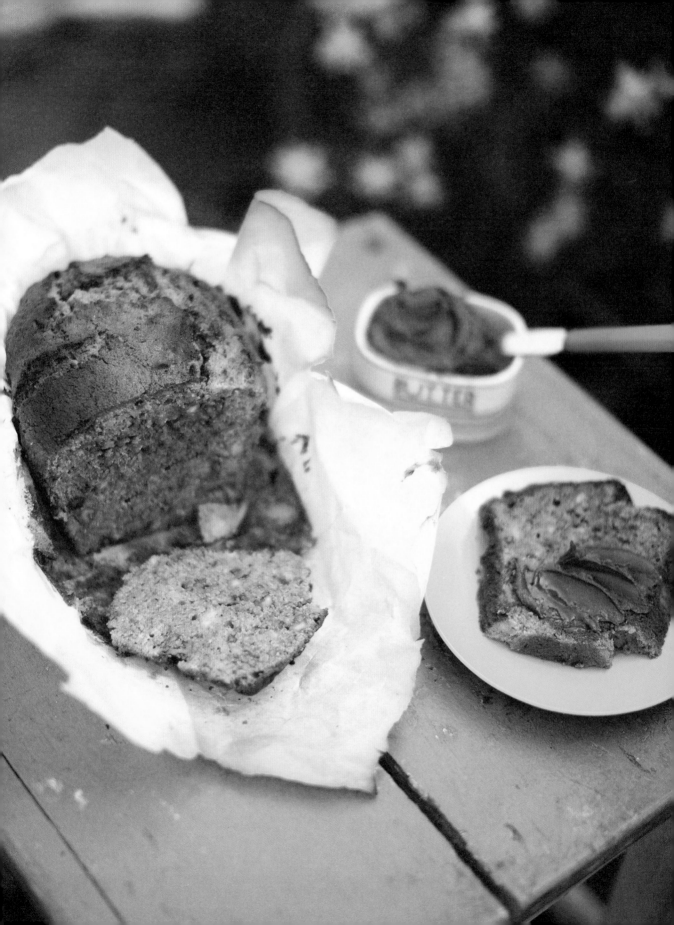

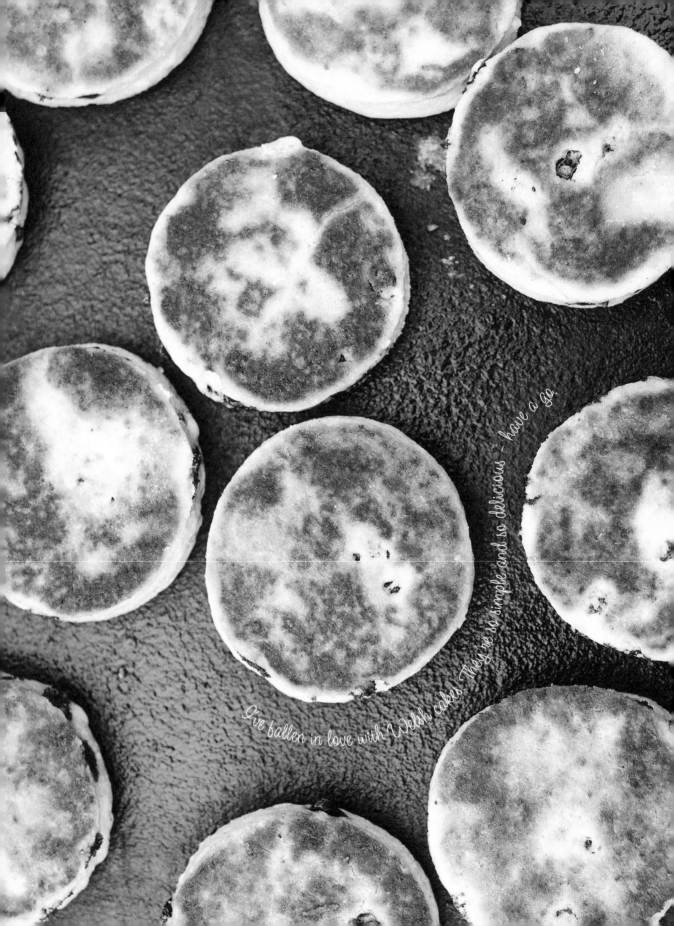

I've fallen in love with Welsh cakes. They're so simple and so delicious - have a go.

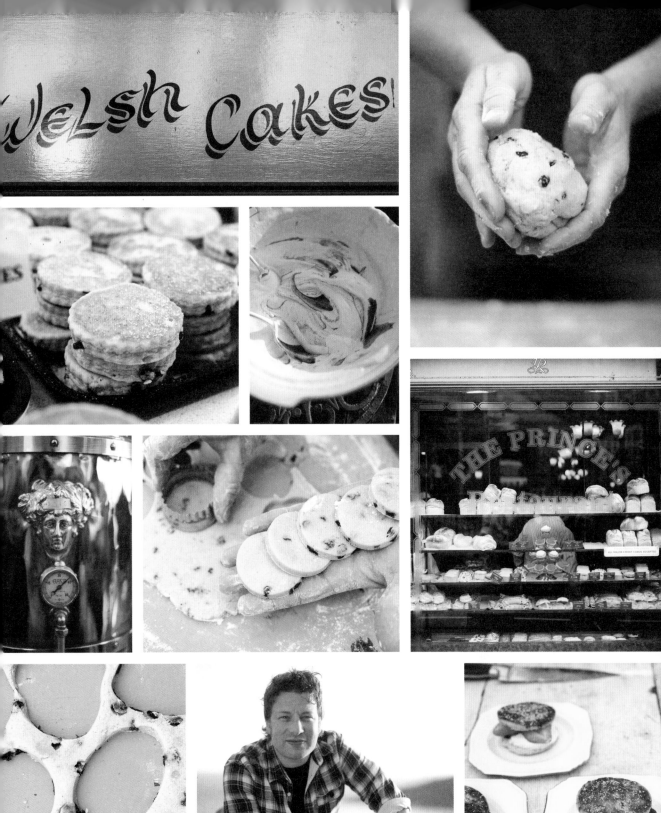
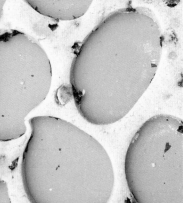
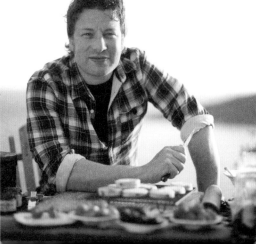

WONDERFUL WELSH CAKES
JAMMED WITH SUMMER BERRIES & VANILLA CREAM

I completely fell in love with Welsh cakes after Jim gave me my first taste of one in Pontypridd market. The Welsh cooks of old did a lot of cooking on bakestones, which are essentially round cast iron skillets. They'd place them over a fire in their home, and use them for things like these sweet little cakes, which have a crisp outside and a soft, slightly crumbly inside that is to die for. You can replicate that bakestone style of cooking using a heavy-bottomed non-stick pan. I love serving these warm as they are or filled with a spoonful of cream and a few berries. Jim was using chunks of chocolate, different dried fruits and even sprinkles of desiccated coconut, so feel free to experiment once you've mastered the basic recipe.

MAKES 35 TO 40 WELSH CAKES

For the Welsh cakes
- 500g self-raising flour, plus extra for dusting
- 75g caster sugar, plus extra to serve
- 1 heaped teaspoon mixed spice
- 250g cold, unsalted butter

- a pinch of sea salt
- 150g mixed raisins and sultanas
- 1 large free-range egg
- a couple of splashes of milk

For the filling
- 300ml double cream

- 1 heaped tablespoon caster sugar, plus extra for sprinkling
- 1 teaspoon vanilla bean paste
- 400g fresh berries, such as raspberries, strawberries, blackberries
- 1 lemon

Sieve the flour into a large mixing bowl and add the sugar and mixed spice. Cut up the butter and add to the bowl with a pinch of salt. Use your hands to rub it all together until you get a fine breadcrumb consistency. Toss in the dried fruit, then make a well in the centre of the mixture and crack in the egg. Add a splash of milk and use a fork to beat and mix in the egg. Once combined, use your clean hands to pat and bring the mixture together until you have a dough. It should be fairly short, so don't work it too much.

Put a large heavy-bottomed non-stick frying pan on a medium heat. While it's heating up, dust a clean surface and a rolling pin with flour and roll the dough out until it's about 1cm thick. Use a 5cm pastry cutter to cut out as many rounds as you can. Scrunch the remaining scraps of dough together, then roll out and cut out a few more. To test the temperature, cook one Welsh cake in the pan for a few minutes to act as a thermometer. If the surface is blonde, turn the heat up a little; if it's black, turn the heat down – leave for a few minutes for the heat to correct itself, then try again. When you've got a golden cake after 4 minutes on each side, you're in a really good place and you can cook the rest in batches. It's all about control.

As soon as they come off the pan, put them on a wire rack to cool and sprinkle them with caster sugar. You can serve them just like this, as they are. Or, if you want to do what I've done, gently cut each cake in half while turning so you get a top and a bottom. Whip the cream, sugar and vanilla paste together until you have soft peaks. Put the berries into a bowl, slicing up any big ones, and toss them with the juice of 1 lemon and a sprinkling of sugar. Open the cakes up, and add a little dollop of cream and a few berries to each one.

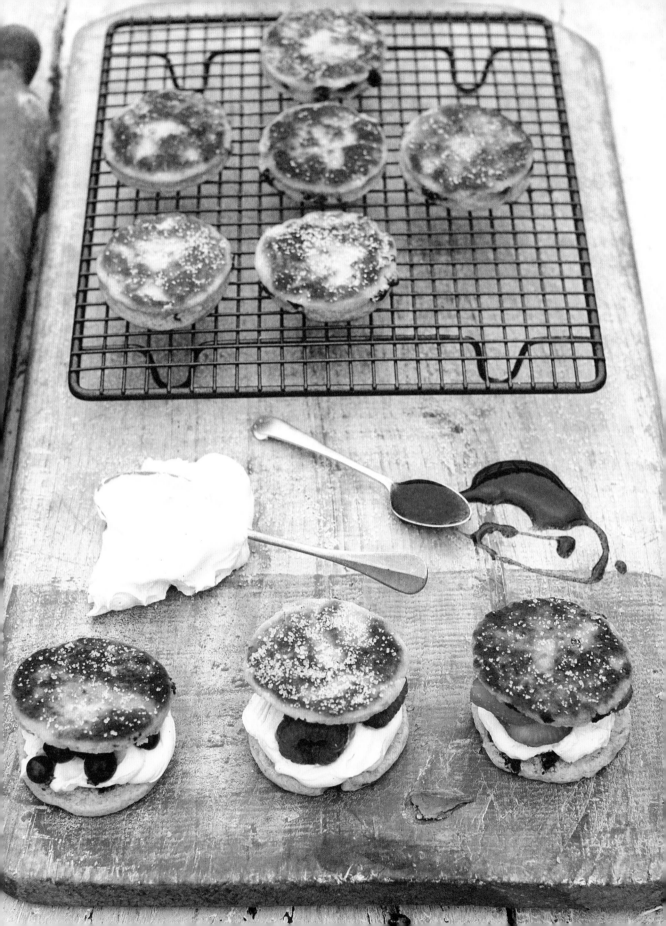

JAMMY COCONUT SPONGE

This is a classic school dinner dessert that many of us Brits have loved with a passion: warm soft sponge smeared with delicious sour jam and covered in coconut. A little slice of this is brilliant with a pot of tea for a midday treat, or as a dessert with a splodge of hot or cold custard. Just pure nostalgia through and through.

SERVES 16

For the cake
- 225g unsalted butter, softened, plus extra for greasing
- 225g caster sugar
- 4 large free-range eggs
- 225g self-raising flour
- ½ a level teaspoon baking powder
- a splash of milk
- 1 teaspoon vanilla extract
- 75g desiccated coconut

For the blackberry jam
- 250g blackberries
- 125g caster sugar
- ½ a lemon

Grease and line the bottom of a 30 x 20cm cake tin. Preheat the oven to 180°C/350°F/gas 4.

Cream the butter and sugar together until lovely, pale and fluffy, then beat in the eggs, one at a time. Fold in the flour and baking powder, add a splash of milk and the vanilla extract, and mix again. Pour into the lined tin and cook in the oven for 25 to 30 minutes. While your cake is cooking, get on with making the blackberry jam.

Mash the blackberries and sugar together in a small pan, using a fork or a potato masher, then add a squeeze of lemon juice and bring everything to the boil. Turn down to a medium heat and simmer for about 20 minutes, stirring occasionally, until lovely and thick. Skim away any foam that rises as the jam cooks, then take off the heat and leave to cool slightly.

By now, the sponge should be golden and cooked through, so remove it from the oven and leave to cool for 5 to 10 minutes. Turn it out on to a board, then pour the jam all over the sponge and use a palette knife to move it all around the sponge and the sides. Sprinkle over the desiccated coconut and serve.

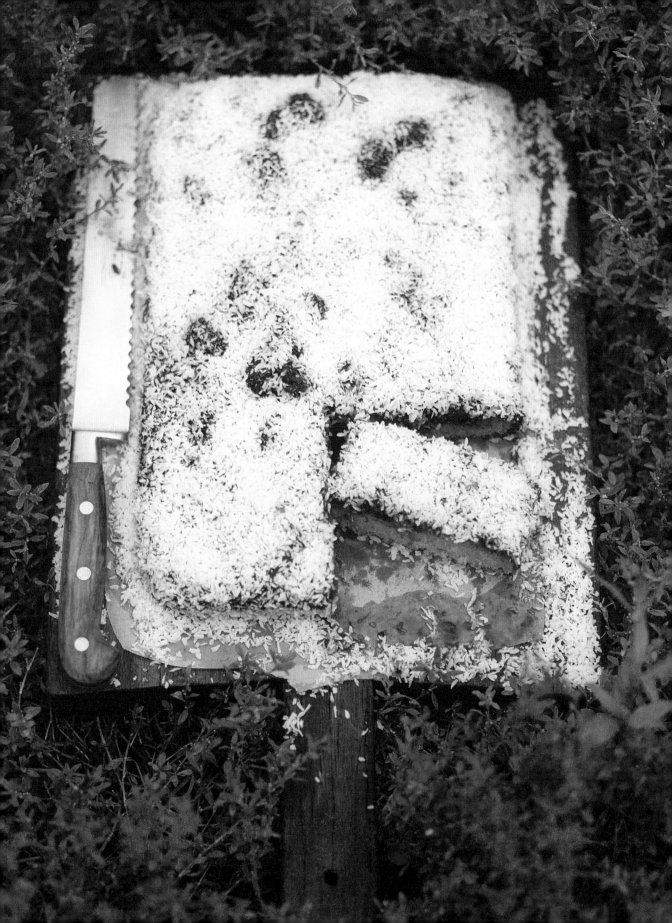

LEGENDARY CLOOTIE DUMPLING

This is an incredible creation. It's a tea-cakey, loafy, bun-type dumpling that I was introduced to in Scotland by a lovely lady named Lisbeth. Clootie is a Scots word for cloth, and this beauty is wrapped in cloth and steamed to perfection – hence the name. When I saw it in the middle of a tableful of cakes with a tartan bow sitting proudly on top, it was love at first sight. You can treat it like a fruit cake and keep it for weeks in a tightly sealed tin, or use it as a base for savoury dishes – even breakfast – and have it sliced up and grilled or toasted with bacon and eggs. I love it forty minutes out of the saucepan with a little smear of butter, and so do my wife and kids.

SERVES 24

- 500g mixed dried fruit, such as sour cherries, blueberries, cranberries, apricots, currants
- ½ teaspoon baking powder
- 1 level teaspoon ground ginger
- 1 level teaspoon ground cinnamon
- 1 level teaspoon ground mixed spice
- 1 tablespoon black treacle
- 1 Granny Smith apple, cored and coarsely grated
- zest and juice of 1 clementine
- 1 large free-range egg
- 125g unsalted butter
- 500g self-raising flour, plus extra for dusting
- 200ml whole milk
- olive oil

Put all the ingredients except the butter, flour, milk and olive oil into a large bowl. Squelch and scrunch everything together with your clean hands, then squash the butter in your hands to soften it up and mix it up with all that spiced fruit. Tip in the flour and keep squeezing and mixing with your hands. Once everything has come together, wash your hands, then pour in the milk and mix with a spatula until you get a fairly stiff consistency.

Now to wrapping it up: I've done a video for *www.jamieoliver.com/how-to*, so have a look at that if you need a little extra help. Wet a large tea towel and two 1m sheets of crumpled greaseproof paper. Lay the tea towel out flat with the greaseproof on top so the sheets overlap in a cross shape. Drizzle over some olive oil and use your hands to rub that all over the paper. Dust over a thin layer of flour from a height so it covers the paper, then spoon the pudding mixture into the centre. Dust the top with a little flour and then gently (so it doesn't tear) bring the greaseproof up round the pudding. Scrunch it together at the top and tie tightly with string. Trim away the excess paper from the top, then bring up the sides of the tea towel and again tie it at the top with string. Tie it tightly, but leave a little bit of room for it to expand at the top. If you can get someone to help you do this, that's even better.

We're going to steam this pudding, so place a small side plate upside down in a very large deep saucepan. Pour in enough cold water to just cover the plate by 1cm, then place a second small plate on top, facing upwards. Put the clootie dumpling on the plate, making sure it doesn't touch the water, and cover the pan with a lid. Bring the water to the boil, then turn down to a gentle simmer and steam for 3½ hours exactly, checking every 30 minutes (set your timer!) and topping up with water, if needed.

Once the time is up, take the pan off the heat. Carefully move the dumpling to a board and let it cool for 40 minutes. Remove the tea towel and paper, and serve with anything you like.

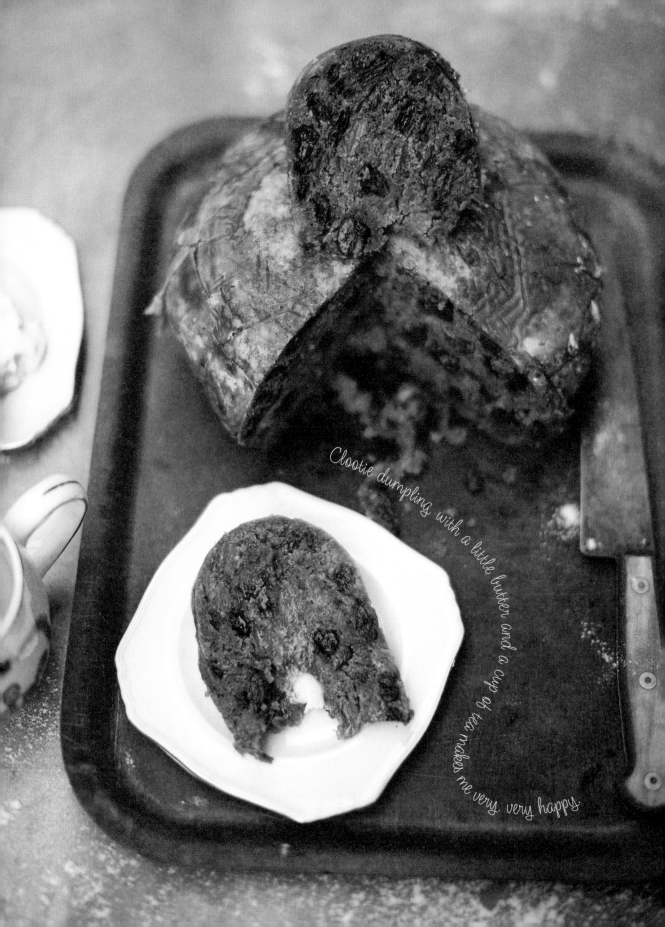

Clootie dumpling with a little butter and a cup of tea makes me very very happy.

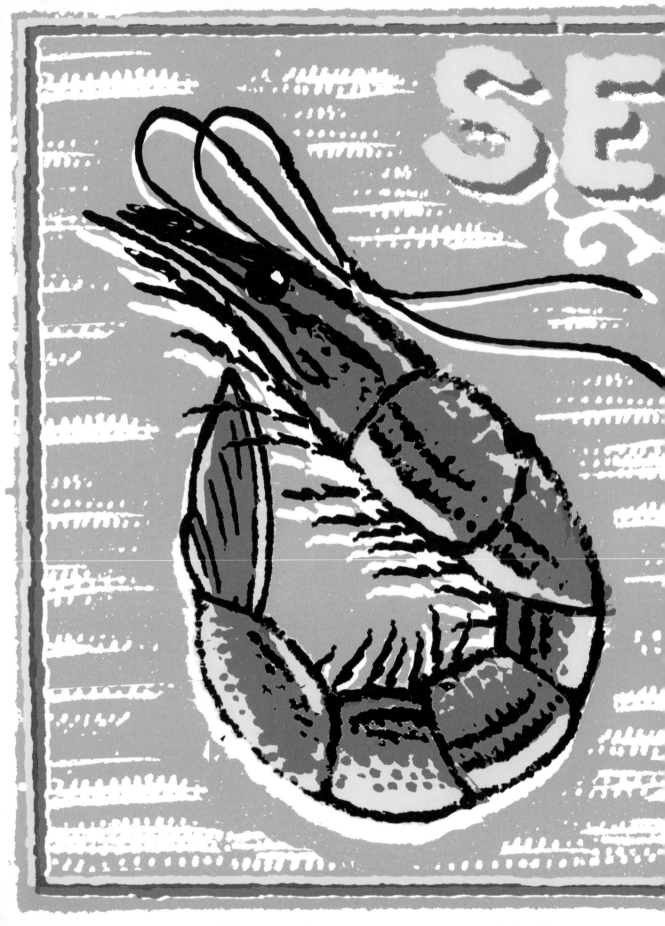

♛

There's something quite kitsch about the British seaside. It has its own personality, and wherever you go in the world, there's nothing quite like it. It's had its good and bad days, but we're an island, so wherever you are you're never too far away from a stretch of beach. We have absolutely beautiful fish and shellfish being landed all over the UK, but much of it is packed up and shipped off to Europe, where they go mad for it – it's time we made more of a fuss about our wonderful fish. These days we have to be aware of sustainability issues. You'll notice I've mentioned the Marine Stewardship Council (MSC) in some of these recipes. That's because they're the best organization out there measuring sustainability, so look for their logo when you buy your fish, or ask your fishmonger to tell you about the fish you're buying. As long as you're buying stuff that's responsibly sourced you're doing absolutely fine. This chapter is light, fresh and takes me back to holidays I took with my family as a kid.

LEIGH·ON·SEA SOLE

This is a great dish I made near my family's historical stomping ground on the Essex coast: Leigh-on-Sea. I used Dover sole, but any sustainable or MSC-approved flatfish like plaice, dab or lemon sole would also be fantastic. Dover sole can be a bit on the pricey side, but they are so tasty that they are a wonderful treat every now and then. You want them skinned, with the heads left on, so either ask your fishmonger to do this for you, or watch the video at *www.jamieoliver.com/how-to*. I've used fresh cockles and peeled brown shrimps, which are deliciously sweet, but way underrated. This dish is best made for two so you can cook everything together quickly in one large pan. There's something about the way these ingredients work together that makes it such a luxurious dinner. Hope you love it.

SERVES 2

- 125g fresh cockles or small clams (or mussels)
- 2 rashers of quality smoked streaky bacon
- olive oil
- 2 sprigs of fresh rosemary
- a small knob of butter
- 2 x 450g Dover sole, skinned
- 50g peeled brown shrimps or small prawns
- a small bunch of fresh chives
- 2 lemons
- sea salt and ground pepper

OK, here's a quick pep talk for you: every house needs an extra-large non-stick frying pan, so if you don't have one, go and get one, otherwise you won't be able to cook two fish at the same time. You will also need a large fish slice. Cooking flatfish like this is very simple, but you mustn't overcook it. How do you know when it's cooked perfectly? Simple: gently try to pull the meat away from the thickest part next to the head. If it moves, it's cooked. If it doesn't, it's not.

Sort through the cockles or clams and tap them. If any stay open, throw them away. Give them a wash and slush about in a bowl of cold water. Put a large frying pan on a medium heat and slice the bacon into matchsticks, then add to the pan along with a drizzle of olive oil and fry until lightly golden. Strip the leaves from the sprigs of rosemary and add to the pan. Fry for a few more minutes, then remove everything to a plate with a slotted spoon. Add a small knob of butter to the bacon fat, give it a little shake and carefully lay both fish in the hot pan, head to tail. You're going to cook them at a medium high heat, so it won't take long, but the cooking shouldn't run away from you. Cook the fish for about 4 minutes, then carefully and confidently turn each one over with a large fish slice. Quickly return the rosemary and bacon to the pan and add the shrimps and the cockles or clams. Using a tea towel to protect your hands, cover the pan immediately with a lid or tinfoil, making it as airtight as you can. Cook for another 4 minutes, or until the cockles have all opened.

Finely slice the chives, then remove the foil when the time is up. Squeeze in the juice of a lemon, scatter over the chives, add a good pinch of salt and pepper, then chivvy the pan around with a sense of urgency and remove the fish to a warm platter or two plates, pouring over all the juices and seafood from the pan. Nice served with wedges of lemon on the side and a simple pea and spinach salad, some buttered asparagus or new potatoes.

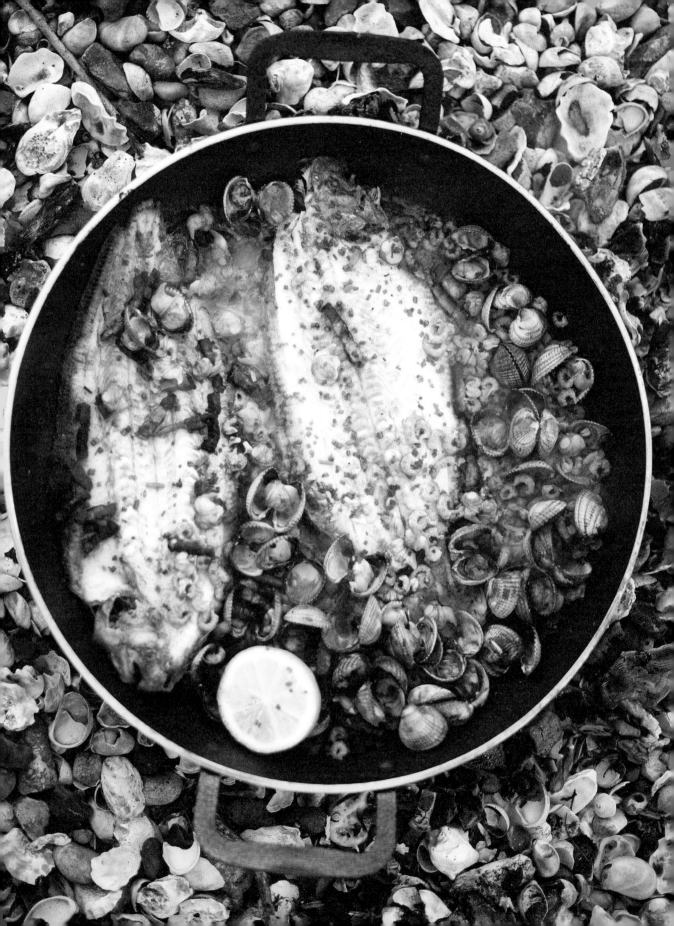

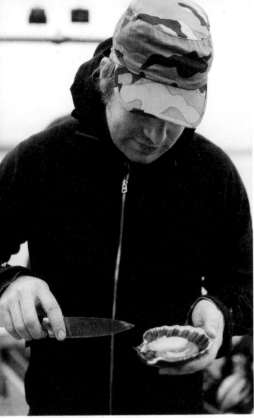
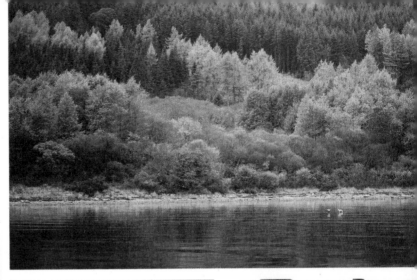
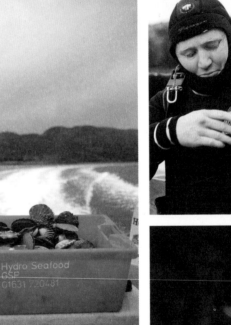
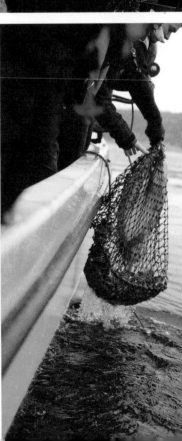
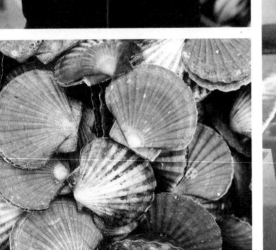
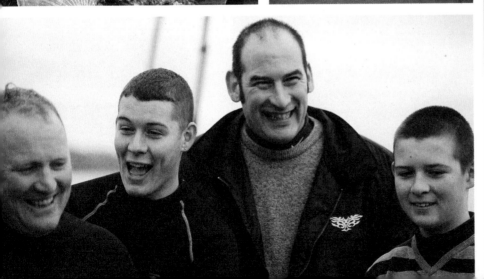

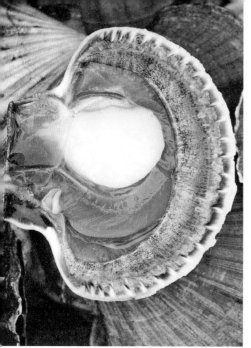

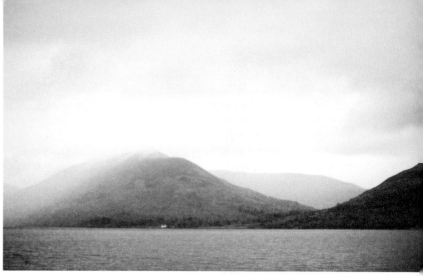

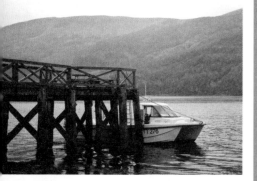

Scallop Diving

I went diving with Hector, his sons Bobby and Sean, and his mate James. Up in Scotland they have some wonderfully dramatic coastlines, with cold clean waters that are a breeding ground for mighty scallops and langoustines – such a delicacy and a treat. Like any kind of fishing – as long as it's done with respect, in harmony with the surrounding area – diving can be beautiful and sustainable. The divers catch and handpick the scallops on the seabed, then box them up, and put them on the overnight train from Inverness to London so chefs like me can get our hands on them while they're still alive and clapping – what a pleasure. Ask your fishmonger to order you live ones, then prepare yourself for a truly epic meal.

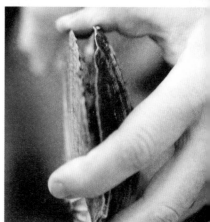

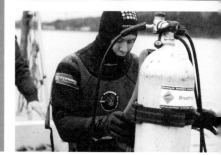

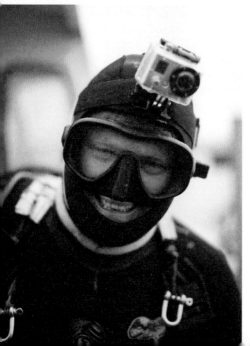

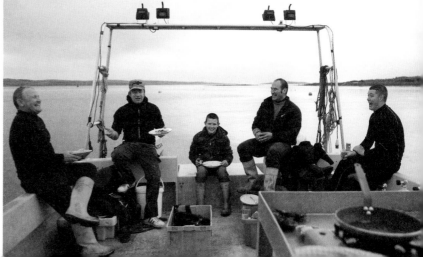

SEARED SCALLOPS

CRISPY BLACK PUDDING • CREAMY CLAPSHOT

Delicate scallops and quality black pudding is a guaranteed successful combo, and clapshot, smoky bacon and crispy sage only make them more mouthwatering. If you haven't heard of clapshot, don't let the name scare you off – it's just turnip mash with finely chopped chives that resemble lead shots from a rifle mixed through it – humble, simple and very tasty. Try and get lovely large fresh scallops about 30g in weight from your fishmonger; they'll be slightly bigger than the little ones you get in the supermarket. If you're able to get big ones you'll only need two for a main course. If they're much smaller, just use your common sense and scale the quantity up. The method will still be the same, they might just cook slightly quicker.

SERVES 4

For the clapshot
- 500g Maris Piper potatoes, peeled and cut into 4cm chunks
- 500g turnips, peeled and cut into 3cm chunks
- sea salt and ground pepper
- a bunch of fresh chives
- 2 knobs of butter
- 1 teaspoon cider vinegar

For the scallops
- 12 large or 16 medium scallops, shelled, trimmed and roes removed
- olive oil
- fennel seeds
- 12 rashers of quality smoked streaky bacon, cut into thick lardons

- 8 thick slices of quality black pudding, roughly 150g
- a knob of butter
- 12 fresh sage leaves
- 1 lemon

Put the potatoes and turnips into a large pan of boiling water and add a generous pinch of salt. Cook for 10 to 15 minutes, or until tender. Meanwhile slowly and carefully slice the chives as finely as you can. Once the vegetables are cooked, drain and allow to steam dry in a colander. Put the pan back on a low heat and add the 2 knobs of butter, a teaspoon of cider vinegar, a good pinch of salt and pepper and your finely chopped chives. As the mixture bubbles and foams, add your drained vegetables and mash until you have the consistency you like. Taste and adjust the seasoning, then cover with a lid and leave on a very low heat to keep warm.

Score each scallop halfway through in a crisscross pattern (like the picture). Season each one on both sides with salt, pepper, a drizzle of olive oil and a few fennel seeds. Get a large frying pan on a high heat and add a drizzle of olive oil. Add the bacon to the pan and fry for 5 minutes, or until lightly golden, then move the bacon to a plate and add the slices of black pudding. Cook until crisp on both sides, then divide the clapshot between four hot plates and top with the bacon and black pudding. Put the frying pan straight back on the heat and add a lug of fresh olive oil, a small knob of butter and the scallops, scored side down, and turn the heat down to low. Cook for just 2 minutes, then turn them over and give them no more than 1 minute. Add the sage leaves to the pan to crisp up and, once ready to serve, squeeze over the juice of half the lemon and shake everything about.

Divide the scallops and crispy sage leaves between everyone and spoon some of the delicious cooking juices from the pan over each plate. Serve with some steamed greens and a few wedges of lemon for squeezing over, and it's happy days.

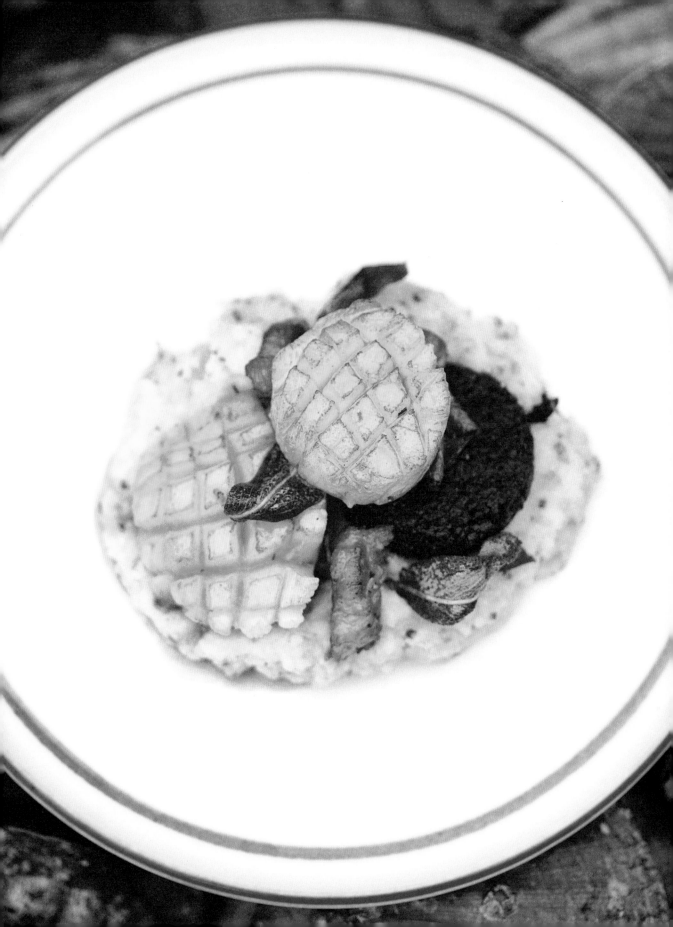

FRESH OYSTERS THREE WAYS

There are two types of oyster: native and rock. Natives only grow in specific climates and are best during colder months (basically any month with an 'r' in it). Rock oysters are more oval in shape and can be farmed in many different locations, which is why they're a bit cheaper. I think the natives from Mersea are kind of special: the nutrients that wash off the marshland become part of them, giving them a fresh zincy saltiness. But of course there are also some amazing oysters to be had in Scotland and Ireland. Purists will say shuck them and eat them raw, which I do with my first two or three. But then condiments come into their own and make your fourth, fifth and sixth ones just as exciting as the first three.

The story of oysters is a rags-to-riches tale: in Victorian times, poor English folk would feed their whole families on these babies, known then as 'the pigeons of the sea' because there were so many of them and they cost next to nothing. Now they're on posh menus all over Britain. My team has done a video to help you get that shucking technique down pat, so go to *www.jamieoliver.com/how-to* and watch that first. Just prise a shucking knife near the hinge of the shell, twist and rock it until it pops open, then dislodge the oyster while keeping it in its shell. Ultimately practice makes perfect, so check out that video and get shucking.

MAKES SAUCE FOR 30 OYSTERS

Sweet Onion Vinegar
Put 1 heaped tablespoon of grated **red onion** into a bowl with a couple of pinches of **sugar** and a pinch of **sea salt**, then cover with **red wine vinegar**. Stir, taste and balance with a little more sugar if needed. Really cute served in a jam jar.

Kinda Bloody Mary
Halve a **ripe tomato** and grate each half finely into a bowl. Discard the skin and seeds. Add a teaspoon of **jarred horseradish**, a few drips of **Worcestershire sauce**, 2 drips of **Tabasco**, a tiny swiglet of **vodka** and one of **extra virgin olive oil**, a few pinches of **celery salt** and the juice of half a **lemon**. Mix up, season with **sea salt and pepper** to taste, then adjust the flavour to give it the personality your Bloody Mary requires.

Yin and Yang
Finely slice the leaves from 2 **coriander sprigs**. Squeeze in the juice of half a **lime** and add a pinch of **sugar**. Peel a clove of **garlic** and finely grate in the littlest amount. Grate in a few scrapings of **fresh red chilli** - just a few scrapings. Then add a couple of drops of **extra virgin olive oil** and a few drips of **soy sauce** or **sesame oil**.

Butter some bread and lay it out on a platter with a few wedges of lemon, a bottle of Tabasco and the sauces. Rest the shucked oyster shells on top, then tuck into them. Don't fall prey to that 'down in one' mentality. These are beautiful little mouthfuls, so chew and savour them.

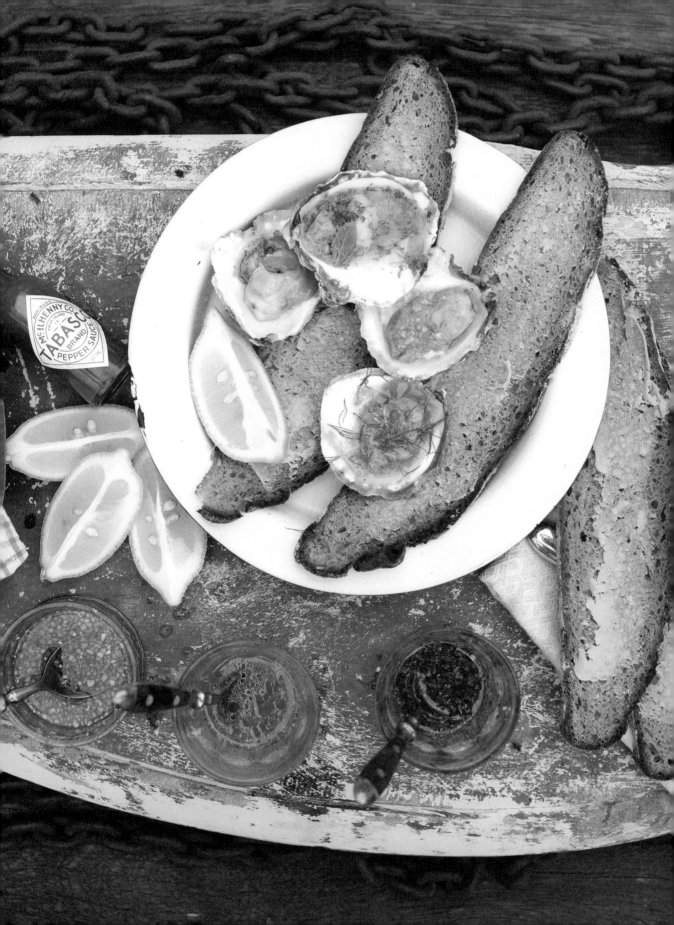

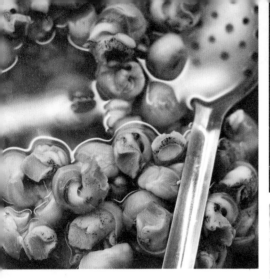

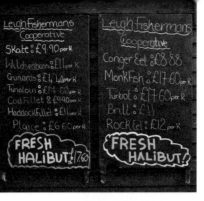

Leigh Fishermans Cooperative
Skate £9.90 per k
Wild seabass £11 per k
Gurnards £4.40 per k
Tuna loin £17.60 per k
Cod Fillet £9.90 per k
Haddock Fillet £11 per k
Plaice £6.60 per k
FRESH HALIBUT! £7.60

Leigh Fishermans Cooperative
Conger Eel £8.88
MonkFish £17.60 per k
Turbot £17.60 per k
Brill £11
Rock Eel £12 per k
FRESH HALIBUT!

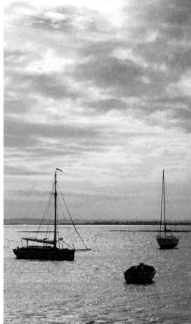

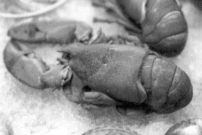

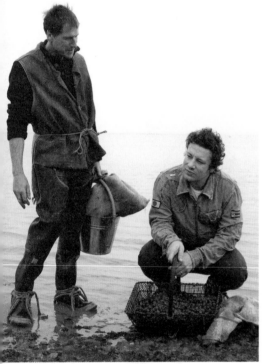

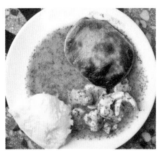

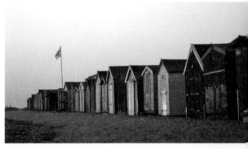

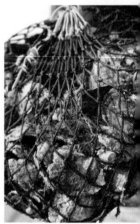

Mersea Island

Picking winkles with my mate Ben on Mersea Island in Essex was brilliant. My family is local to the area, so appreciating the world-quality West Mersea oysters and shellfish is second nature. If you're in that part of the world, get yourself to the cockle sheds in Leigh-on-Sea for some seafood and a pint.

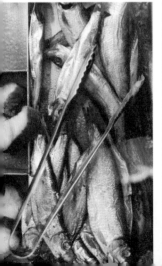

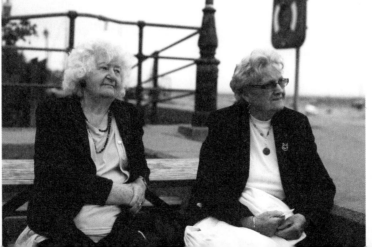

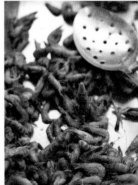

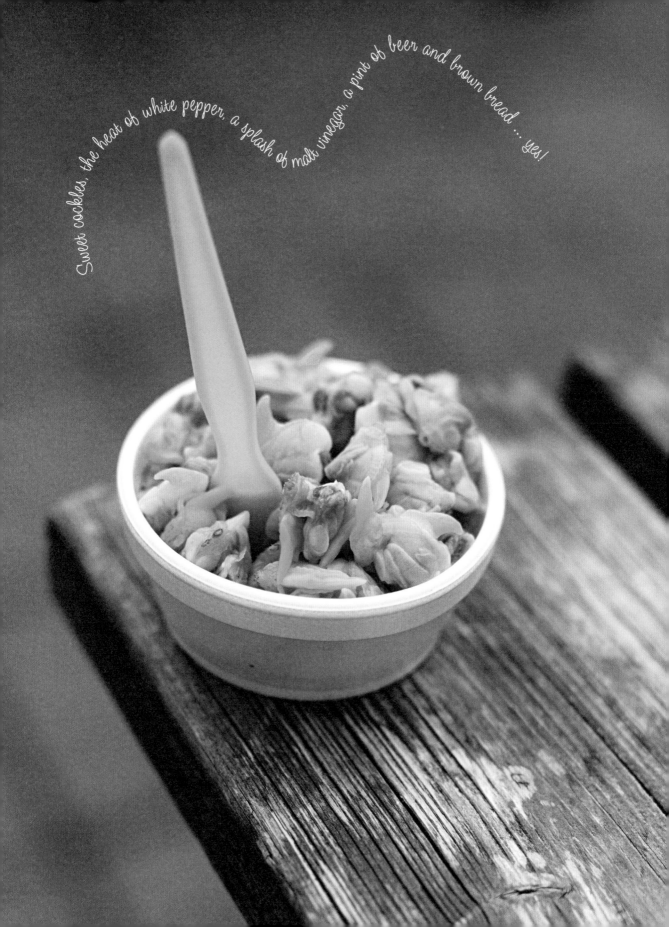

Sweet cockles, the heat of white pepper, a splash of malt vinegar, a pint of beer and brown bread … yes!

WHITE PEPPER SKATE
... ON A BED OF FRESH MINTED PEAS

A lovely wing of skate every now and again is such a pleasure. I used to eat this quite a lot when I was a kid, and I remember how cool it was to pull the flesh off the bones in spaghetti-like strips. Depending on where you live, skate may be plentiful, or it might be a little overfished. Ask your fishmonger, and if he doesn't have any sustainably caught skate, ask for ray wings instead – they are also delicious. Using fennel and copious amounts of white pepper helps create a really tasty crust with attitude and heat that contrasts nicely with the delicate flavour of the fish and the minted peas. This is the kind of dish I only really cook when it's just me and the missus – it makes a really generous dinner.

SERVES 2

For the minted peas
- a knob of butter
- rapeseed or olive oil
- 3 spring onions, trimmed and finely sliced
- 400g frozen peas
- a handful of mint leaves

- 1 lemon
- sea salt and ground pepper

For the skate
- 2 skate or ray wings (about 400g each)
- 2 heaped teaspoons fennel seeds

- 1 level teaspoon white peppercorns
- ½ a mugful of plain flour
- 1 large free-range egg, beaten
- rapeseed or olive oil
- a knob of butter

Put a medium-sized pan on a medium heat and add a knob of butter and a splash of oil. Add the spring onions and cook for a few minutes until softened, then add the frozen peas and half the mint leaves. Add a swig of water, pop the lid on and leave to cook for 10 to 12 minutes.

Use scissors to trim the ruffled outer edges (skirt) of the skate wings, and use a knife to cut off the backbone (if you want to see how this is done, go to *www.jamieoliver.com/how-to* and you'll find a video to guide you). Grind the fennel seeds and white peppercorns in a pestle and mortar or in a liquidizer until you've got a fine powder, and put aside. Tip the flour on to one large plate and the beaten egg on to another. Sprinkle, rub and pat the peppery mixture all over each skate wing, then quickly dip each one into the egg to coat really well on both sides. Let any excess egg drip off, then put each wing straight into the plate of flour and pat and coat really well on both sides until you have a good covering.

Put a large non-stick frying pan, big enough to hold both the wings (cut them in half if need be), on a high heat. Once hot, add a good lug of oil, a knob of butter and the skate wings. Cook for roughly 3 minutes on each side, then an extra minute on each side to finish them off, until the meat comes off the bone at the thickest part of the fish and you've got a nice golden crust.

Add a squeeze of lemon juice and the remaining mint leaves to your peas, then stir and season to taste. If you want to smash or purée them you can, but I like sprinkling them over a warm platter and simply placing the sizzling golden skate wings on top. Sprinkle over a pinch of sea salt and serve with the rest of the lemon, cut into wedges. An absolute joy.

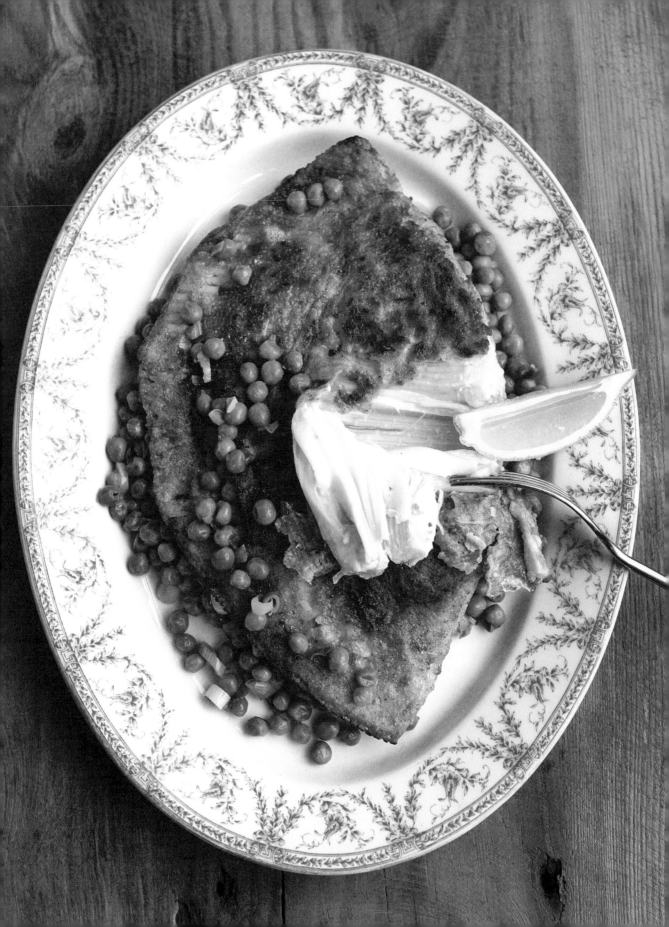

HEAVENLY POTTED SHELLFISH

Whether you use crab, tiny shrimps, lobster, prawns or even smoked fish, this recipe is really easy and never fails to impress. Just a few simple flavourings complement the delicate shellfish sealed and trapped under the clarified butter lid. Ultimately you're making a spread; a mixture that will keep in the fridge quite happily, then melt into a plain piece of toast in the most luxurious way when you serve it. This is something you can make well in advance of a dinner party to make your life easy, and it's also great for picnics, or for sandwiches when shoved between some nice bread with lettuce leaves.

Good fishmongers will have peeled prawns and shrimps as well as picked crabmeat, so why not have fun with this and make up a few pots using different kinds of shellfish? I guarantee if you put a dish of potted crab, and one of lobster, and one of shrimps out on the table with a few different rustic breads, a bowl of crunchy salad and a bottle of chilled white wine, your guests will be blown away by how classy you are.

SERVES 8 TO 10

- 180g unsalted butter
- 1 lemon
- 1 teaspoon fennel seeds
- 1 small dried chilli
- 1 whole nutmeg, for grating
- 400g cooked and picked crab, brown shrimps, lobster, prawns or smoked trout
- sea salt and white pepper
- 1 heaped tablespoon fennel tops or fresh dill

Get a packet of butter out of the fridge and cut off a 60g chunk. Put it into a small pan over a very low heat and slowly melt it so the golden part separates from the milky part. Don't let it boil! Cut off another 120g chunk and chop it into 1cm dice, then leave it to soften at room temperature. Grate the zest of the lemon into a mortar, add the fennel seeds and dried chilli, and bash everything together really well. Add the softened butter, grate in about a third of the nutmeg and mix until everything is combined.

If you're using delicate shellfish like picked crab or little shrimps, simply fold them in now. If you're using chunkier shellfish, like lobster or large prawns, take a minute to chop them up into smaller pieces before folding them in. Mix everything together, then toast a bit of bread, smear a little of the mixture on the toast and have a taste. This is your opportunity to really get those seasonings perfect, so adjust with a pinch of salt and pepper, a squeeze of lemon juice or a pinch more dried chilli if needed.

When you're happy with the flavours, spoon the mixture into a serving dish (roughly 18cm in diameter and 5cm deep) or divide it between eight little teacups or bowls and spread it out in an even layer. Angle the pan of melted butter and carefully spoon the clarified butter (not the milky stuff underneath) all over the seafood. Use the bottom of the spoon to spread it around and make sure the butter coats every bit of it, then tear over some pretty dill or fennel tops. This clarified butter will create a natural seal and allow you to keep the potted shellfish in the fridge for a few days, as long as that seal completely covers the seafood mixture.

Serve with a stack of little hot toasts, a green salad or some nice salad cresses.

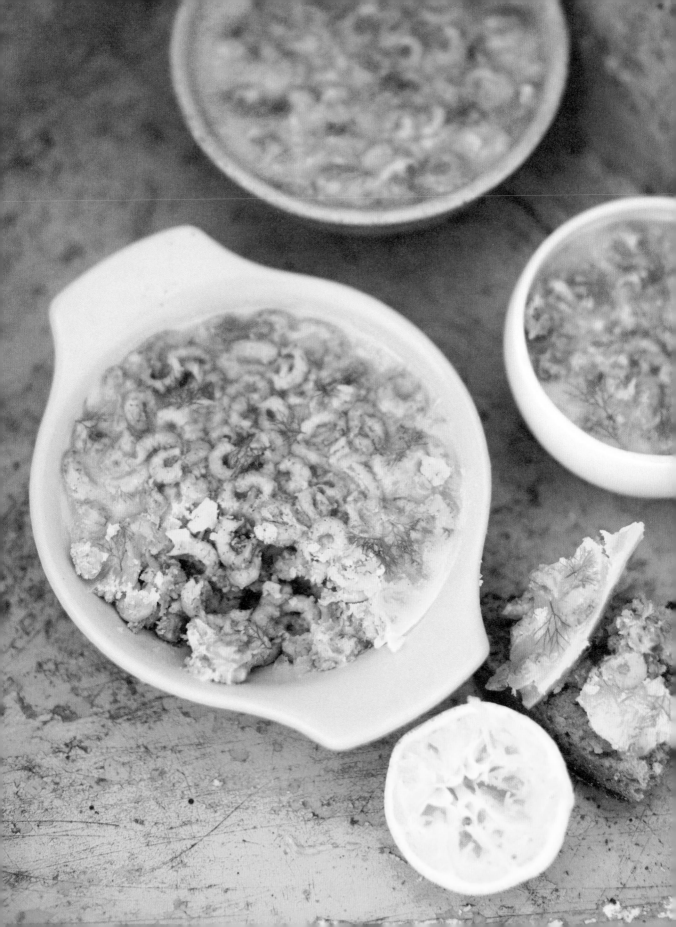

I must say I've got a soft spot for quaint British seaside towns: quiet, peaceful and idyllic.

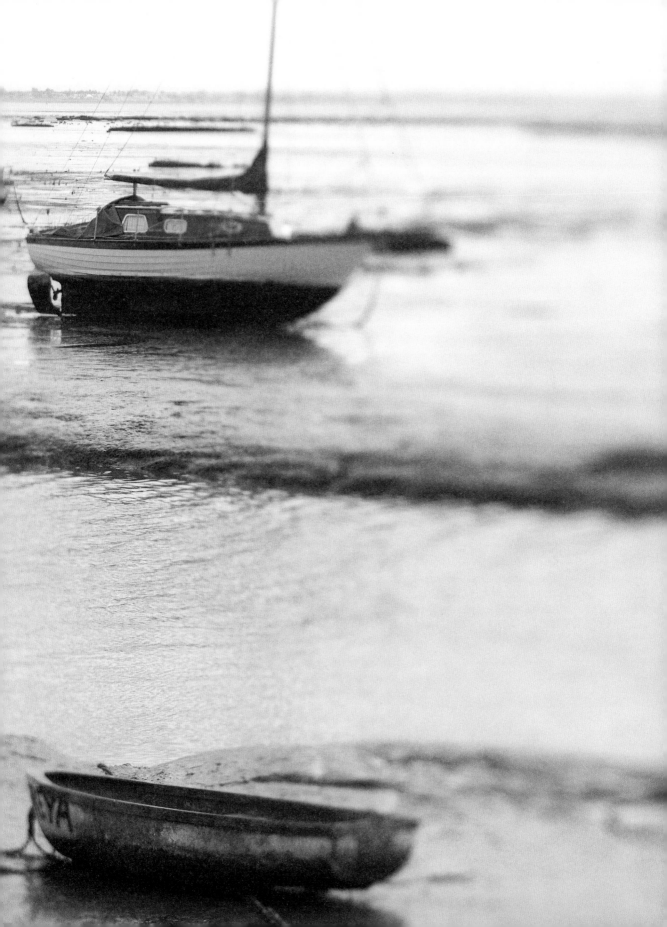

CRISPY ROASTED PRAWNS

People love prawns, and this recipe is so easy for dinner parties. If you can, look for prawns that are MSC-approved. The sauce is a brilliant mixture of sticky flavours that clings to their thin outer shells, and when you roast those prawns it will flavour the meat inside and make the shell crispy and delicious at the same time. Put a few of these on a board with some fingerbowls nearby and let everyone dive in and share. There will be hands everywhere, bits of shell flying about and lots of finger-licking, but nobody will knock you for that.

SERVES 4

- a loaf of brown bread, to serve
- a small bunch of fresh curly parsley
- 2 lemons
- olive oil

- a knob of butter
- 12 raw whole king prawns, shells on
- sea salt and ground pepper
- 4 cloves of garlic, peeled
- 2 teaspoons English mustard

- 2 tablespoons tomato ketchup
- I whole nutmeg, for grating
- 2 tablespoons Worcestershire sauce

Preheat your oven to full whack (about 240°C/475°F/gas 9). Wrap the loaf of bread in tin foil and place it at the bottom of the oven to warm up. Roughly chop the parsley and halve one of the lemons. Put a lug of olive oil and a knob of butter into a large roasting tray. Throw the prawns into the tray with half your chopped parsley and season well with a few good pinches of salt and pepper. Crush in the peeled garlic with a garlic crusher, then squeeze over the lemon halves and add the mustard and ketchup. Quickly grate over a few scrapings of nutmeg, then mix and toss everything around until all the prawns are really well coated. Put the tray under the hot grill for around 5 minutes, or until lightly golden. If you have smaller prawns they might need less time.

When you take the prawns out of the oven, quickly stab and squeeze their heads so the delicious juices run out. Shake over the Worcestershire sauce for some wicked flavour, and jiggle the tray at the same time so the prawns get flipped over and all the flavours mix together. Put them back in the oven for another few minutes while you take the bread and slice it up, then arrange the crispy sizzling prawns on a board with the bread. Sprinkle over the rest of the parsley and wedge up the remaining lemon for squeezing over. Make sure you've got a big empty bowl for shells, a few fingerbowls with warm water and lemon slices at the table and, if you're common like me, some kitchen paper. Perfection.

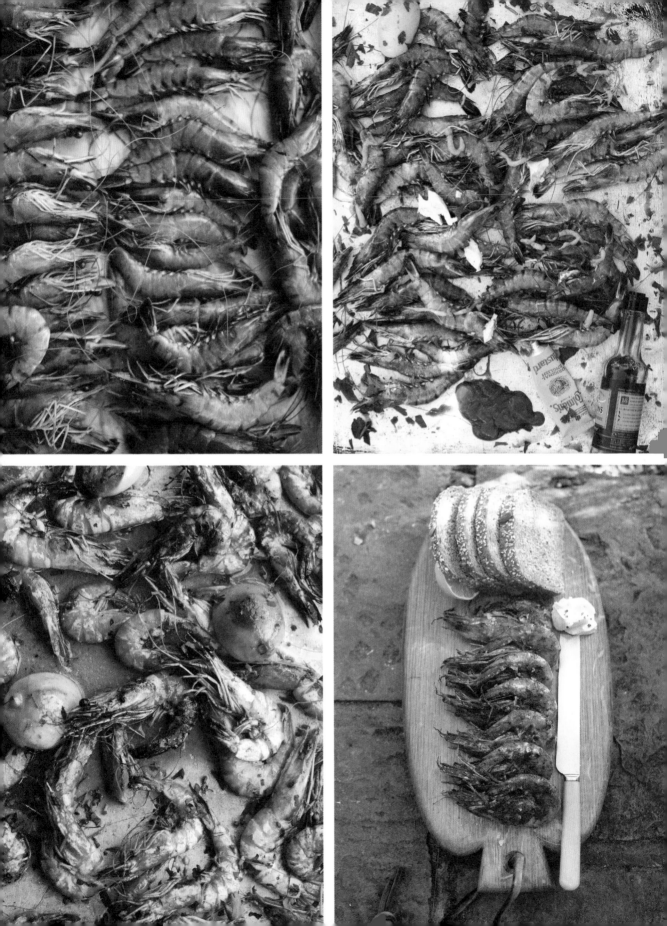

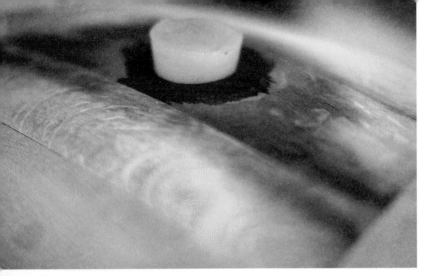

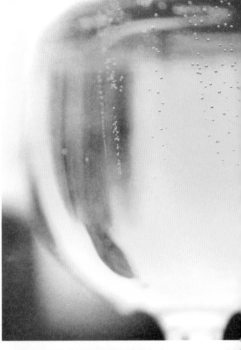

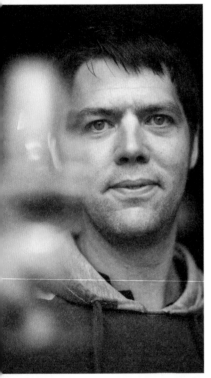

Chapel Down Winery

Who would have thought that Britain would ever get into serious wine production? Over the last ten years it's been really exciting to see the quality of our wine go up and up, so much so that French vineyards are buying up land on our south coast. Kent is often called 'the garden of England' and the local Chapel Down winery is in my opinion one of the best British winemakers. They've got some great wines, special editions, sparkling rosés, and exceptional ciders and beers. I went there for a tasting and had to pinch myself because in just an hour and a half I'd gone from the hustle and bustle of London's streets to this beautiful, quiet country vineyard. Well worth exploring.

www.englishwinesgroup.com

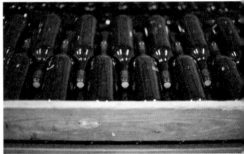

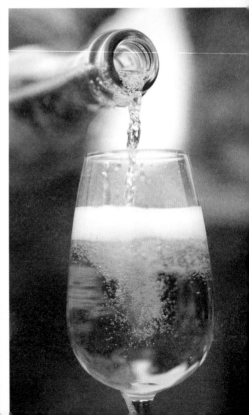

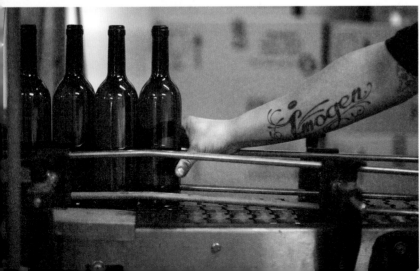

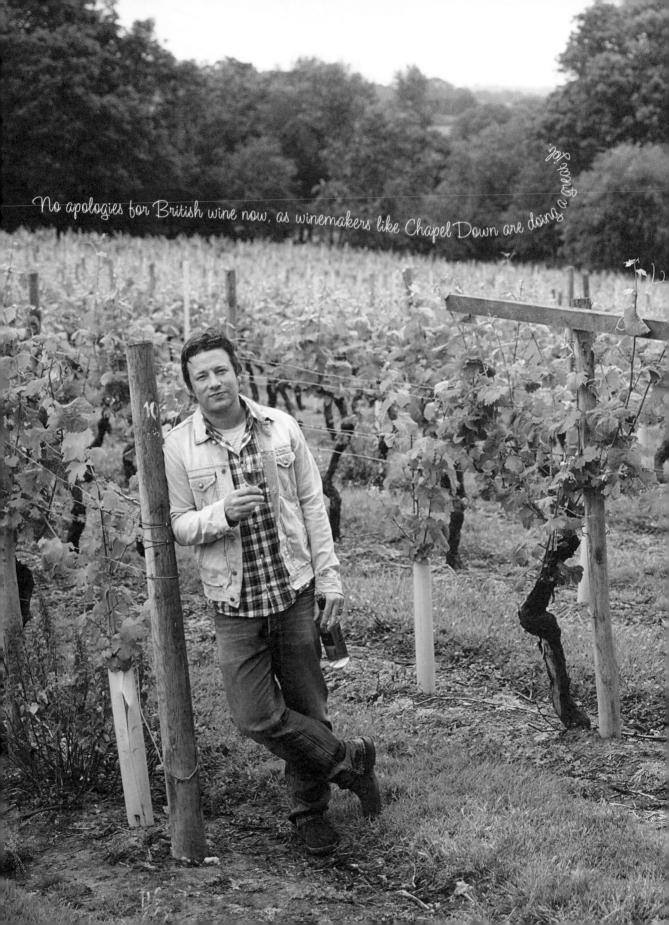

No apologies for British wine now, as winemakers like Chapel Down are doing a great job.

HIGHLAND MUSSELS
JUICY • LEEKY • WHISKY • CREAMY • SMOKY

I tasted my first mussel at the age of eight. I remember looking at the pile of shells and thinking, I'm never going to eat those, but my mum said, 'Don't look at them, darling, just eat them,' so I did. Once I figured out how to use an empty shell as pincers to grab the meat from the other shells, I went through the whole bowl in no time flat. Mussels are one of the most sustainable types of seafood. They can be cultivated on a large or small scale, they clean the water around them, take literally 4 minutes to cook and are nutritious and wonderful to eat … I can't think of any negatives! What are you waiting for?

SERVES 6

- 2kg mussels
- 1 large leek
- 1 stick of celery
- olive oil
- 2 small knobs of butter
- 250g undyed smoked haddock, skin off and pin-boned

- 6 shots of whisky (25ml each)
- 200ml double cream
- a small bunch of flat-leaf parsley
- extra virgin olive oil, to serve
- 6 hunks of sourdough bread, to serve

Quickly wash and debeard all the mussels (pull off any bits that look like wire wool), discarding any that won't close (your fishmonger will do this for you if you ask in advance).

Trim, wash, then finely slice the leek and the stick of celery, reserving any of the delicate yellow leaves for sprinkling over later. Put a really wide, deep pot on a medium heat and add a lug of olive oil and a knob of butter, along with the sliced leek and celery. Cook and stir for 10 minutes, or until the vegetables have softened, then flake in the smoked haddock and pour in the whisky - feel free to light it with a match to burn off the alcohol if you want. I think this adds to the flavour, but don't set yourself on fire.

Next, add the mussels and double cream. Stir and shake the pan, put the lid on and cook for 4 to 5 minutes, or literally just until the mussels have all popped open - discard any that haven't. Use a slotted spoon to move them to a large serving platter or bowl. Leave the pan of cooking liquor on the heat and let it bubble away until it thickens to a consistency you're happy with. While that's happening, roughly chop the parsley, then add it to the pot and shake it about. Have a quick taste of the sauce, correct the seasoning if it needs it, and pour all over the mussels. Scatter over any celery leaves, drizzle with extra virgin olive oil and serve straight away with fresh or toasted hunks of bread for a beautiful hearty lunch or dinner.

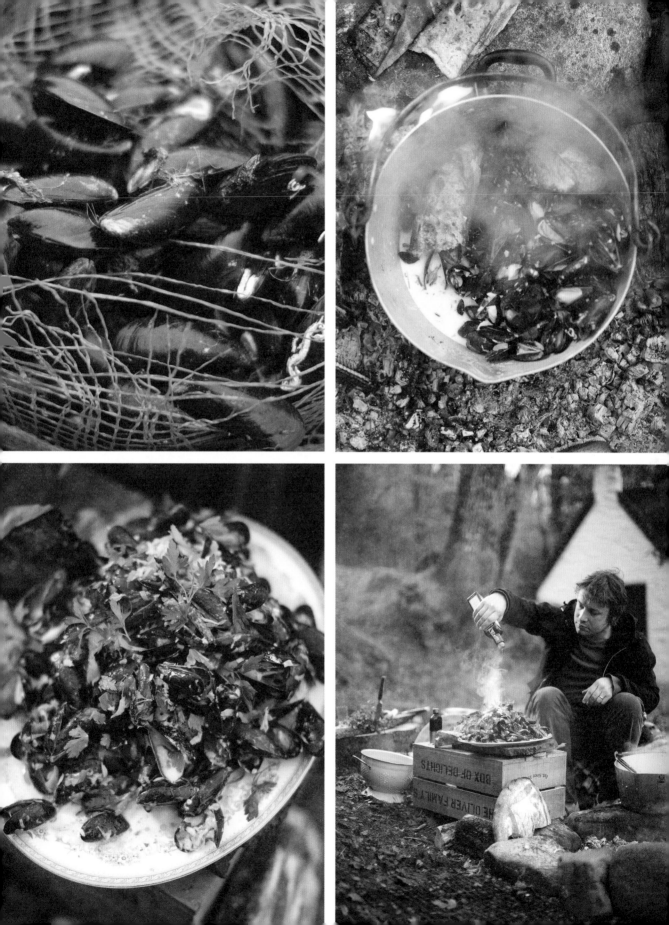

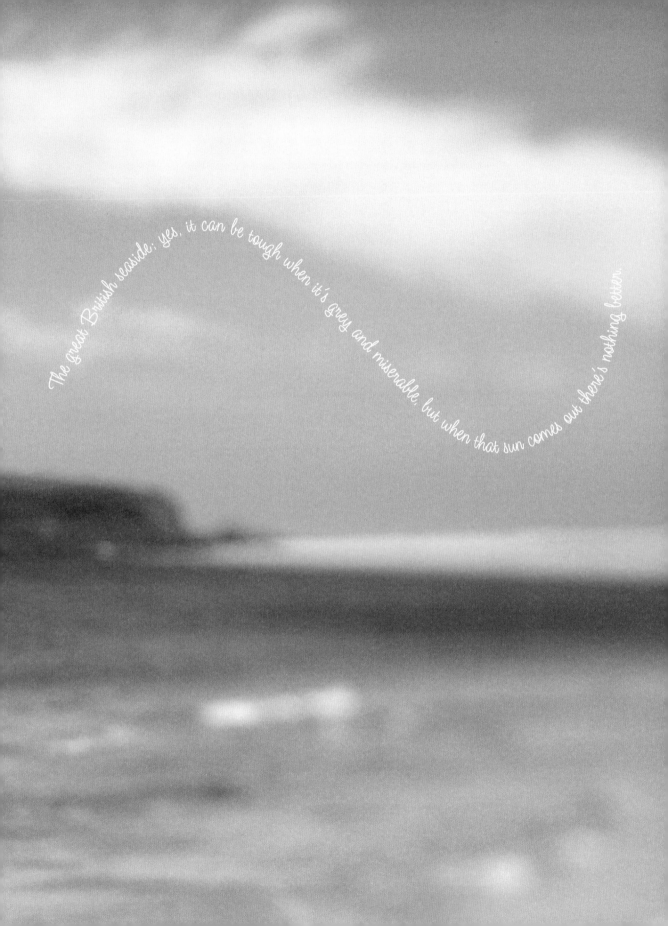

The great British seaside; yes, it can be tough when it's grey and miserable, but when that sun comes out there's nothing better.

SUMMER CRAB SALAD
HERBY AVOCADO • SOURDOUGH SOLDIERS

You can knock this recipe out of the park with pre-picked brown and white crabmeat, which you can get in most good supermarkets or fishmongers these days. But you can also invest in the experience of cooking by picking your own crabmeat, which will take the flavours of this salad to a whole new level. It is one of the most scrumptious ways to eat crab at its best.

SERVES 4

- 2 x 1kg live brown crabs

or

- 300g picked white crabmeat
- 150g brown crabmeat

For the brown crabmeat
- 2 lemons
- a whole nutmeg, for grating
- sea salt and ground pepper

- 3 tablespoons extra virgin olive oil
- 2 tablespoons natural yoghurt
- ½ a crumbled dried chilli

For the platter
- 1 ripe avocado
- 2 tomatoes
- a few yellow celery leaves

- a few sprigs of fresh flat-leaf parsley, leaves picked
- a few sprigs of fresh mint, leaves picked
- extra virgin olive oil
- 1 loaf of sourdough bread
- butter, to serve

If you've already bought pre-picked meat, go straight to 'Making your Salad'. If you're going to cook and pick your own, read on …

Cooking and Picking Crab

Put the live crabs in the sink and cover them with a cold wet cloth. Get your biggest pan (large enough to fit both crabs), fill it three-quarters of the way up with water and add enough salt so that it tastes like seawater. Bring to a fast boil on the highest heat, adding any fragrant herbs or veg you like (parsley, dill, onions, carrots and celery work well) and a squeeze of lemon juice. You can kill the crabs by putting a skewer or knife through their skulls, but as not everyone can do this properly I always think it seems more efficient to simply pop them into fast boiling water and put the lid on. Cook for exactly 12 minutes for a 1kg crab, then drain and leave to cool for around 15 to 20 minutes. Once cooled, remove the legs and claws by twisting them from the body. Watch the video demonstration before you start picking the meat (*www.jamieoliver.com/how-to*). Once you're done, put the empty shells into the pan and smash them up with a rolling pin. If you like, you can then make the tomato soup recipe from page 46 in the pan; just make sure you pass it through a sieve right at the end. The crab shells will give it the most kick-ass flavour. You've paid for them, so you may as well enjoy every last bit!

Making your Salad

Spoon the brown meat into a liquidizer and squeeze in the juice of half a lemon. Add a few gratings of nutmeg, a good pinch of salt and pepper, the extra virgin olive oil, yoghurt and the crumbled dried chilli. Liquidize everything so you get a nice smooth brown meat purée. Have a taste and add more salt and pepper and lemon if need be. Pour on to a large platter or board and sprinkle the delicate, flakey white meat all over. Halve, stone and peel a ripe avocado, and chop into 1cm dice. Chop the tomatoes into 1cm dice and scatter everything over the platter. Sprinkle over the celery, parsley and mint leaves, and drizzle with extra virgin olive oil. Cut the sourdough into thick slices and grill or toast them, spread with butter and cut into inch-wide soldiers. Pile on a plate with some lemon wedges and serve. Delish.

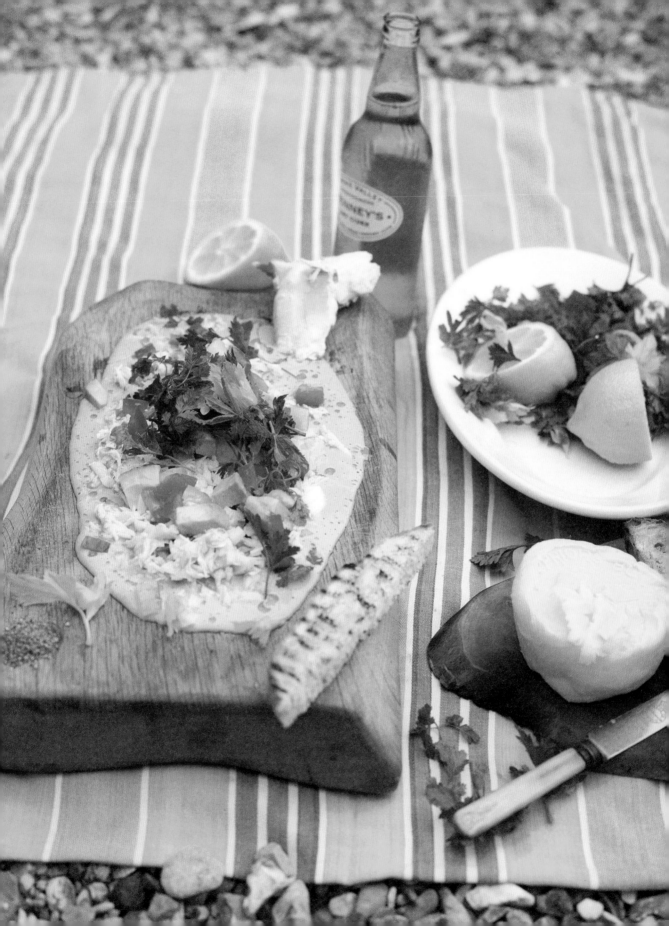

CRISPY ROASTED FISHCAKES
...WRAPPED IN SMOKED STREAKY BACON

There are a few stages to making these fishcakes, but each step is dead easy and so worth it, because the end result just seems to make people happy. I think you have to accept that sometimes in life even something humble, like a fishcake, requires effort. The reaction to these fishcakes has been amazing, and interestingly, whenever homemade fishcakes are on a restaurant menu, they always shift. The difference with making your own is that you get flavours and texture suited to your own particular tastes. So I'll happily give this recipe to you, knowing that a kid could make them ... mine have, with a little help.

SERVES 6

- 2 leeks
- a knob of butter
- 1 whole nutmeg, for grating
- sea salt and ground pepper
- 500g potatoes
- 3 large free-range eggs

- 240g smoked salmon, smoked trout, or (even better!) a mixture of the two, roughly chopped
- 2 lemons
- 6 sprigs of fresh flat-leaf parsley, leaves picked and finely chopped
- a few handfuls of plain flour

- 6 slices of white bread, crusts removed
- 1 dried red chilli
- olive oil
- 6 rashers of quality smoked streaky bacon
- watercress, to serve

Top and tail the leeks, then peel back the tough outer green leaves. Cut them lengthways, wash under the tap and finely slice. Put them into a large pan on a medium heat with a knob of butter and a few scrapings of nutmeg, and season with salt and pepper. Cook gently with the lid on for around 25 minutes, or until softened, then take the pan off the heat and leave to cool.

While your leeks are cooking, peel the potatoes, halve or quarter them depending on their size, and whack them into a pan of salted boiling water for about 15 minutes, or until cooked through and mashable. Drain them, then return them to the saucepan, smash them up so the mixture is smooth but also has chunks, and put to one side to cool down a bit. Crack the eggs into a wide, shallow bowl, then carefully remove one of the yolks and stir it into the potato mixture, followed by the sweet leeks and smoked fish. Add the zest of 1 whole lemon and the juice of half, and two-thirds of the parsley. Leave to one side.

Whisk up the eggs remaining in the bowl and tip into a shallow dish. Put a few handfuls of flour on a plate. Pulse the bread and chilli in a food processor with a tiny swig of olive oil until you have coarse breadcrumbs, then stir in the remaining parsley and tip the crumbs on to another plate. Divide your fishcake mix into 6 little balls. Dust each one in flour, shaking off the excess, then dip them in the egg until completely coated. Let the excess drip off, then move them to the tray of flavoured breadcrumbs. Wash your hands, and spend a bit of time patting, shaping and hugging them into nice-looking patties around 2cm thick. Cover and leave in the fridge until you're ready to cook them.

Preheat the oven and a large baking tray to 220°C/425°F/gas 7. Lay the bacon rashers out side by side on a board and lay a sheet of clingfilm over them. Use a rolling pin or a wine bottle to roll and stretch the rashers out a little bit lengthways so they're longer and thinner (sounds cheffy, but it's dead simple). Wrap one rasher around the circumference of each fishcake and secure with a cocktail stick. Place the fishcakes on the hot baking tray and roast in the oven for around 20 minutes, or until golden and crispy. Serve hot from the oven, with some lemony dressed watercress and a few wedges of lemon for squeezing over.

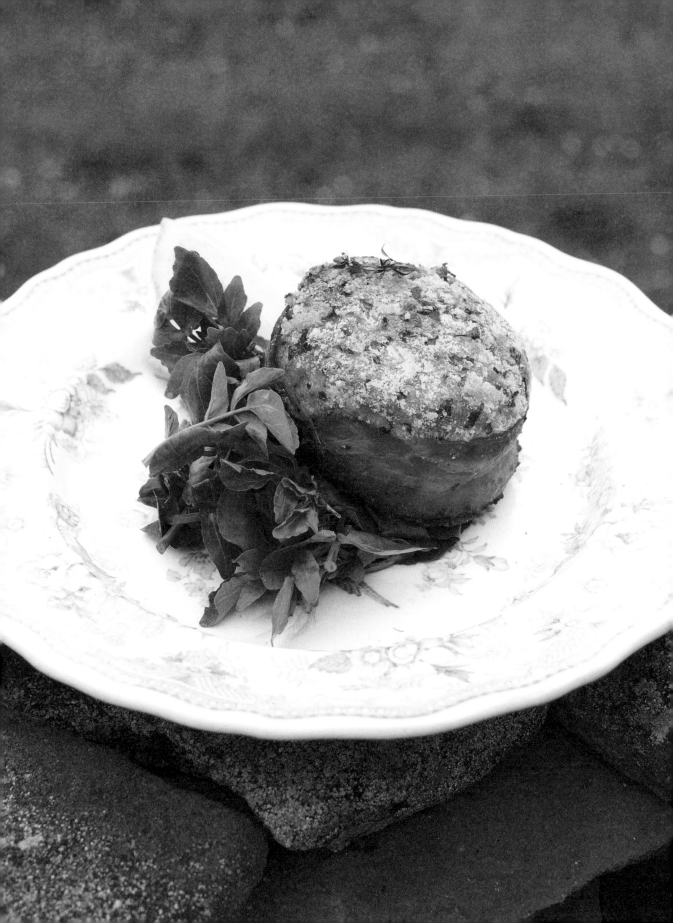

BAKED SEA BASS IN A BAG

If you want a fish recipe that's always exciting and always an event, this is it. The steam from all the lovely things cooking inside the foil bag will puff the bag up, and when you cut it open before serving, your kitchen will be filled with the most amazing smells. I used a line-caught sea bass for this and admittedly it was fairly large, but if you contact a good fishmonger in advance they'll be able to sort you out. Ask for MSC-approved fish and if they don't have one that size, you can always cook two smaller fish or another variety of fish the exact same way – just adjust the time accordingly. Ultimately, you know it's cooked when the meat behind the head flakes apart easily. One thing I will say is that even though this is an elegant dish, it's difficult to be elegant when you're fighting over the cheek meat (the best bit, by the way) and mopping up the juices with hunks of bread or buttery potatoes.

SERVES 6

- 1 x 2kg whole sea bass, scaled, gutted and gills removed
- a bunch of mixed fresh herbs, such as basil, rosemary and flat-leaf parsley
- 2 lemons
- sea salt and ground pepper

- olive oil
- a bunch of spring onions, trimmed
- 1 bulb of fennel, herby tops reserved in cold water
- 4 anchovy fillets in oil
- a few little knobs of butter

- 1 large free-range egg
- 250ml white wine
- 50ml double cream
- 1 x 200g bag of washed baby spinach

Preheat the oven to full whack (about 240°C/475°F/gas 9) and move the shelves to the top of the oven so you have lots of space at the bottom. Lay your fish on a board and score it on both sides at 2cm intervals. Stuff the herbs into the cavity of the fish, then finely slice the lemons and put a few slices in with the herbs. Sprinkle both sides of the fish with a few pinches of salt and pepper and drizzle over a little olive oil.

Tear off a piece of extra wide tin foil that's double the length of your fish (be generous!). Get your largest roasting tray and place the foil on top, leaving half hanging off one end of the tray. Finely slice the spring onions, fennel and anchovies, then arrange on the tray end of the foil and lay your fish on top. Dot little knobs of butter around the fish. Lay the remaining lemon slices on top. Quickly beat your egg and use a pastry brush to brush 2cm of egg along the edges of the foil. Fold the overhanging foil over the fish and seal the two long sides, folding them up tightly so they're about 2cm away from the fish inside. Pour the wine into the open end of the bag, making sure it doesn't spill out, then fold and seal up that end. Put the roasting tray right at the bottom of the oven and cook for 35 minutes for a 2kg bass, around 25 minutes for a 1.5kg fish and so on. Don't open the door during the cooking time.

When the time is up, take the tray out of the oven and carefully cut open the top of the puffed-up bag. Go straight to the thickest part of the fish, right behind the head; if the flesh comes away from the bone easily, that's brilliant. Simply pour in the cream and let it mix and mingle with all the juices, then sprinkle the spinach into the juices and mix it around gently to help it wilt down. Scatter over the reserved fennel tops. You can serve the fish in the roasting tray, or snip it out of the bag and move it carefully to a serving platter. Serve it in nice pieces, or pull it apart like you haven't been fed for a month; just remember to pop a bowl for the bones, skin and head nearby. Serve with simply boiled new potatoes, minted peas or asparagus.

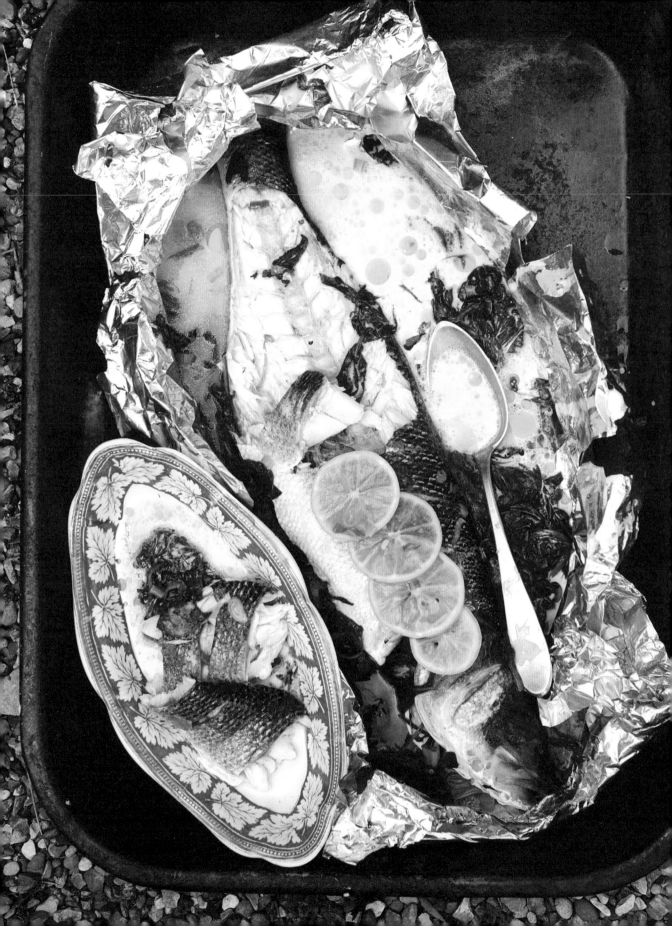

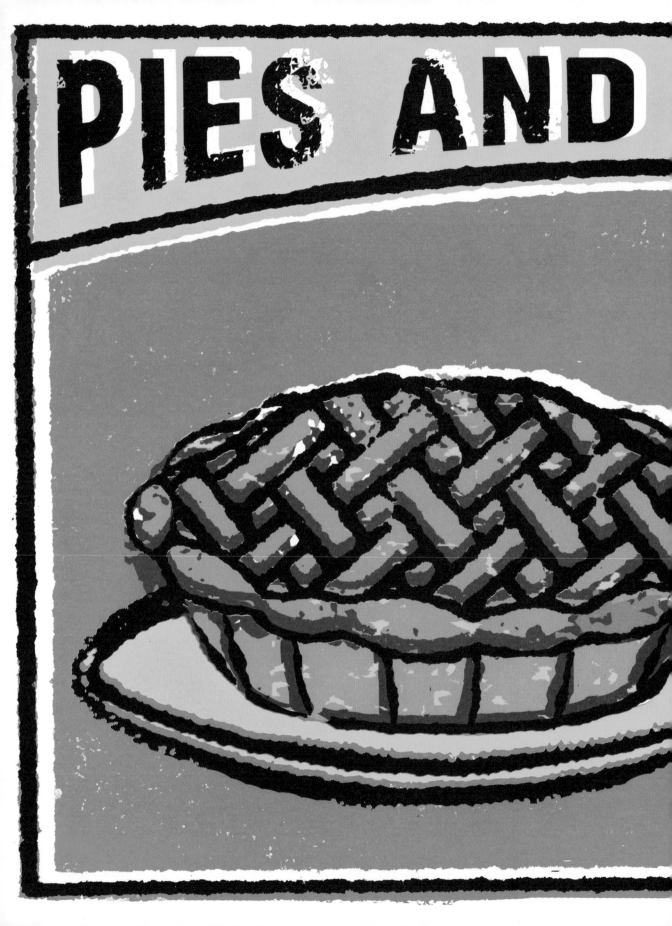

PIES AND

PUDDINGS

You haven't lived until you've enjoyed a savoury pie with golden flaky pastry, a steamed meat pudding, or a beautiful Cornish pasty. The dishes in this chapter are very British and have been part of our food landscape for a very long time. The Romans first brought the concept of pies with them when they marched on to this little island around AD 43. From there, our pie-making traditions developed and we became resourceful, using cheaper cuts of meat to create impressive and filling dishes and, in the case of the Cornish pasty, a portable food that miners could take to work and eat for their lunch. But not many of us are miners or marching soldiers these days, and if you eat a pasty or a big slice of pie every day your waistline will be in real trouble. I had to practically wrestle my nutritional adviser to the ground to get her to let me put this chapter in the book. She was talking to me about the amount of saturated fat in pastry, and I was talking about sheer happiness. The sad truth is that none of the pie fillings are bad for you, but the minute you introduce pastry into any equation the calories and fat content skyrocket. But you know, my grandad would have eaten something like this once a week, every week – so the best advice comes from him: everything in moderation, and a little bit of what you like.

KATE & WILLS'S WEDDING PIE
BEEF & BEER FILLING • UNBELIEVABLE PASTRY

I got really excited about the royal wedding. So much so that I was inspired to dedicate my favourite pie to the happy couple. Without being soppy, pies are about sharing; they're comforting, down-to-earth, humble and luxurious at the same time, and this one in particular is definitely fit for a (future) king and queen. One of the best things about our great British pies is that they look so grand, yet they're also a great way of using up the less-loved cuts of meat, which are so delicious when they're given time and a little attention. If you want to cook the pie from cold another day cook at 170°C/325°F/gas 3 for 1 hour 10 minutes.

SERVES 10

For the filling
- 2 tablespoons olive oil
- 1 knob of butter
- 3 sprigs of fresh rosemary, leaves picked and chopped
- 3 sprigs of fresh thyme, leaves picked
- 3 fresh bay leaves
- 3 medium red onions, peeled
- 1kg shin of beef (ask the butcher to cut it into 2.5cm dice and give you the bone)

- sea salt and ground pepper
- 2 tablespoons tomato purée
- 400ml good local smooth stout
- 2 heaped tablespoons plain flour
- 1.5 litres organic beef or chicken stock
- 140g pearl barley
- 3 teaspoons English mustard
- 2-3 tablespoons Worcestershire sauce, to taste
- 100g good Cheddar cheese

For the pastry
- 300g plain flour, plus extra for dusting
- 100g Atora shredded suet
- 100g butter
- sea salt
- 1 large free-range egg, beaten

Put the olive oil, butter and herbs into a large casserole-type pan (roughly 24cm in diameter and 12cm deep) on a high heat. Roughly chop and add the onions, with the diced meat, the shin bone and a couple of pinches of salt and pepper. Mix well, and cook for 10 minutes, stirring occasionally. Add the tomato purée, stout, flour and stock and stir until everything comes together to a simmer. Turn the heat down very low, pop the lid on and let it cook for 1 hour, stirring occasionally. When the hour is up, stir in the pearl barley. Put the lid back on and simmer for another hour, then remove the lid and simmer for a further 30 minutes, or until the meat shreds easily and the gravy is thick. Spoon away any oil from the top, then stir in the mustard and Worcestershire sauce and finely grate in the cheese. Season to taste.

While the stew is ticking away, put the flour, suet and butter into a bowl with a good pinch of salt. Use your thumbs and forefingers to rub the butter into the flour until it resembles cornflake shapes. Lightly stir in 125ml of cold water, then use your hands to gently pat and push it together into a rough dough. Do not overwork it. Wrap the dough in clingfilm and put into the fridge until needed.

Preheat the oven to 180°C/350°F/gas 4. Discard the shin bone and ladle the hot meaty stew into the pie dish (24 x 30cm, and about 4cm deep, is about right). Use some of the beaten egg to eggwash the edges of the pie dish, then dust a clean surface and a rolling pin with flour and roll out the pastry about 1cm thick and a little bit bigger than your pie dish. Carefully place on top of the pie, then trim off any overhanging pastry. Pinch and squash the edges of the pastry to the dish. Eggwash the top, and cook the pie right at the bottom of the hot oven for around 45 to 50 minutes, or until your pastry is golden and gorgeous. Serve with steamed drained greens.

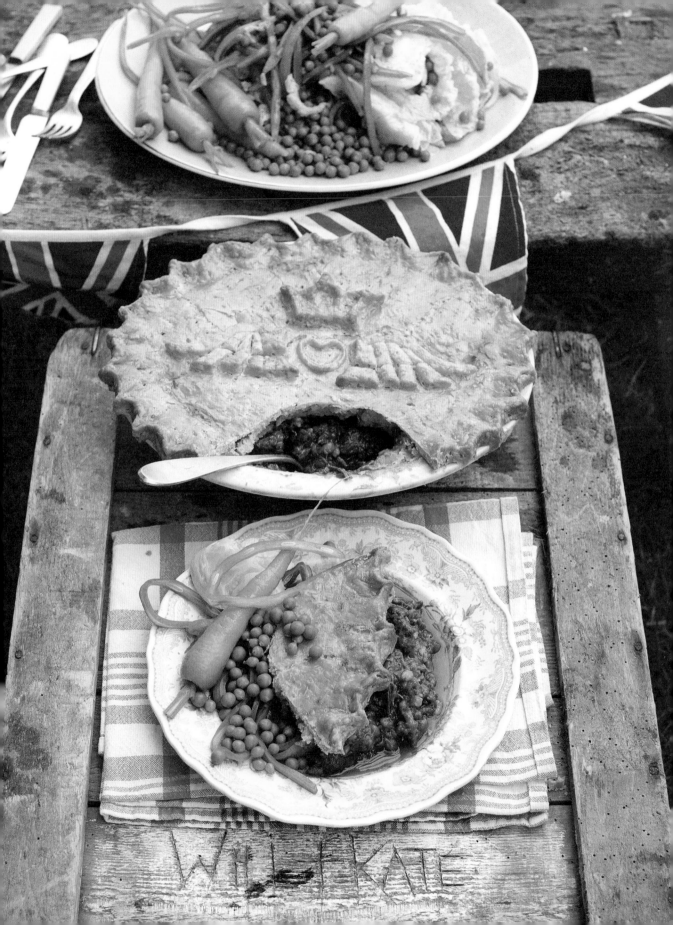

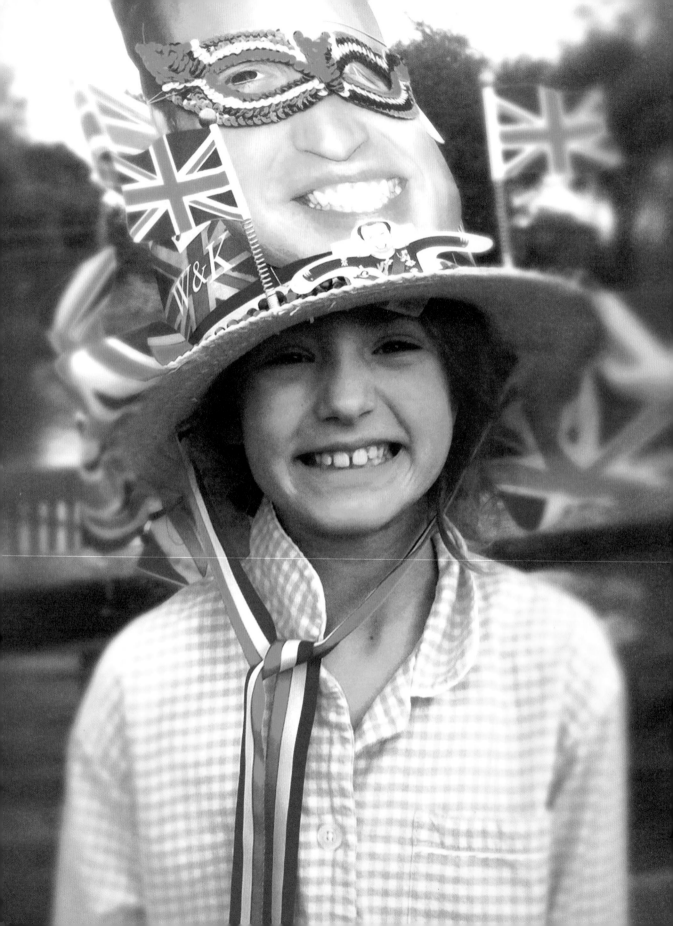

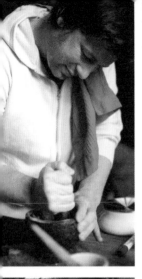

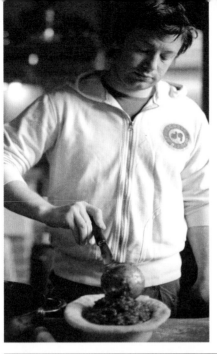

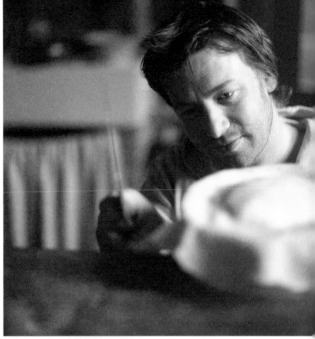

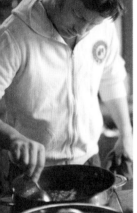

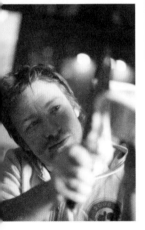

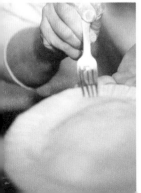

Pie Making

For some reason, whatever you put into a pie gets eaten. You can turn leftover meat or a hearty stew into the most incredible filling, and once that's been topped with beautiful homemade pastry you know the end result will get you massive brownie points with friends and family, not to mention the kids. I get mine involved in making decorations for the pastry lid. If you're anything like my little Daisy, you'll tuck in so fast most of the pie will end up around your mouth and you won't even know it - bless her.

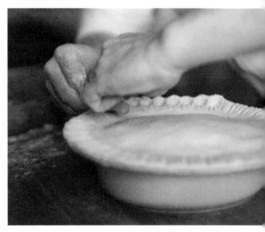

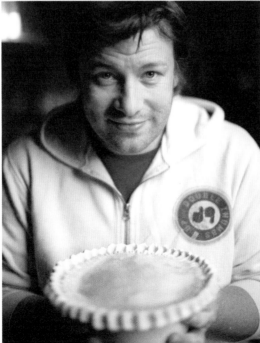

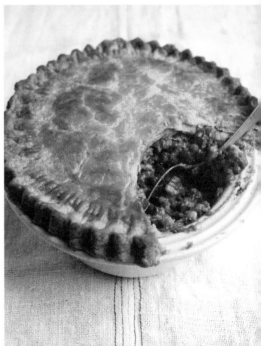

LINCOLNSHIRE POACHER PIE
MINTED COURGETTE STUFFING • ROASTED SHALLOTS

You won't believe how tasty the courgettes get with this method of cooking – it really does take them to another level. You've got to find some Lincolnshire Poacher, it's an amazing cheese made by the very talented Jones brothers, Simon and Tim (see *www.lincolnshirepoachercheese.com*). The pastry is rich and amazing, so embrace the fact that it's really crumbly and will definitely break as you're making it. I'm serving this with a lemony salad and sweet salt-baked shallots, which will get caramelized and gorgeous and pick up the seasoning from the bed of salt. This method is also a great one for beetroots, so if you like this, try that.

SERVES 12

For the pastry
- 500g plain flour, plus extra for dusting
- 250g cold unsalted butter, cubed
- sea salt and white pepper
- 1 large free-range egg, beaten

For the filling
- olive oil
- a bunch of fresh thyme
- 1 whole nutmeg, for grating
- 1 lemon
- 1.5kg courgettes, a mixture of yellow and green if you can get them, finely sliced

- sea salt and ground pepper
- 300g Lincolnshire Poacher cheese
- a small bunch of fresh mint, leaves picked
- 250g rock salt
- 24 shallots
- a few sprigs of fresh thyme

Preheat the oven to 180°C/350°F/gas 4. Blitz the flour and butter in a food processor with a pinch of salt and a few good pinches of pepper until the mixture resembles breadcrumbs. Tip on to a work surface, make a well in the centre and add 100ml of cold water. Gently mix until it starts to come together, then – most importantly for a short, crumbly pastry – have the confidence to only just press, pat and almost hug it together to form a rough scruffy ball. Please don't be tempted to knead the dough or it won't be short and crumbly. Pop it into a floured bowl, cover with clingfilm and put into the fridge to chill while you make the filling.

Put a drizzle of olive oil into a large pan on a medium heat and pick in the leaves from half the bunch of thyme. Add a few gratings of nutmeg, the zest of half the lemon, the sliced courgettes and a good pinch of salt and pepper. Cook gently (the courgettes will cook down and become easier to handle), stirring occasionally, for around 25 minutes. Then turn the heat down to low and cook for another 20 minutes, so the courgette mixture becomes dense and the flavours really intensify and sweeten. Allow to cool a little, finely chop and crumble in the cheese, then chop and add the mint leaves. Set aside.

Halve the pastry and roll each half into a circle just under 1cm thick and slightly larger than the pie dish you've chosen (roughly 23cm diameter x 4cm deep). Don't worry if the pastry breaks up – that's normal. Just patch it. Roll one of the circles around the rolling pin and carefully unroll it over the pie dish. Gently press the pastry into the corners and sides of the dish, then spoon and spread all your courgette mixture into the dish. Carefully unroll the pastry lid over the top, then flour your thumb and forefinger and gently pinch and crimp the edges together. Trim off any excess pastry and brush the top of the pie with the beaten egg.

Now simply throw the rock salt into a roasting tray with the shallots, still with their skins on, and a few thyme tips. Put the pie right at the bottom of the oven, with the tray of shallots above. Cook for 1 hour, or until the pie is golden, then allow to cool and serve with those soft roasted shallots.

PS: All the leftover salt from baking the shallots can be bashed up and reused.

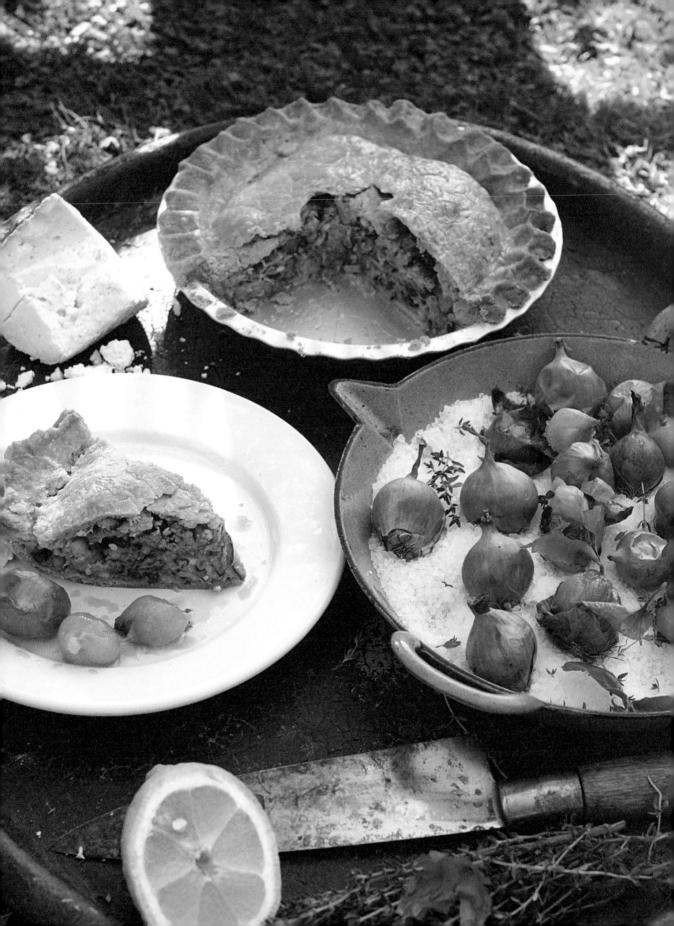

SHEPHERD'S PIE Vs MILKMAN'S PIE

Everyone loves shepherd's pie and this recipe has its heart in exactly the same place, but it's a homage to our long-suffering dairy farmers. Sadly, two are going bankrupt every day in the UK. It's just as tasty and comforting to tuck into, but the inspiration for this dish comes from veal. For many years, no one wanted to buy veal because there were some cruel practices involved in that industry; however, those practices have been out of favour for decades now in the UK and veal is a wonderful meat, light, delicate and so underused. If we ate more of it, it would be an incredible lifeline for our great British dairy farmers, who make a loss when their cows give birth to male calves. I've used butter, a swig or two of cream, a splash of milk, some cheese and Mr Veal to celebrate the best of the British dairy farms. Try it out, and I promise it will become a new family classic. Remember to buy British!

SERVES 6 TO 8

- 2 onions
- 2 carrots
- olive oil
- 50g unsalted butter
- sea salt and white pepper
- 8 sprigs of fresh thyme, leaves picked

- 2 fresh bay leaves
- 450g British veal mince
- 1 heaped tablespoon plain flour
- 1 lemon
- 1 organic chicken stock cube
- ¼ of a tin of John Smith's Bitter (110ml)

- 800g fluffy potatoes, such as Maris Piper
- milk
- 150g button or chestnut mushrooms
- 200ml single cream
- 50g Cheddar cheese

Peel the onions and carrots, cut roughly into 1cm pieces, then gently fry in a large pan with a couple of drizzles of olive oil, a knob of butter, a few good pinches of salt and white pepper, the thyme leaves and bay leaves. Cook on a medium to high heat for about 8 to 10 minutes, stirring often, until the vegetables have softened. Add the veal mince and flour, grate in the lemon zest, and crumble in the stock cube. Keep cooking, stirring and breaking up the mince, until the liquid from the meat starts to evaporate. Once it starts to fry again and takes on a little bit of colour, pour in the bitter and just enough water to cover the mince by 1cm. Bring everything to the boil, then turn down to a low heat and simmer with the lid askew for 1 hour. Keep your eye on it and stir occasionally.

When the mince has been cooking for about 30 minutes, preheat the oven to 180°C/350°F/ gas 4. Peel and quarter the potatoes and cook them in a pan of boiling salted water for 10 to 15 minutes, or until tender and cooked through. Drain, allow to steam for 2 to 3 minutes, season well, then mash with a good splash of milk and a few knobs of butter. Put aside.

At this point, finely slice the mushrooms and add to the mince, then pour in the cream. Season to taste and bring back to the boil for a few minutes, or until the mixture has thickened up a bit. Pour it into an earthenware dish, tin or casserole-type pan (roughly 24 x 24cm) that you're happy to have in the middle of the table. Grate over the Cheddar, then use a fork to dollop and drop a mountain range of mashed potato over the pie so it looks rustic. Or use a fork to squash it down and make squiffs and quiffs. Put the pie into the oven and cook for around 40 minutes, or until golden on top. Serve with some sprouting broccoli, spring greens and fresh peas.

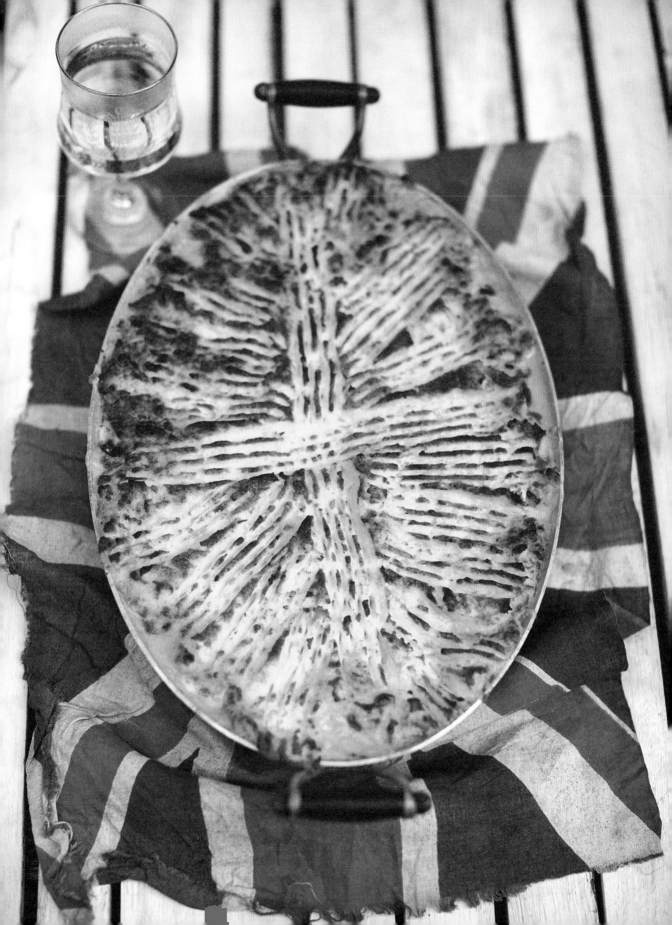

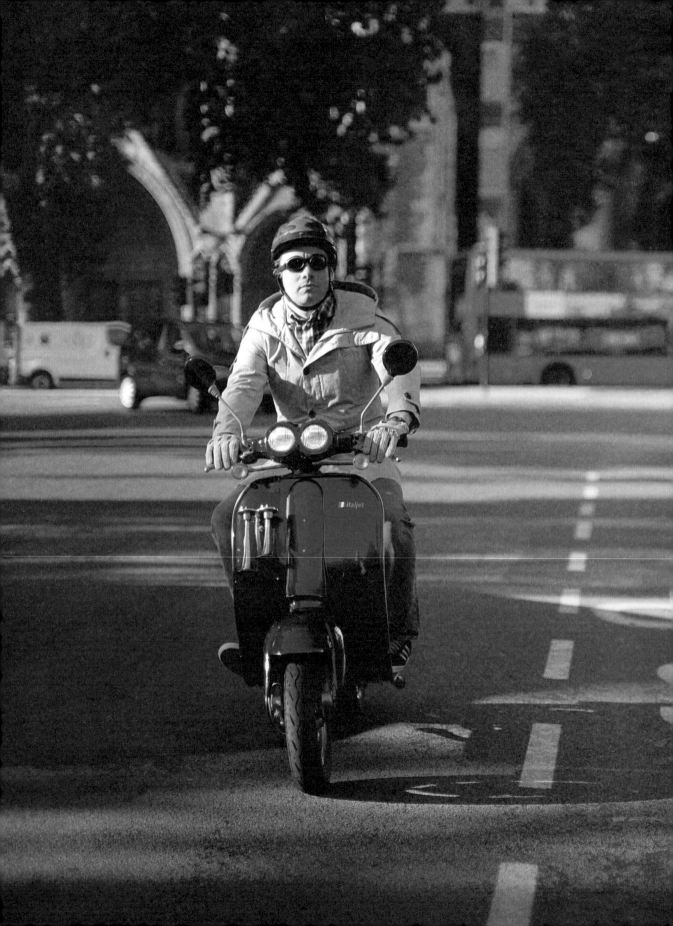

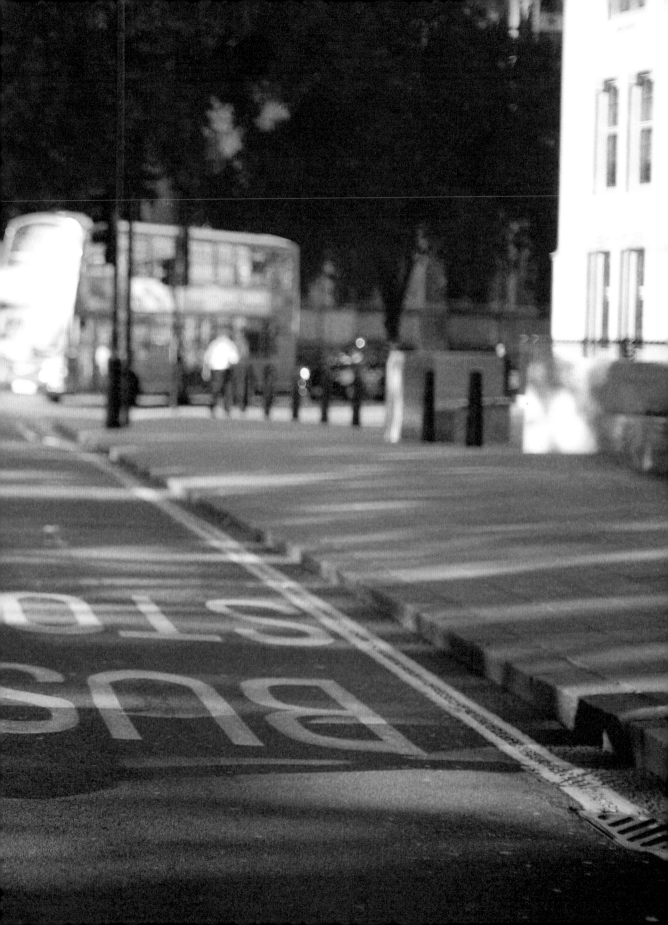

EARLY AUTUMN CORNISH PASTIES

These pasties are guaranteed to put a smile on your face. They're delicious, homely, and light years away from the everyday ones on the high street. The recipe isn't difficult at all, but please make sure you use skirt steak and chop up the meat and veg exactly how I've said, because that is going to create the perfect equation for what happens inside the pastry case and ensure that all the filling ingredients cook at the same time. Feel free to swap out some of my key autumn veg to reflect the season you are in, using peas, broad beans or asparagus in spring and other root veg in the winter. One of these with salad, mustard and beer is pure happiness, just go easy with the rest of the day's meals to balance out that rich pastry.

SERVES 6

For the pastry
- 500g plain flour, plus extra for dusting
- sea salt
- 250g cold unsalted butter
- 1 large free-range egg, beaten

For the filling
- 350g skirt steak
- 1 white onion, peeled
- 1 white potato, peeled
- 1 small courgette
- 1 small carrot, peeled
- 200g butternut squash, cut into 1cm cubes
- 1 whole nutmeg, for grating
- sea salt and white pepper
- a few sprigs of fresh rosemary and thyme, leaves picked
- olive oil

Pour the flour into a bowl, season it with a pinch of salt, then use your thumbs and forefingers to rub in the butter. Add 200ml of water and use your hands to quickly mix it up. As it comes together, squeeze, hug and pat it together crudely and imperfectly. Add a splash more water here if need be, but please don't overwork it.

Preheat the oven to 200°C/400°F/gas 6. Cut the steak and the vegetables into 1cm dice, then put into a bowl, finely grate over a quarter of the nutmeg and add a generous pinch of salt and pepper. Finely chop the rosemary and thyme leaves together and add them to the bowl of filling mixture. Drizzle in a little olive oil, then mix well and put aside.

Cut the pastry into 6 equal pieces and roll each one into a ball. Dust a clean surface and a rolling pin with flour, then pat and push each piece of pastry out to the thickness of a pound coin, dusting and turning as you go. Repeat until you have 6 rounds roughly 22cm in diameter. Get a little filling, compact it in your hand, and place it in the middle of one of the pastry rounds, leaving a border around the edge. Drizzle with a little olive oil, then brush the edges of the pastry with beaten egg and confidently fold the pastry over the meat and vegetables to make a semicircle. Make 5 more pasties the same way and put them on a baking tray dusted with flour.

Pep talk: Look at the picture next door. You can either put the filling right in the middle and bring both sides of the pastry up and together, or you can put it to one side then pull the other half of the pastry over. Once you're done, feel where the filling is and use your thumb to press down and seal it around the edges. You might make a mistake and make a few holes, but you can patch those up and it will still taste nice.

Brush the pasties all over with egg wash and cook in the oven for around 30 to 35 minutes, or until golden and delicious.

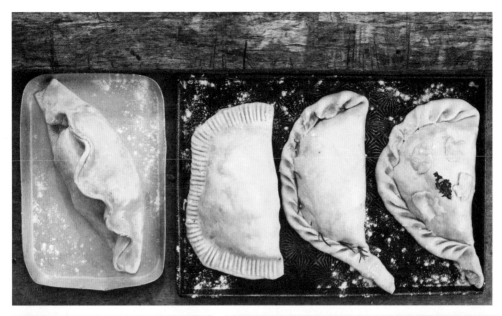

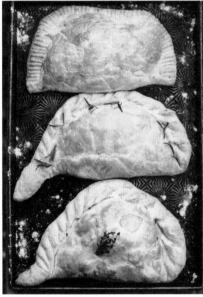

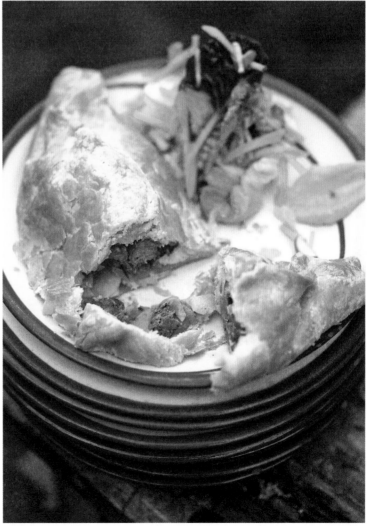

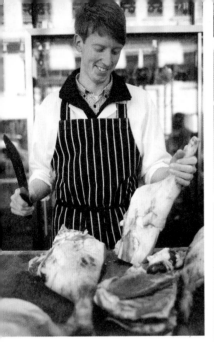
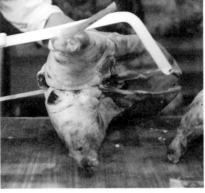
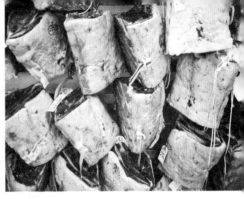
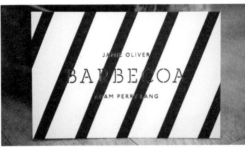
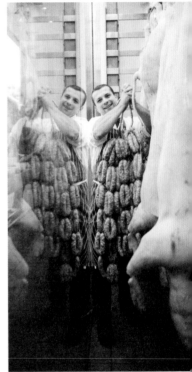

Barbecoa Butcher's Shop

I opened Barbecoa restaurant with my mate, American chef Adam Perry Lang, in 2010. The butcher's shop downstairs really is a sight to behold. It almost looks like a Damien Hirst installation, with its massive see-through fridge of whole cows and ageing ribs of incredible beef. If you're ever near St Paul's Cathedral, come and find us and have a chat to our lovely talented butchers. Look how friendly they look!

www.barbecoa.com

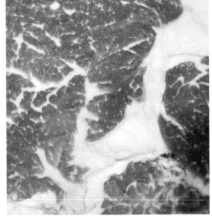
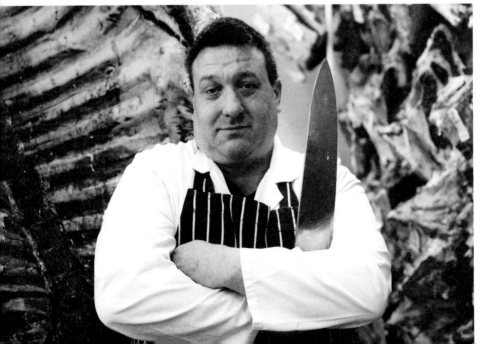
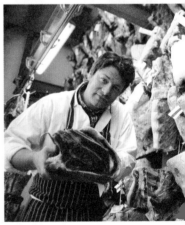
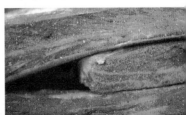

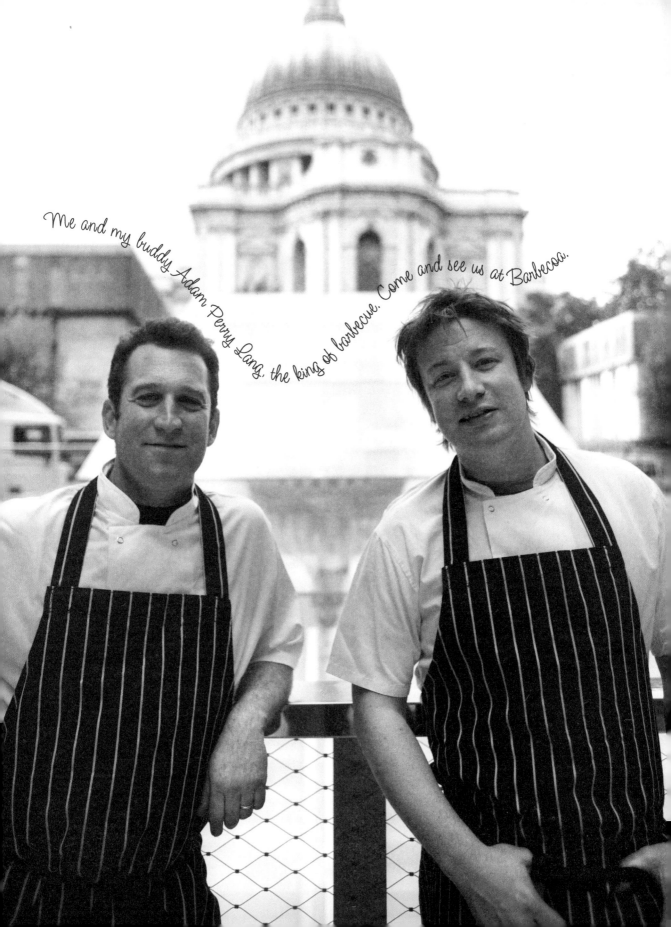

Me and my buddy Adam Perry Lang, the king of barbecue. Come and see us at Barbecoa.

STEAK & KIDNEY PUDDING

SERVES 6

For the filling

- 2 rashers of quality smoked streaky bacon, roughly chopped
- olive oil
- ½ a whole nutmeg, for grating
- 1 heaped teaspoon ground allspice
- 4 fresh bay leaves
- 4 sprigs of fresh rosemary
- 2 onions, peeled and roughly chopped
- 1 tablespoon marmalade
- 2 tablespoons plain flour
- 4 tablespoons Worcestershire sauce
- 750ml organic beef stock
- 2 tablespoons tomato purée
- 500g chuck steak, cut into 2.5cm dice
- a little butter, for greasing
- 250g kidneys, pork or lamb, halved, trimmed and cut into 1cm dice
- 2 carrots, peeled and cut into 1cm dice
- 6 button mushrooms, wiped clean and quartered
- sea salt and ground pepper
- 50g Cheddar or Stilton cheese

For the pastry

- 350g self-raising flour
- 75g unsalted butter
- 100g Atora shredded suet
- sea salt

A steamed meat pudding is so traditional, so comforting and so completely British I just love everything about it. I'm revisiting the classic savoury combo of steak and kidney for this one.

Put a large casserole-type pan on a high heat and add the bacon and a lug of olive oil. When lightly golden, add the nutmeg, allspice, bay, rosemary sprigs and chopped onions, turn the heat to medium and cook for 10 minutes, stirring often. As the onions soften, add the marmalade, plain flour and Worcestershire sauce. Fry and stir until it is quite dark, then add your stock, tomato purée and diced steak. Simmer for 1 hour with the lid on.

Put the self-raising flour, butter, suet and a couple of pinches of salt into a bowl and use your fingers to rub the fat into the flour. Once the mixture resembles breadcrumbs, add roughly 100ml of cold water to bring it together until you have a soft dough. Cover with clingfilm and place in the fridge. When the stew has had an hour, pour it into a large colander over another large pan, so the gravy drips into the pan below. Discard the herb sprigs. Tear off a large sheet of greaseproof paper and rub both sides with butter, then push and flatten it inside a 1.5 litre pudding bowl.

Dust a clean surface with flour and roll out 80% of your dough so it's about 0.5cm thick. Loosely drape it over the rolling pin, then unroll it over the pudding basin. Push and pat it in, letting a couple of centimetres hang over the edge. Gently mix the diced kidneys, carrots and mushrooms into the stew that's in the colander, season with salt and pepper, crumble in the cheese, then pour that dense stew into your pudding basin – don't worry if it doesn't quite fill it. Put the pan of gravy aside. Roll out the last bit of dough, put it on top of the filling, fold over the overhanging pastry to seal and pack it down, then put a sheet of buttered greaseproof face down on top, followed by a piece of tin foil. Get 2 metres of string, wrap it round the rim of the bowl twice, tie it in a double knot twice, then attach the other end to the opposite side with a double knot to make a handle – this will make pulling the bowl out at the end much easier. Go to *www.jamieoliver.com/how-to* for a quick tutorial on this if you like. Put the pudding into a large pan that the pudding basin will fit inside with the lid on, then half fill it with water. Put the lid on, boil, then simmer with the lid on for 3 hours. Set a timer, and top up with water every now and then.

When ready, carefully pull out the basin, cut away and discard the string, greaseproof paper and foil, and place a nice serving platter on top. Carefully and confidently turn over and leave upturned while you warm up the reserved gravy and get any veggies ready. When you're ready to serve, carefully ease the basin off, peel away the paper and pour over a little of the hot gravy. Take to the table with your seasonal veg.

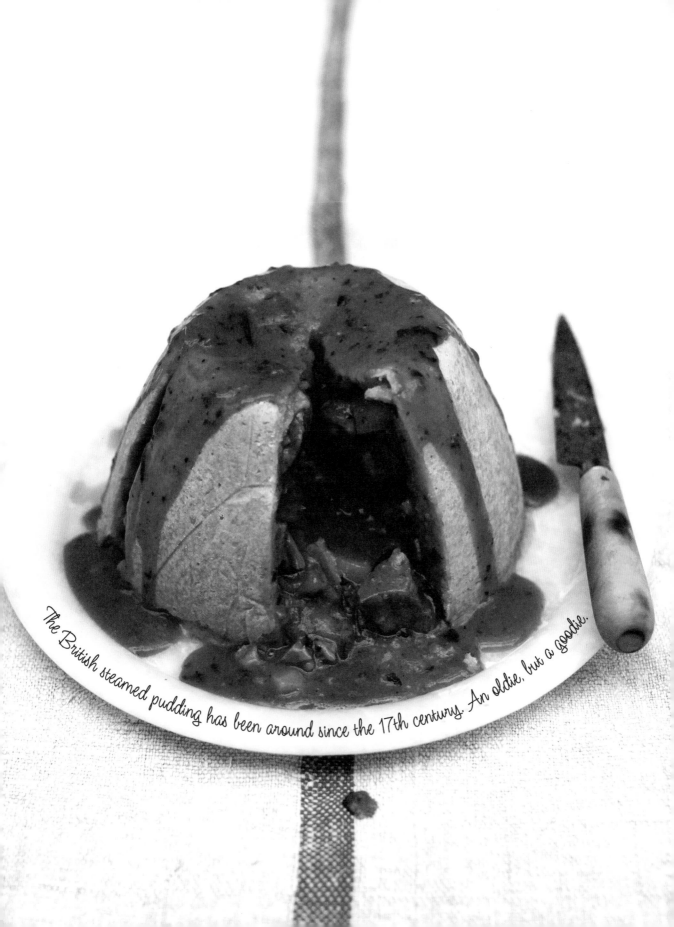

The British steamed pudding has been around since the 17th century. An oldie, but a goodie.

SWEET LEEK & RABBIT PIE
CIDER • CREAM • FLAKY PUFF PASTRY • PEAS • SPINACH

Even fussy eaters who say they don't like rabbit love this pie (my family!). And why not? It's a complete joy to eat (I just tell them it's chicken). Rabbit used to be one of the big meats of Britain before the supermarkets took over, and you can still buy it from good butchers. Farmed rabbits are often sweeter and milder in flavour than wild rabbits, which are usually a bit smaller and stronger, and so sometimes need a bit more cooking time. Ask your butcher to joint the rabbit into eight or ten pieces, and to give you the offal. I'm chopping this up and adding it to the pie – please, please don't omit it because it absolutely makes the flavours. You chop everything up so finely you'll never know it's there, but the end result will be incredible. I've turned this into a pie, but you could simply make the stew and top it with mashed potato, spoon it over a jacket potato, or toss it through pasta for a quick dinner. It's so flexible.

SERVES 8

- 6 rashers of quality smoked streaky bacon
- olive oil
- 4 large leeks, trimmed
- 3 sprigs of fresh rosemary
- 1 rabbit, skinned and jointed into 8-10 pieces (ask your butcher to do this for you), including offal

- 3 heaped tablespoons plain flour, plus extra for dusting
- a knob of butter
- 600ml organic chicken stock
- sea salt and ground pepper
- 500ml good-quality cider
- 200g frozen peas
- 100g baby spinach
- 100ml single cream

- 1 lemon
- 1 x 500g all-butter puff pastry
- 1 large free-range egg, beaten

Heat a large casserole-type pan on a medium heat. Finely slice and fry the bacon with a few lugs of olive oil while you wash the leeks. Finely slice them and add to the pan. Pick in the rosemary leaves. Stir and fry for around 20 minutes. Chop all the offal together until fine and stir it into the pan with the flour, butter, rabbit pieces, stock, a good pinch of salt and the cider, pop the lid on and cook for around 1½ hours on a low heat, or until the meat falls off the bone.

Once ready, put on some clean rubber gloves and pull out the pieces of rabbit, then strip all the meat off the bone and put it back into the sauce. Really use your eyes and fingers to help you get rid of any bones or gnarly bits. Stir in the peas, spinach and cream and simmer for 5 minutes. Correct the seasoning to taste, then add a few gratings of lemon zest.

Preheat the oven to 200°C/400°F/gas 6 and get yourself a deep baking tray or pie dish, roughly 25 x 30cm. If the casserole dish you cooked the stew in is nice, use that. Pour all the stew into the dish, then dust a clean surface and a rolling pin with flour. Roll the puff pastry out so that it's less than 0.5cm thick and large enough to cover the pie dish. Use some of the beaten egg to eggwash the sides of the pastry dish. Roll the pastry loosely over the edges of the pie dish, press down on the edges to seal, and pull off or trim away any excess pastry with a knife. If you're feeling a bit creative, you can roll out any extra pastry, cut it into long strips and sort of crisscross it on the top. Egg wash the top of the pie, then put it into the oven and cook for around 25 to 30 minutes, or until the pastry lid is golden and delicious. Serve with steamed carrots and lovely fresh greens.

PS: To get ahead, make the stew and keep it in the fridge overnight. To cook, top with pastry and cook on the bottom of the oven for around 40 minutes at 180°C/350°F/gas 4.

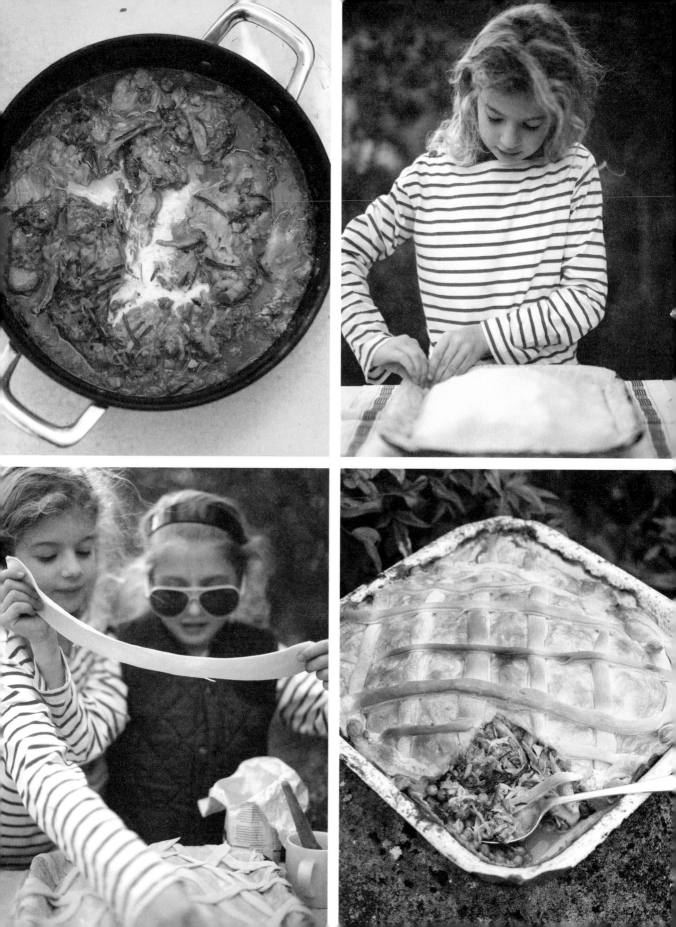

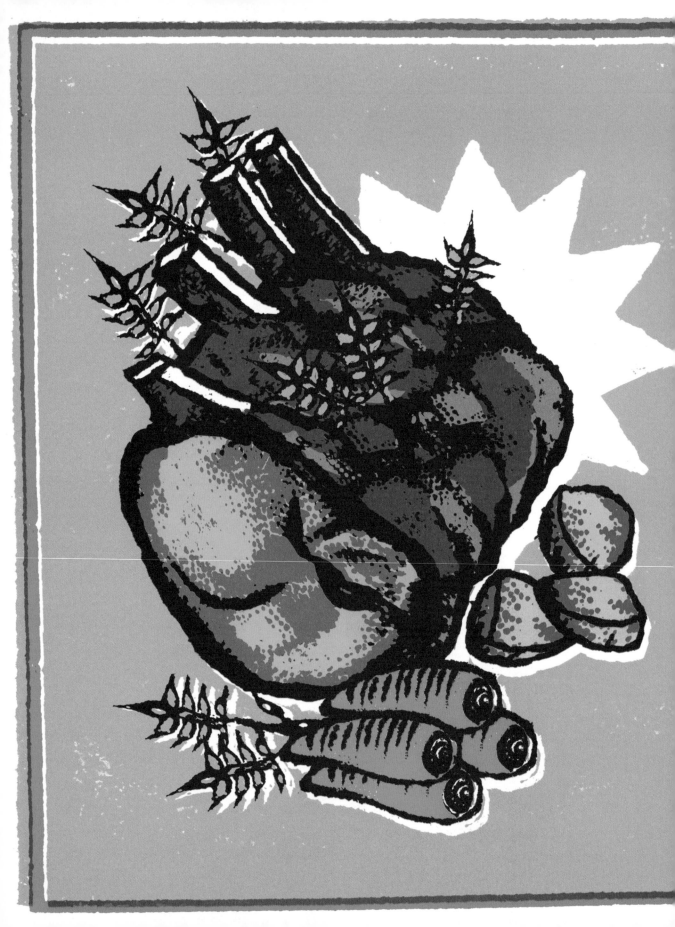

SUNDAY LUNCH

I honestly don't know anybody who doesn't look forward to, and love, Sunday lunch. This wonderful tradition of sitting down with your family for a classic roast dinner (or Sunday lunch) has stuck like glue, regardless of the many changes in our food culture. Because of that, in this chapter what I've tried to do is bend the concept of what a Sunday lunch can be by giving you some of the different options I use in my home. Because of Britain's climate, we've always had access to amazing meat, and there are so many ways to enjoy it – whether it's choosing a different cut of roast beef and slicing it up in a totally new way, butterflying a leg of lamb and cooking it on a barbecue with lobster, or revisiting an old classic, like goose, the recipes I'm giving you here will give you plenty more excuses to sit down with your family and enjoy the end of the week together.

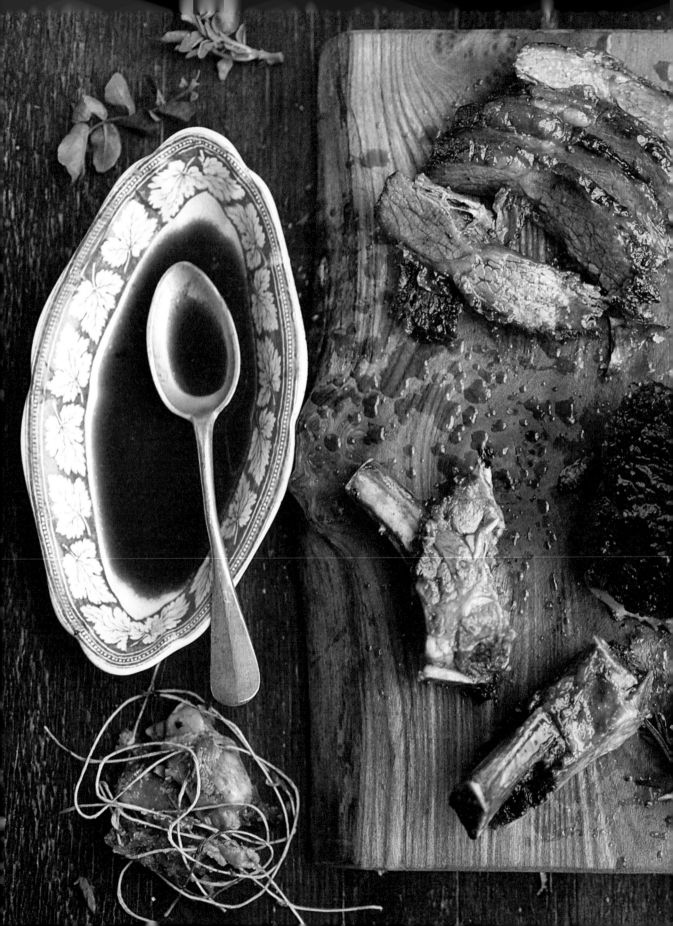

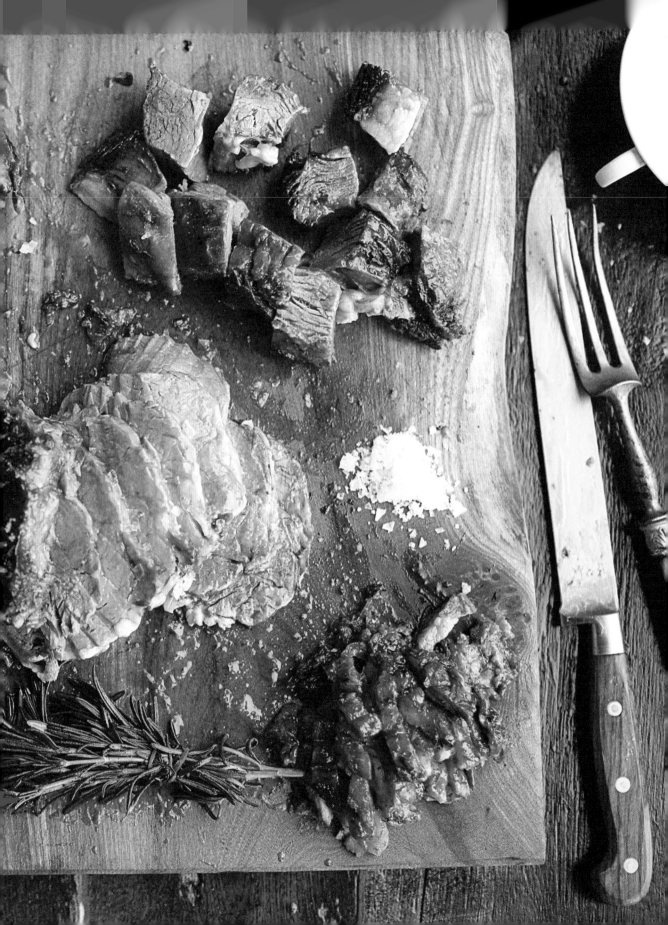

SUNDAY ROAST STEAK

The brilliance of this meal lies in confidently slicing up each element of the forerib in a different way (flick back a page to see what I mean). This encourages people to think about the individual parts of the meat. It's a special alternative to your traditional roast beef dinner.

SERVES 6 (WITH LEFTOVERS)

- 1 x 2.25kg forerib of beef (with 2 bones)
- a bunch of fresh rosemary
- sea salt
- 1 heaped teaspoon white or black peppercorns
- olive oil

- 1.2kg Maris Piper potatoes
- 500g turnips
- 50g butter, at room temperature
- 2 tablespoons runny honey
- 1 whole bulb of garlic, separated into cloves

- 20 fresh bay leaves
- 6 tablespoons red wine vinegar or cider vinegar

To serve
- jarred horseradish
- English mustard

Take the beef out of the fridge 30 minutes before cooking it. Preheat the oven to full whack (240°C/475°F/gas 9) and put your largest, sturdiest roasting tray in it to heat up. Bash the leaves from 2 sprigs of rosemary to a paste with a heaped teaspoon of salt and the peppercorns, then rub this paste all over the beef, with a drizzle of olive oil. Place the beef straight in the hot roasting tray and cook in the oven for 50 minutes (set the timer).

Meanwhile, put a large pan of salted water on to boil. Peel the potatoes and turnips, then halve or quarter them to give you rough 2.5cm chunks. Add them to the water once it's boiling, bring back to a fast boil, then cook with the lid on for 10 minutes. Drain the veg in a colander, toss a few times to chuff them up, then leave them to steam dry.

Once the beef is ready, carefully move it to a plate and put the roasting tray aside. Dot half the butter on top, then use the remaining rosemary sprigs to drizzle and brush the honey all over the meat. Cover with a double layer of tin foil and a tea towel and leave to rest for 30 minutes. Put the rosemary sprigs aside.

Quickly bash the unpeeled cloves of garlic, then add them to the fat in the hot roasting tray with the rest of the butter and the 20 (yes, 20!) bay leaves. Pour in the vinegar and place the tray over a high heat. Add the potatoes and turnips. Keep moving everything around, season well, and when everything is frying away, pop the tray straight back into the hot oven for 30 minutes, or until the veg are crisp and golden. Once cooked, transfer to a serving platter, put in the oven and turn off the heat. When the potatoes and turnips are nearly perfect, carve the beef. Get two boards: one to carve on, one to serve on. Discard any string, then pour the resting juices from the plate into a little heatproof dish and pop it into the oven. Slice and separate the rib bones, then gently pull the two cap bits away from the eye meat. Trim away any wobbly fat. Put the ribs on the serving board. Dice the largest piece of cap meat into roughly 2.5cm cubes. Thickly slice the other cap, toss the meat in any juices. Slice the blushing eye meat thinly and pile it in the middle of the serving board.

Use the rosemary brush from earlier to dab and paint the meat with all the flavourful juices, then serve with the hot crispy platter of vegetables, the little dish of hot resting juices and a lemony watercress salad if you like. This, with a good smear of mustard and horseradish, has to be my ultimate Sunday lunch.

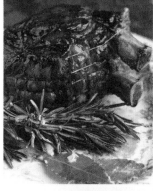

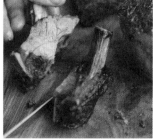

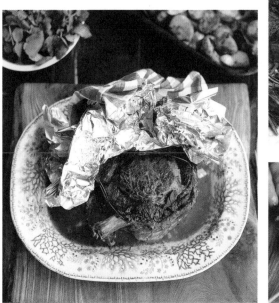

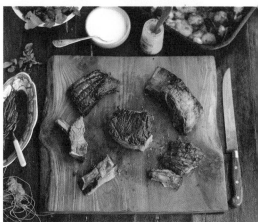

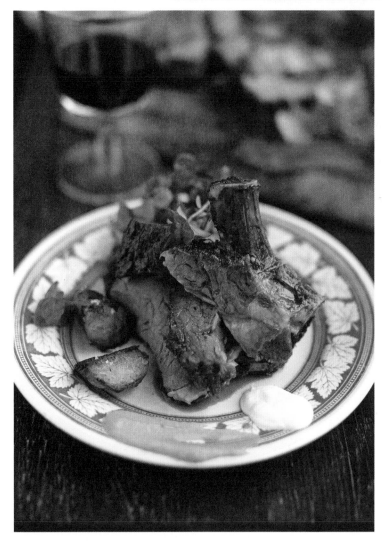

HEARTY OXTAIL STEW
SPINACH DUMPLINGS • CREAMED HORSERADISH

I've got a little feeling in my stomach that tells me a dark black kick-ass soup-stew with beautiful dumplings is where it's at. I'm trying to achieve deep dark gravy and melt-in-the-mouth meat, then contrasting that with these vibrant green spinach dumplings.

SERVES 6 TO 8

For the stew
- 5 tablespoons white caster sugar
- a few cloves
- 500ml good-quality bitter ale
- 2 tablespoons Worcestershire sauce
- 1 x 400g tin of plum tomatoes
- 2kg oxtail
- sea salt and ground pepper

- 2 carrots, peeled and roughly chopped
- 2 celery sticks, trimmed and roughly chopped
- 2 onions, peeled and quartered
- 2 sprigs of fresh rosemary, leaves picked
- 2 fresh bay leaves
- 1 tablespoon creamed jarred horseradish

For the dumplings
- 200g baby spinach
- 1 whole nutmeg, for grating
- 75g unsalted butter
- 500g self-raising flour
- a good pinch of sea salt
- 1 heaped teaspoon mustard powder
- ½ teaspoon bicarbonate of soda

Put your largest, widest pan on a medium heat and add the sugar and cloves. Cook for a few minutes until the sugar starts to caramelize and go dark golden, then add the ale, Worcestershire sauce and tinned tomatoes. Bring to the boil, then plop in the pieces of oxtail. Give the pan a jiggle and season generously. Put the carrots, celery, onions and a good pinch of salt and pepper into the food processor with the rosemary and bay leaves and pulse until finely chopped. Tip the vegetables into the pan, stir, then cover tightly with a lid or a double layer of tin foil. Turn the heat down to low and leave to simmer slowly for about 4 to 5 hours, or until the meat can easily be pulled away from the bone. Stir occasionally during this time, and add a splash of water if needed.

Pile all the spinach into the clean food processor and pulse until finely chopped. Grate in half the nutmeg, then add the rest of the dumpling ingredients and pulse again until you have fine crumbs. Add around 100 to 150ml of cold water, until everything comes together and you have a sort of firm dough. Dust a clean surface with flour and roll the dough into a long sausage. Clank it up into small dumplings (you should end up with around 30 small ones, which I think are a bit more delicate than the big ones I've done in the pic), roll them into rough balls and leave covered with a damp towel while your stew ticks away.

Once the meat on your oxtail pulls apart really easily, you have a choice: do you want to go old school and serve the meat on the bone? Or, do you want to spend a few minutes shredding the meat off? It's totally up to you. Once the meat is back in the pan, add a splash of water and stir in 1 tablespoon of horseradish sauce before plopping in the dumplings. Put the lid or foil back on the pan and cook for 25 to 30 minutes, until the dumplings have plumped up and are nice and fluffy inside (break one open to test if you like). Serve with a few spoonfuls of jarred horseradish. Delicious.

PS: Cooking this dish over the hob steams the dumplings, but if you want them to be soft and fluffy underneath and crisp and golden on top, feel free to drop in the dumplings, then put the pot (uncovered) into a hot oven at 180°C/350°F/gas 4 for the same amount of time.

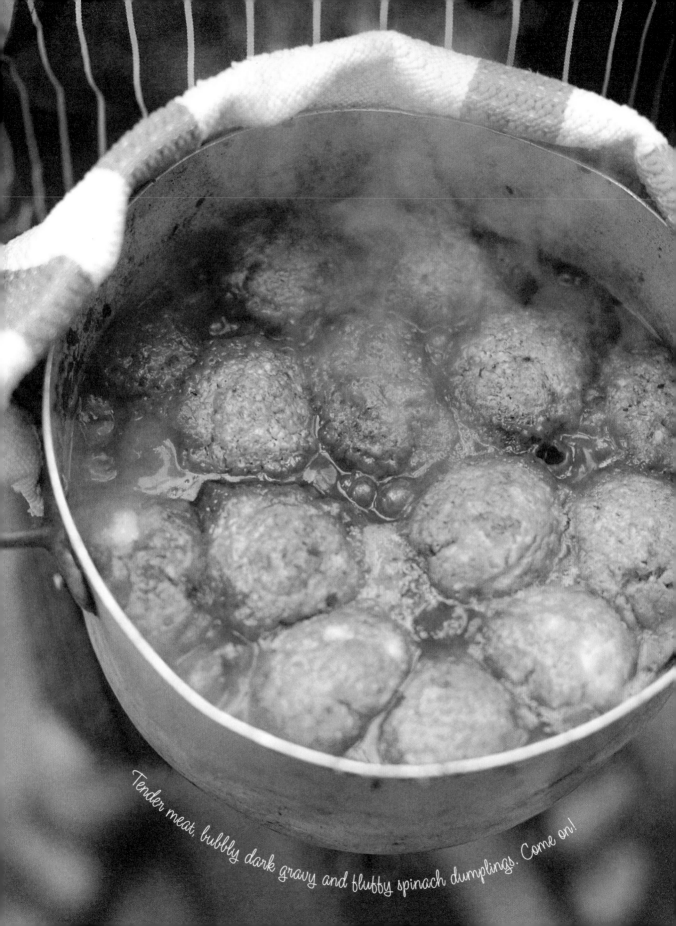

Tender meat, bubbly dark gravy and fluffy spinach dumplings. Come on!

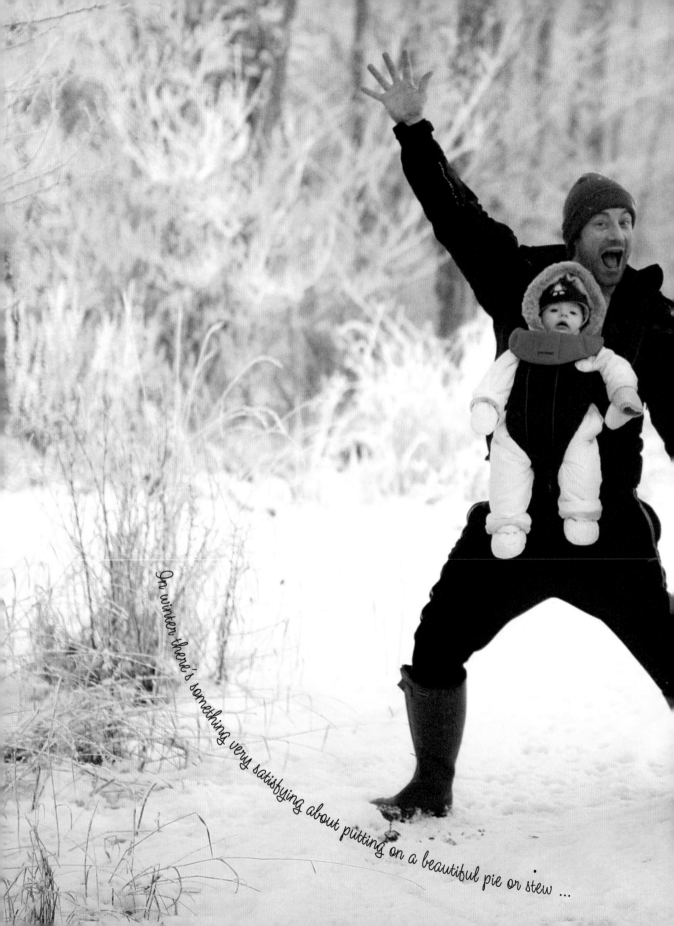

In winter there's something very satisfying about putting on a beautiful pie or stew ...

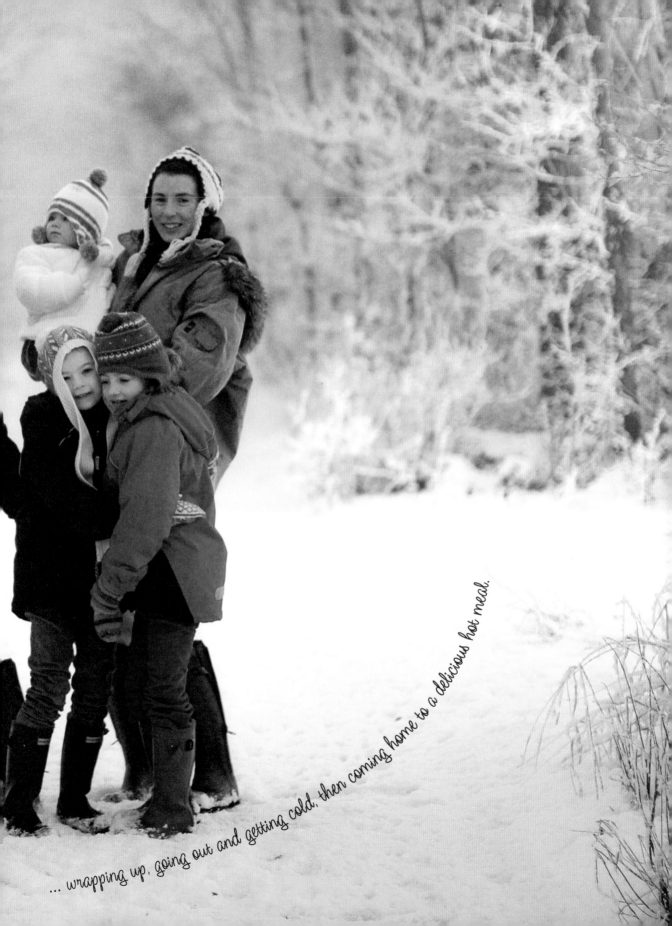

... wrapping up, going out and getting cold, then coming home to a delicious hot meal.

INCREDIBLE ROAST GOOSE

Goose was, traditionally, the most highly respected bird for important family occasions. But when turkeys started arriving from America, the poor old goose was quickly shoved out of the mainstream market because it couldn't ever be intensively farmed the way turkeys could. And because of that, it couldn't compete from a price point of view either. But it is beautiful to eat, and this way of cooking allows you to eat it whenever you like. It will sit happily in its baking tray in the fridge for a few days; so long as it's completely submerged in its own fat, the fat will act as a natural seal, trapping in flavour and moisture. When you're ready to reheat, simply roast it in a hot oven for thirty minutes, or until it's piping hot and crispy again. The fat left behind can be spooned into a Kilner jar and kept in the fridge. Just a little bit of this fat, added to a tray of potatoes or other root veg, will give you the most mind-blowing crispy veg.

SERVES 8 TO 10

- 6 large cinnamon sticks
- 6 star anise
- 2 teaspoons cloves
- a thumb-sized piece of fresh ginger, peeled and finely sliced
- sea salt and ground pepper
- 1 large free-range goose (roughly 4-5kg), halved lengthways by your butcher
- 2 oranges, sliced
- red wine vinegar

Preheat your oven to full whack (about 240°C/475°F/gas 9) and clear a space in the fridge large enough for your biggest roasting tray. Bash 3 cinnamon sticks, 3 star anise, 1 teaspoon of cloves and the sliced ginger in a pestle and mortar along with a good pinch of salt and pepper, and rub these flavours into the skin of the goose halves. Put both skin side up, into a very large deep-sided roasting tray, along with the remaining cinnamon sticks, star anise and cloves. Put the tray into the oven and immediately turn the temperature down to 160°C/325°F/gas 3. Cook for 3½ to 4 hours (depending on the size of your goose), basting carefully once or twice. After the goose has been in for around 2 hours, add the orange slices.

Once the goose is cooked the leg meat should fall off the bone easily, so take it out of the oven and spoon all the spice-infused fat over the top so it's really well coated. This is important. Allow to cool then smear the thickened fat all over. Cover the roasting tray with clingfilm and pop it into the fridge, where it will sit happily for 2 to 3 days as long as all the meat is really well covered with the solidified fat.

When you're ready to serve the goose, preheat your oven to 190°C/375°F/gas 5. Remove the goose to a board, then spoon nearly all the fat left behind in the roasting tray into a clean jar and keep sealed in the fridge to use when you make roast veg. Place the goose back in the roasting tray, skin side up, to reheat and crisp up in the oven – this should take about 30 minutes. Once cooked, take the goose out of the oven and put it back on the board again. Shred the crispy leg meat and slice the breast meat so everyone gets a bit of everything. Add a good swig of red wine vinegar to the roasting tray and mix with the melted fat left behind, making sure you scrape up all the gnarly goodness from the bottom of the pan. Toss the meat in this mixture to really bring all those gorgeous flavours to life. This is absolutely delicious as part of a roast dinner, but also rockin' in a salad, or even in iceberg lettuce wraps. Enjoy.

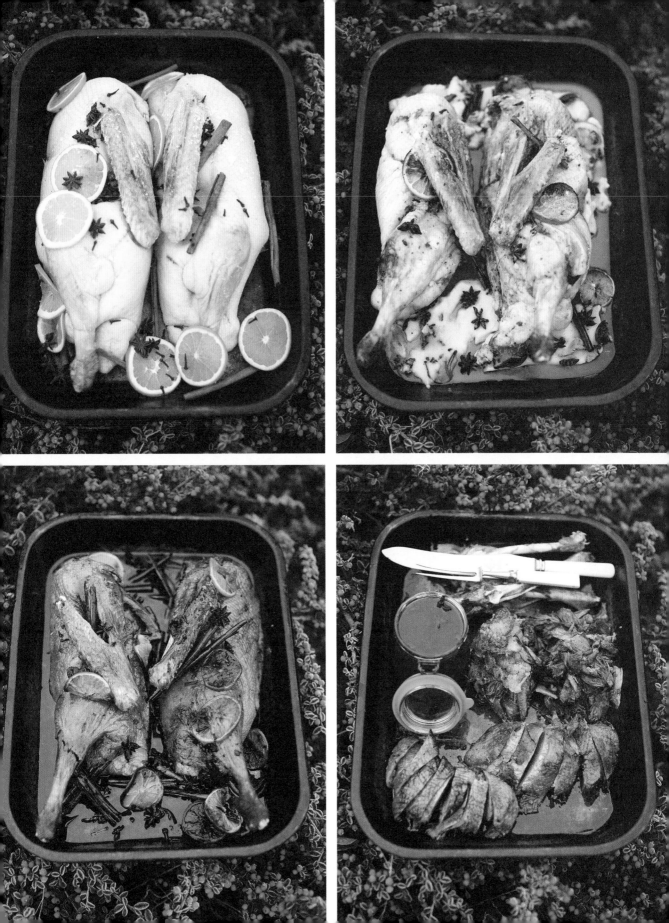

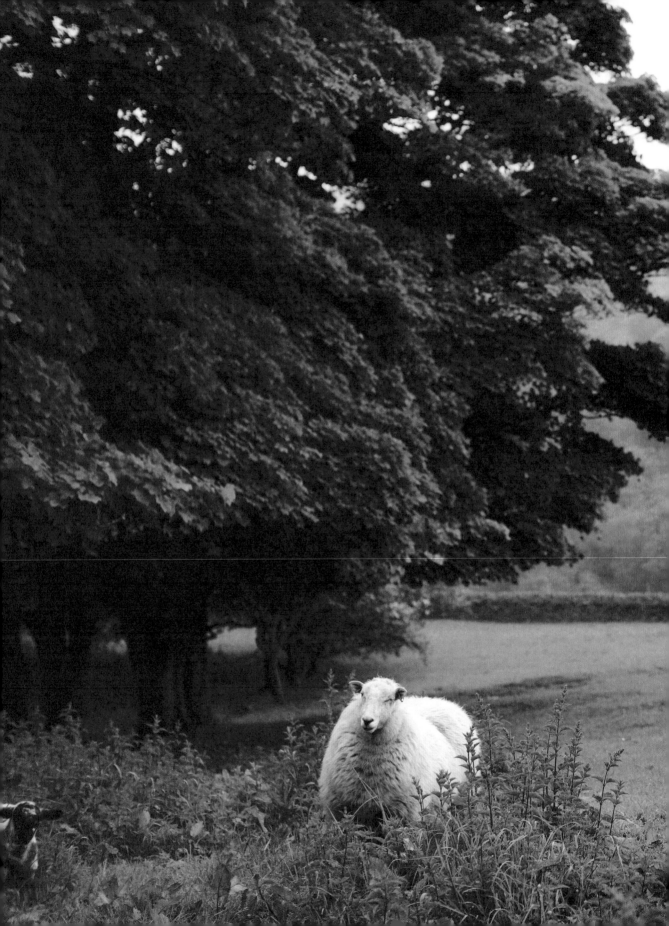

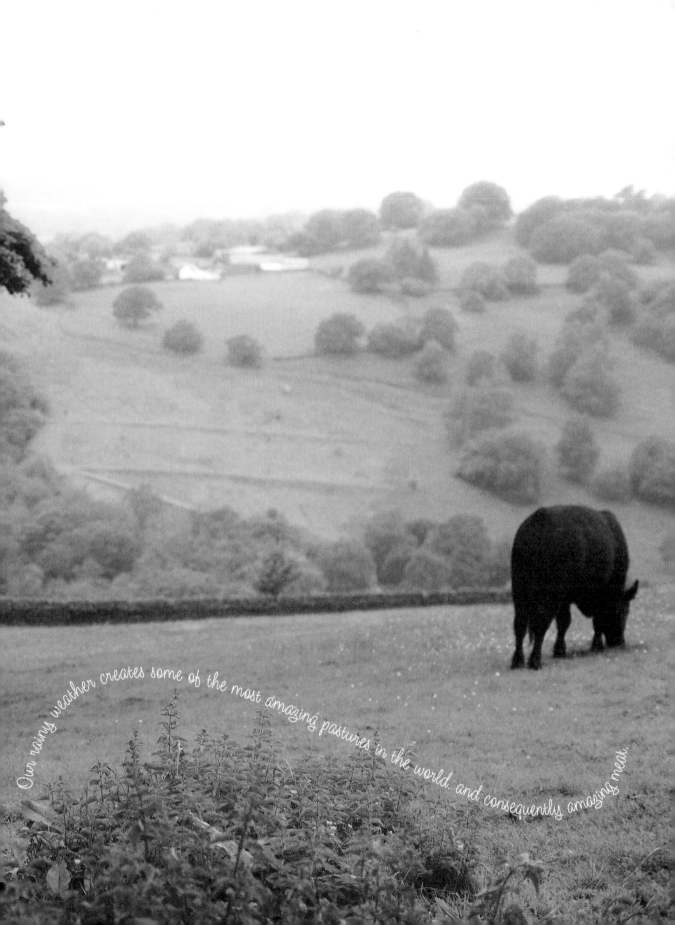

Our rainy weather creates some of the most amazing pastures in the world, and consequently amazing meat.

GUINNESS LAMB SHANKS
STICKY DARK GRAVY • FRESH MINT DRESSING

People absolutely love lamb shanks. You cook them until they're just falling apart and they develop the most amazing flavours. This recipe is all about investing in dark sticky sauce and tender meat. We're spoiled for choice when it comes to interesting ales, and adding a good dark ale or even Guinness to the onions creates the most brilliant depth of flavour. The sauce here makes enough for ten lamb shanks, so if you want to make this recipe serve more people, just plop a few more shanks into the pan and top up with a little more stock if need be. Whatever you do, do NOT skip the mint oil or spring onions. It's like switching on a light, and just that simple little touch makes the whole dish sing.

SERVES 6

- 3 red onions, peeled
- olive oil
- sea salt and ground pepper
- 2 handfuls of raisins
- 3 heaped tablespoons thick-cut marmalade
- 1 heaped tablespoon tomato ketchup

- 2 tablespoons Worcestershire sauce, plus extra for serving
- 200ml Guinness or smooth dark ale
- 6 lamb shanks, roughly 350g each
- 8 sprigs of fresh rosemary
- 1 litre organic chicken stock

To serve
- potato and celeriac mash (see page 334)
- a small bunch of fresh mint leaves
- a few tablespoons rapeseed or olive oil
- 2 spring onions, trimmed
- cider vinegar

Finely chop the onions and put them into a really large casserole-type pan (roughly 26cm in diameter and 12cm deep), with a lug of olive oil and a good pinch of salt and pepper. Cook over a medium to high heat, stirring as you go, until the onions start to caramelize. Add the raisins and marmalade, then add the ketchup, Worcestershire sauce and booze. Give it all a good stir, then leave to gently simmer.

Put the lamb shanks into a large frying pan (roughly 30cm wide) on a medium to high heat with a drizzle of olive oil – you can cook them in batches if needed. Turn them every few minutes; once they have some good colour, pick in the rosemary leaves and move them around in the pan to get crispy, but don't let them burn. Use tongs to move the shanks into the pan of onions, then pour in all their juices and the crispy rosemary. Add the stock, put the lid on, turn down the heat and leave to blip away slowly for around 3 hours, or until the meat falls off the bone easily. Try to turn the shanks halfway through so they cook evenly. About 30 minutes before the lamb is cooked, make the potato and celeriac mash from page 334.

When the lamb shanks are ready, carefully move them to a plate, making sure the meat stays intact. Whiz or liquidize the gravy with a stick blender until smooth, then allow to reduce down and thicken. Quickly bash most of the mint leaves in a pestle and mortar with a good pinch of salt and the olive or rapeseed oil, then take to the table. Finely slice up the spring onions and toss on a plate with the remaining fresh mint leaves, a drizzle of cider vinegar and a pinch of salt.

By now the celeriac mash should be ready, so put it on a platter and put the lamb shanks on top (again, be gentle, so they don't fall apart). Add a little splash of cider vinegar and a few more splashes of Worcestershire sauce to the sauce, then ladle it all over the platter and pour the rest into a jug for people to help themselves. Scatter the vinegary spring onions and a few fresh mint leaves all over the top, drizzle the mint oil all around the shanks, and serve. The plate will be clean before you know it.

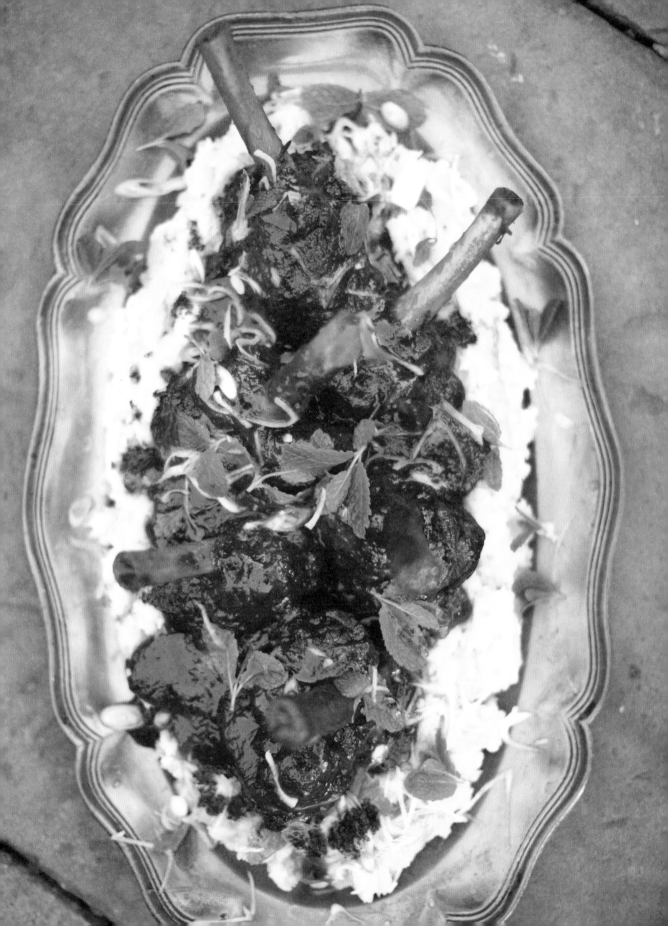

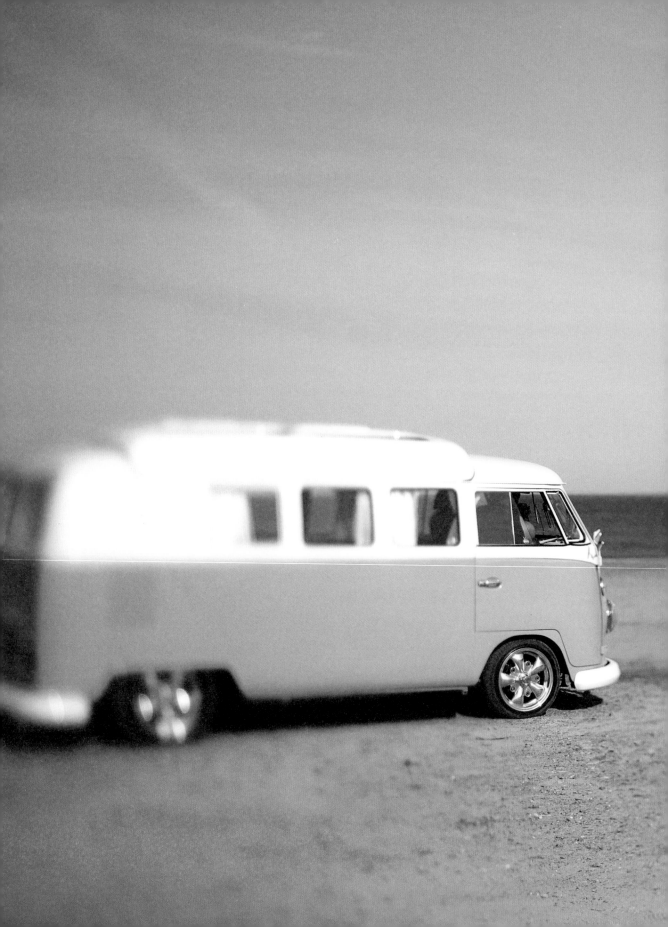

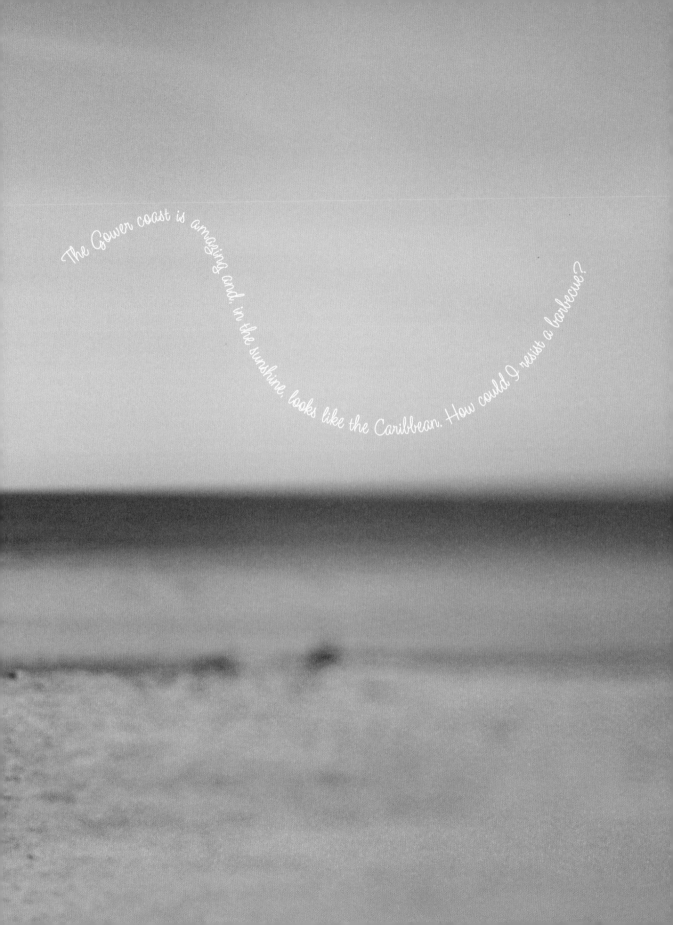

The Gower coast is amazing and, in the sunshine, looks like the Caribbean. How could I resist a barbecue?

WELSH SURF & TURF
BBQ BUTTERFLIED LAMB • POACHED LOBSTER

SERVES 10

For the surf
- sea salt
- a small bunch of fresh dill
- a small bunch of fresh
  flat-leaf parsley
- 1 fresh red chilli
- 1 tablespoon peppercorns
- 3 lemons
- 5 x 1kg live lobsters
- 125g butter

For the turf
- a small bunch of fresh
  rosemary, leaves picked
- 4 cloves of garlic, peeled
- sea salt and ground pepper
- olive oil
- red wine vinegar
- 1 butterflied leg of lamb
  (ask your butcher to do
  this for you)
- a few knobs of butter
- a large handful of fresh
  mint leaves
- 1 fresh red chilli
- extra virgin olive oil

Lamb and lobster go beautifully with fresh summery salads like the ones on page 90, and if you can marinate the lamb the night before to maximize the flavours – even better! To cook the lobsters efficiently, you'll need a 20-litre stockpot – either borrow one or buy one. You can get them on the internet for £24, and it's well worth investing in.

For the Surf
Fill your stockpot three-quarters of the way up with water and season it with enough salt to make it taste like seawater. Bring it to a hard fast boil, then throw in the herbs, chilli and peppercorns. Squeeze in the juice of 2 of the lemons, then chuck in the squeezed halves. At this point, you can kill your lobsters manually with a skewer through the little cross on the back of their head, but to be honest, if you aren't totally confident, you might get it wrong, so I say simply throw them into the fast-boiling water and pop the lid on (leave the elastic bands on the claws). After 5 minutes, turn the heat off and leave them. They'll be beautifully cooked and flavoured in 15 minutes, but will stay hot and lovely for up to 40 minutes. This is by far the most forgiving and efficient way I've ever found of cooking lobster.

Before serving the lobsters, pop a bowl that will float into the stockpot. Put the butter, a pinch of salt and a good squeeze of lemon juice into the bowl and just leave it to melt. As guests come up with their plates, split the lobsters carefully and sensibly down the middle so you have two long halves (there's a video on *www.jamieoliver.com/how-to* that will teach you how to do this). Discard the stomach sac and the digestive vein, then crack the claws open with the heel of a knife. Quickly dip a pastry brush in the melted bowl of butter and paint it all over the lobster meat before serving each person one half.

For the Turf (best marinated overnight, or a few hours before cooking)
Bash the rosemary leaves, garlic and a good pinch of salt and pepper to a paste in a pestle and mortar, then add about 4 tablespoons of olive oil and a little swig of vinegar. Rub this paste all over the butterflied leg of lamb (your butcher will do the butterflying for you, but if you want to learn a new skill, go to *www.jamieoliver.com/how-to*.

Once your meat's marinated, get your barbecue going. Put the lamb on the hot barbecue and cook for around 15 minutes. Turn it over every minute and rub with a little butter as it cooks to help it build up colour. You want it to cook as easily as possible, so score the meat to help the heat penetrate if you need to. If you don't have a barbecue, you can cook the lamb on a very large (at least 25 x 30cm) and screaming hot griddle pan, turning every minute or so for 35 minutes.

Dressing the Board (for the juiciest, most incredible meat)
When your meat is looking close to perfect, finely chop the mint and chilli on your largest serving board. Drizzle over a few lugs of extra virgin olive oil and vinegar, then mix everything on the board. Wipe the meat in the dressing to protect and flavour it. Get a mate on lobster duty, splitting them up and painting them with butter, while you slice up long 1cm-thick slices of lamb. Toss the slices in all the juices on the board before dividing between the plates.

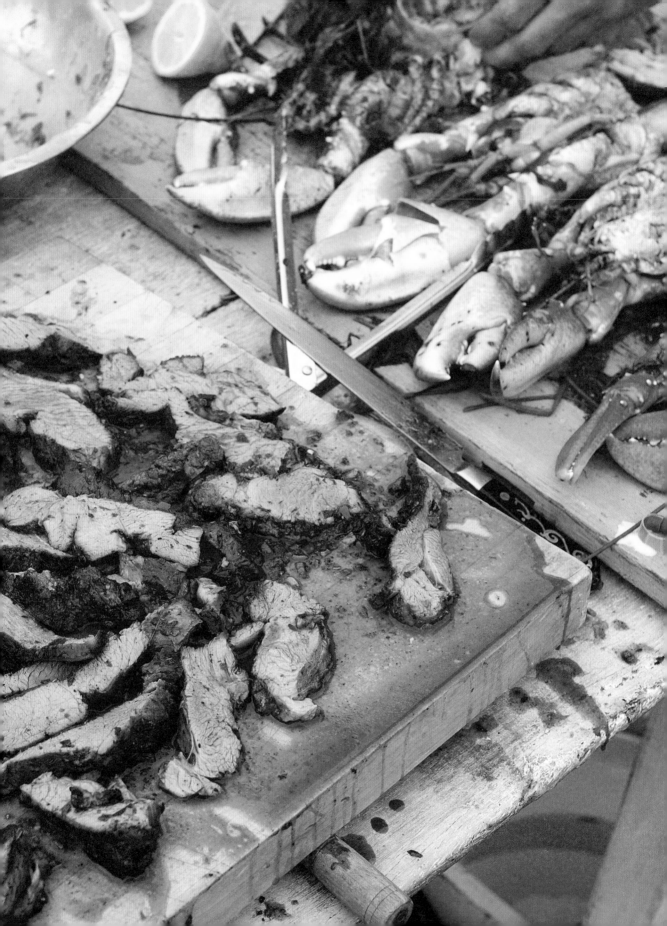

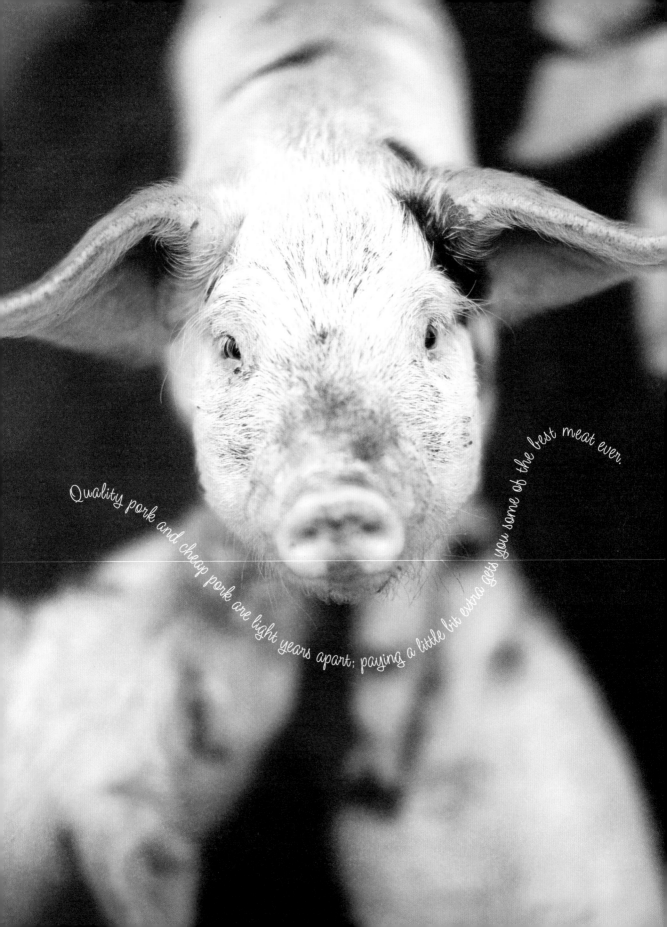

Quality pork and cheap pork are light years apart; paying a little bit extra gets you some of the best meat ever.

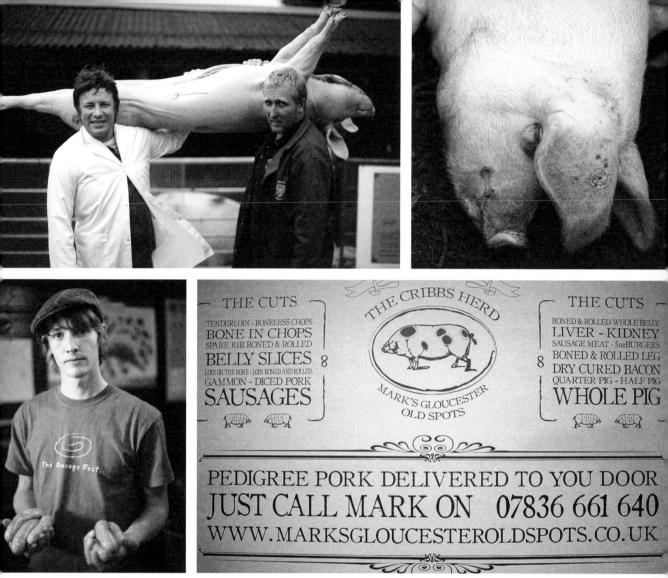

The Cribbs Herd

While in Bristol, I met a farmer called Mark Hook. He breeds Gloucester Old Spot pigs and raises them with care and respect. His pigs are a great example of inner-city, outdoor-reared pork.
www.marksgloucesteroldspots.co.uk

I also met a lad called Ryan Coghlan, who makes award-winning bangers with his company, The Sausage Fest. They use old methods and interesting ingredients to produce lovely sausages to sell at festivals.
www.thesausagefest.co.uk

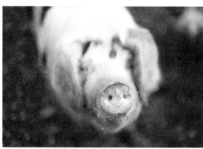

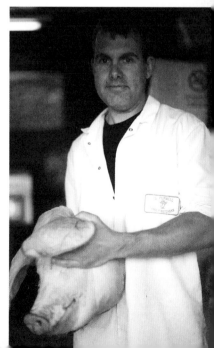

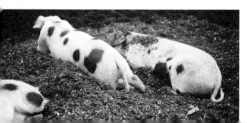

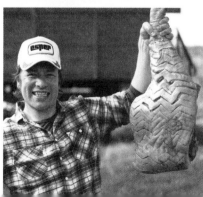

SUPERB PORK LOIN
... BOLDLY COOKED WITH BAY & VINEGAR

This is an epic pork dish that everyone should try. It requires you to have complete faith in me, and in using the bold quantities of bay and vinegar that are required to make the dish work. As it cooks, the vinegar reduces down and you have a balanced, but intense and perfumed, roasted joint. It's nice to cook this much meat, even if there are only four of you eating, because then you'll have lovely meat for epic salads and sandwiches in the week to come.

SERVES 10

- 1 x 2kg piece of boneless free-range pork loin, skin on
- olive oil
- 2 teaspoons sea salt
- 2 teaspoons ground pepper
- 2 teaspoons fennel seeds
- 1 whole nutmeg, for grating
- 20 fresh bay leaves
- 2 red onions, peeled and roughly chopped
- 250ml good-quality cider vinegar

Preheat the oven to full whack (about 240°C/475°F/gas 9). Score the skin side of the pork all over in a criss cross fashion, about 2cm apart and 1cm deep. Drizzle over a little olive oil, then rub in the salt, pepper and fennel seeds and finely grate over half the nutmeg.

Put a snug-fitting roasting tray on a high heat and add a few lugs of olive oil. You need a snug-fitting tray, otherwise the liquid you add will evaporate too quickly and the onions will burn. Put the pork into the tray, skin side down. Leave to cook and crisp up for 4 minutes to get the crackling started, then use tongs to hold the pork up while you add the bay leaves and chopped onions to the tray. Flip the pork over so it's skin side up and drizzle over all the vinegar. Put the tray into the oven, then immediately turn the heat down to 200°C/400°F/gas 6 and cook for 1 hour and 20 minutes. During that time, baste the meat two or three times. Try to maintain a little moisture in the tray and if the vinegar has evaporated, add a splash of water.

This is your opportunity to make something to enjoy with the pork. Ultimately anything white and starchy is going to work well, whether that's a great mashed potato (see page 334), rice, polenta, cheese risotto, butter beans or cannellini beans. Add a green salad or simply steamed greens, and you'll be laughing.

When the pork is ready, use a knife to carefully prise off the crackling. If it's a quality fattier pig, you can pop the crackling into a clean tray and put it back into the oven for 5 to 10 minutes to let the underside crisp up, but don't let it burn. Set a timer. Move the meat to a carving board. Carefully pour any excess fat (not the delicious juices) from the tray into a jam jar and save it for another day. Discard the bay leaves. Put the tray of juices back on the heat, add 250ml of water and bring to the boil, then turn down and simmer until it reduces, making sure you get all the sticky goodness off the bottom. Use a sharp carving knife to slice the pork as thinly as possible, using the whole length of the knife and a long carving action. Pick up the slices and fan them out on a platter. Pour little spoonfuls of juice all over and put it in the middle of the table. Cut or snap up the crackling and place that around the platter as well. I love the idea of people helping themselves to crackling, meat and drizzly juices.

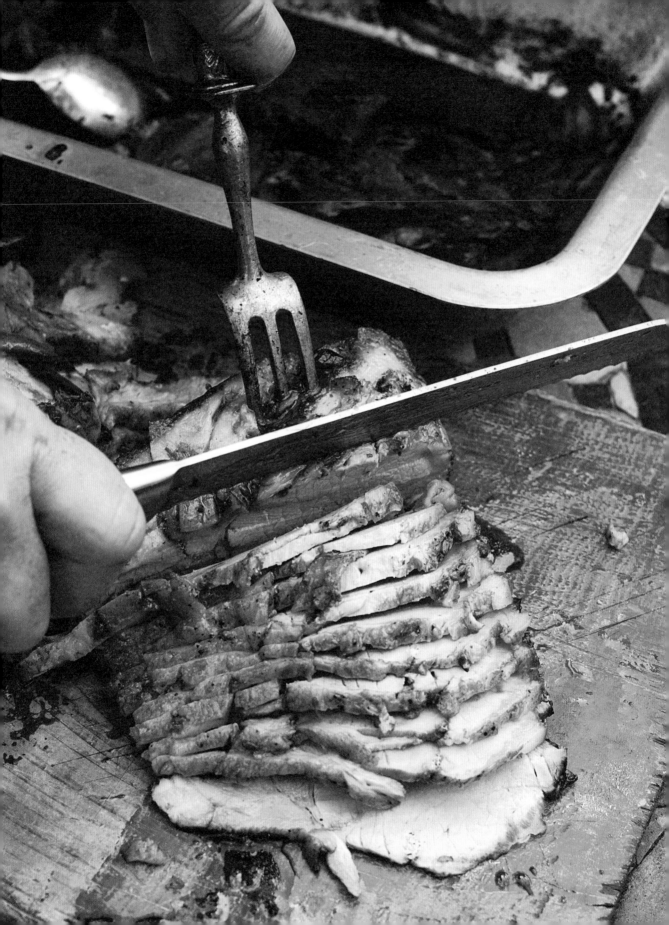

CRACKLED PORK BELLY
... WITH MASH & SWEET ONION SCRUMPY SAUCE

This dish is so simple, and a total pleasure to make. It gives you tender melt-in-the-mouth meat, crispy crackling and outrageous cider cream sauce. If you get your hands on decent British scrumpy (strong, traditionally made cider) and a free-range pig (which is easily done these days), you're laughing. Great served with mashed potato and any nice seasonal greens for a truly memorable dinner.

SERVES 8 TO 10

- a small handful of fresh sage
- 1 tablespoon white pepper
- sea salt
- olive oil
- 4 white onions, peeled

- 2kg free-range pork belly
- 1 x 500ml bottle of good-quality scrumpy
- 2 heaped teaspoons wholegrain mustard

- 100ml single cream
- *optional:* 2 heaped tablespoons light soft brown sugar

Preheat the oven to 160°C/325°F/gas 3. Pick the sage leaves, then pound them in a pestle and mortar with the pepper and a couple of good pinches of salt until you have a green paste (you can use a liquidizer if you like). Loosen with a couple of lugs of olive oil and stir.

Cut the onions into 1cm thick slices. Spread the slices around the base of a snug-fitting roasting tray. Score the skin side of the pork belly every 2cm, then pour over the sage oil and rub it all over the skin with your hands. Place the pork on top of the onions, skin side up. Sprinkle with a pinch of salt and pepper and pour just over half the scrumpy into the tray. Cover with a double layer of tin foil and cook in the hot oven for 3½ hours, or until the meat starts to pull apart easily. Check on the pork half way through cooking and add more scrumpy if needed.

Take the pork out of the oven and turn your grill on to full whack. Transfer the pork to a separate snug-fitting tray, place on the middle shelf under the grill, and crackle your crackling until gorgeous-looking and golden. This really depends on your oven, so just watch it like a hawk and don't let it burn. Sometimes certain parts puff up and colour before others, and I make little folded bits of tin foil to put over those bits so the other areas have a chance to catch up.

Meanwhile, go back to your tray of onions and spend some time skimming away as much fat as you can without getting rid of the beautiful juices underneath. Put the tray over a medium heat, stir in the mustard and a splash of water, then gently bring to the boil. Reduce the heat and keep it at a gentle simmer for 5 minutes, then pour in the cream. Simmer for a further 10 to 15 minutes, or until it's thickened slightly and you've got a good consistency.

I like to add extra glaze to the pork, so if you want to do this, pop the sugar into a small bowl and add just enough scrumpy to make a loose slurry. Spoon this over the pork and pop it back under the grill for a couple more minutes, until even more delicious. Once it's shiny, crackling and beautiful, remove the pork from under the grill and allow it to rest before slicing and serving on top of the creamy onions, with some nice lemony greens to cut through the richness of the meat.

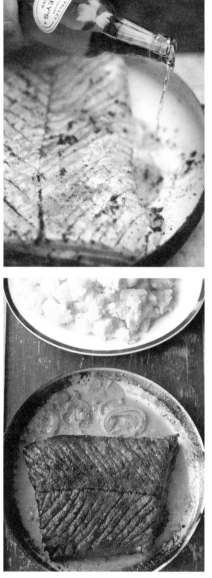

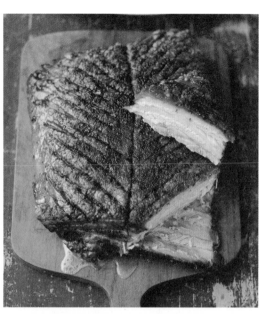

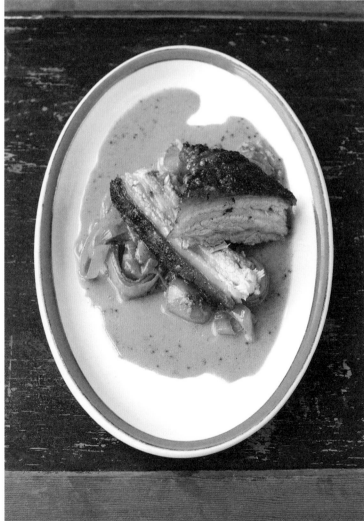

BOILED & GLAZED BACON
PEASE PUDDING · SPRING VEG · MUSTARD

SERVES 8
WITH LEFTOVER MEAT

For the gammon
- 1 x 1.8kg piece of middle-cut free-range gammon, rind on
- 4 each of white and black peppercorns
- 3 or 4 fresh bay leaves
- a small bunch of fresh parsley stalks
- a small bunch of fresh dill
- 2 cloves
- 2 medium white onions, peeled and halved
- ½ a jar of good-quality thick-cut marmalade

For the pease pudding
- 275g yellow split peas
- 1 small potato, peeled
- 1 small onion, peeled
- 1 small bunch of fresh herbs (rosemary, sage, thyme, bay)
- 2 cloves
- Colman's mustard
- sea salt and ground pepper
- a few knobs of butter

For the veggies
- 400g baby carrots, peeled and trimmed
- 400g new potatoes
- 1 bulb of fennel, trimmed and cut into 6 wedges, herby tops reserved
- 200g podded fresh or frozen broad beans (roughly 1kg before podding)
- 200g runner beans, trimmed and sliced
- 200g fresh (shelled) or frozen peas

This recipe is inspired by the happy memories I have of tucking into boiled bacon and pease pudding as a child. My version is a little different, because I'm glazing the ham to build up a character and flavour you don't normally get from boiled meat, but the pease pudding is quite traditional. It's one of the true tastes of Britain, and economical comfort food at its best. It would have filled up hungry bellies back in the days when it was cold and there wasn't much food to go round.

The night before you want to cook this, put the meat into your largest, deepest pan with enough cold water to cover. Put the split peas into a small pan of cold water and leave both meat and peas to soak overnight. The next day, lay a piece of muslin or a clean tea towel (roughly 80 x 80cm) in a large bowl. Drain the peas and put them into the lined bowl. Cut the potato into 1cm chunks and finely chop the onion, then add both to the peas along with the herbs and cloves. Draw up the corners to make a tight bundle and secure tightly with a piece of string, then put aside.

Next drain the meat, and cover it with fresh cold water. Add the peppercorns, herbs, cloves, onions and the bag of pease pudding. Bring to the boil, skimming the surface as needed, then cover with a lid. Reduce to a gentle simmer and cook for 1 hour 20 minutes. When the time is nearly up, preheat your oven to 180°C/350°F/gas 4.

Once the meat is beautiful and tender (try a bit to check), carefully move it to a large roasting tray. Remove any string round the meat, then peel off and discard the skin. Deeply score any fat left behind, then brush over the marmalade and glaze in the oven for about 30 to 35 minutes, basting when you can, until golden and sticky.

Meanwhile, sit a colander on a large pan over a medium high heat. Move the bag of pease pudding to a plate, then pour the cooking broth through the colander. Discard whatever is left in the colander and bring the broth to the boil. Add the carrots, new potatoes and fennel first and cook them for roughly 20 to 25 minutes, or until tender. Add the beans and the bag of pease pudding for the last 5 minutes, and the delicate peas at the very last minute.

When the meat is sticky and golden, move it to a carving board. Spoon 2 ladles of broth into the roasting tray and bring to the boil on the hob to pick up all the sticky pan juices. Stir in a teaspoon of mustard, season with salt and pepper, then reduce to the consistency you like and pour into a gravy boat. Drain the veg, reserving the broth, and tip them on to a platter. Pour over 2 ladles of the broth and season with salt and pepper, if needed. Untie the pease pudding and transfer it to a serving bowl. Mash in the butter and a teaspoon of mustard, and add a splash of broth to loosen if needed. Season to taste, pull out any herb sprigs and serve with the glazed gammon, the beautiful vegetables, with more mustard on the side, and the gravy boat.

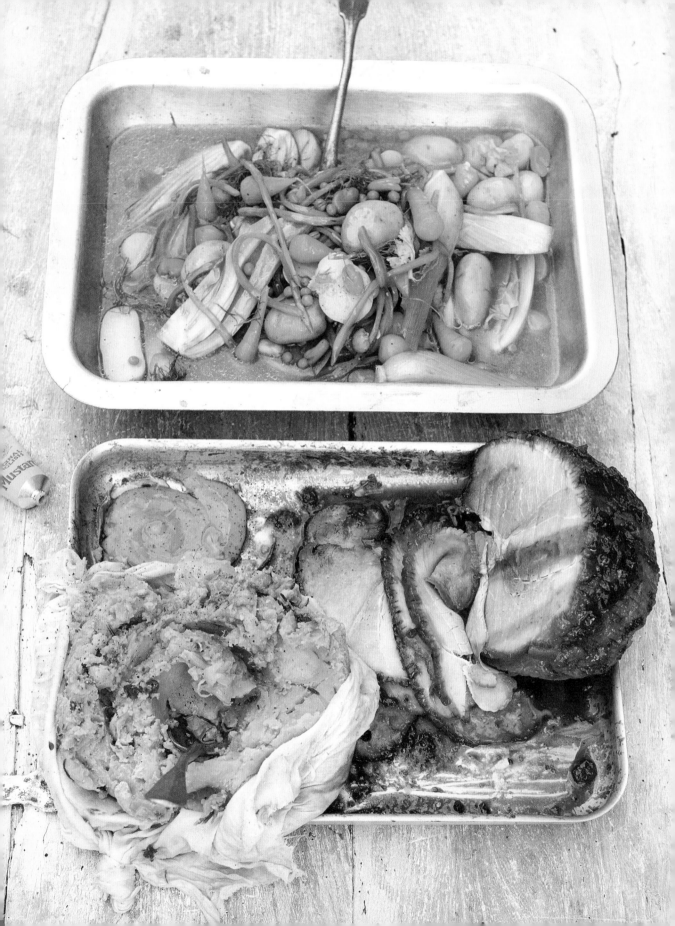

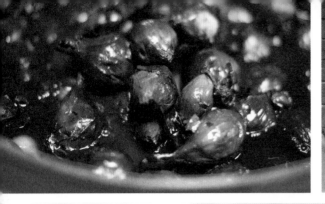

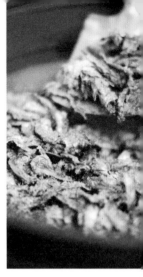

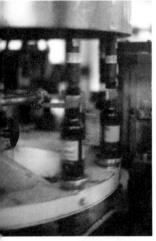

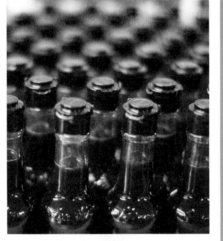

Lea & Perrins

Worcestershire sauce is made in such a small factory. It was amazing to see all the onions and garlic pickling in barrels and whole batches of the finished sauce being bottled up. There are various stories behind the creation of this sauce. One of them is that a nobleman with ties to India had a secret recipe, which he asked local chemists, John Lea & William Perrins, to make for him. It was so successful we now use it in everything from Bloody Marys to cheese on toast. I love it.

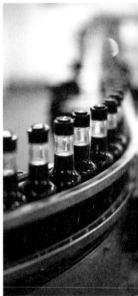

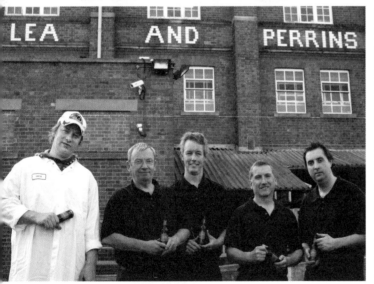

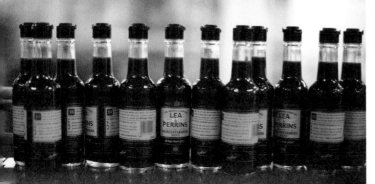

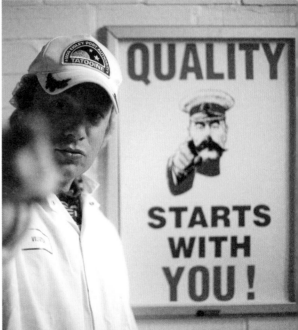

QUALITY STARTS WITH YOU !

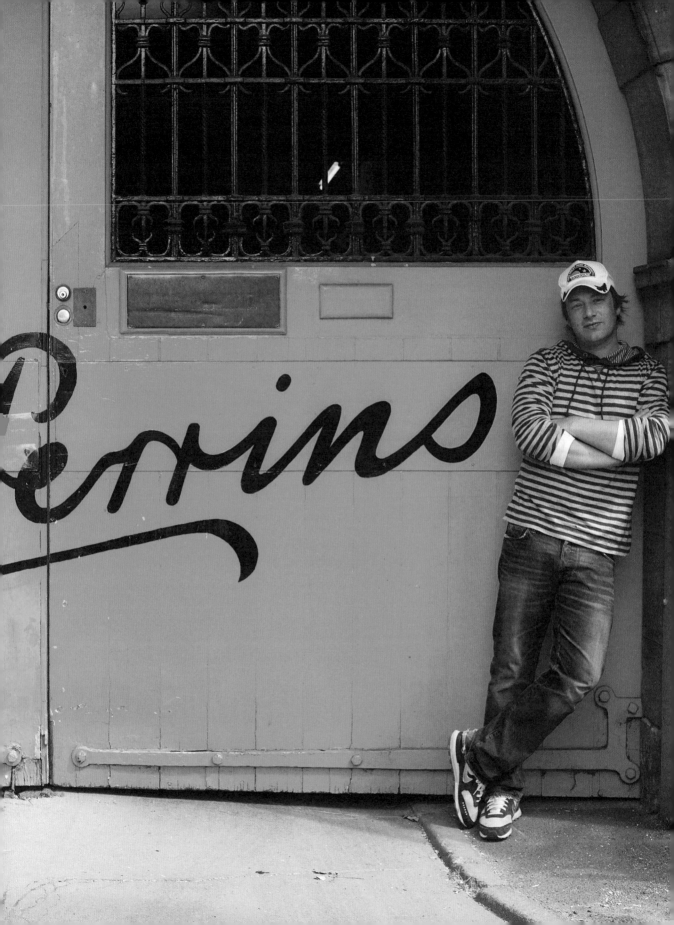

WORCESTERSHIRE BEEF SARNIE

This is one of the most pleasurable and delicious lunches you can make. My lot go mad for it. It uses brisket, one of the cheaper cuts of beef, so it's great value and wonderful comfort food. What can I say? Tender, juicy flavoured beef, thinly sliced into lovely soft sandwiches with pickles and mustard, is just one of the best things ever. And, more than likely, you'll have brilliant leftovers for the days ahead. What I love about this meal is that when you wake up in the morning you can sling it together in three minutes and just let it effortlessly simmer away until lunchtime. I promise you it will be a wonderful, luxurious experience.

SERVES 10

For the beef
- 1kg beef brisket, unrolled
- 1 x 150ml bottle of Worcestershire sauce
- 4 onions, halved

- 4 sticks of celery, halved lengthways
- 4 sprigs of fresh rosemary
- 4 fresh bay leaves
- sea salt and ground pepper

To serve
- a large loaf of soft white bread
- butter, at room temperature
- English mustard, wholegrain mustard, horseradish, etc.

Put your brisket and all the other beef ingredients, including the contents of an entire bottle of Worcestershire sauce, into a large pot with a lid. Add 1 heaped tablespoon of sea salt, then pour in enough water to cover by 2.5cm, pop the lid on and simmer gently for around 2½ hours for juicy meat that's easy to carve, 3 hours for meat that'll pull a little, and 4 to 5 hours for meat that'll just fall apart. There's no right or wrong way - just do whatever makes you happy, then turn the heat off and keep it warm in the pot along with the broth until you need it.

For the most unbelievable sandwich (there is an art to the perfect sandwich, so please bear with me), make the cucumber salad on page 90 and pop the loaf of bread into a warm oven for 10 minutes to heat up - you want it crunchy on the outside and soft in the middle. Use a serrated knife to slice the bread 1cm thick, then put the loaf back together and put it in the middle of the table with the bowl of cucumber salad and any mustards or condiments you fancy. Finely slice or pull the brisket, lay it all on a platter and immediately drizzle over some of that lovely broth to keep the beef moist and hot.

Now all you've got to do is thinly butter each slice of bread from corner to corner, place a pinch of cucumber on one side, and smear the other side with whatever condiment you choose. Add some beef then eat it pretty quick while it's still warm and delicious. Such a heavenly lunch.

PS: The broth will taste amazing, so keep it in the fridge or freeze in sandwich bags and make sure you use it - it'd be a crime to waste it! You can use it for a fantastic onion soup, Scotch broth (see page 54) or even gravy for a Sunday roast.

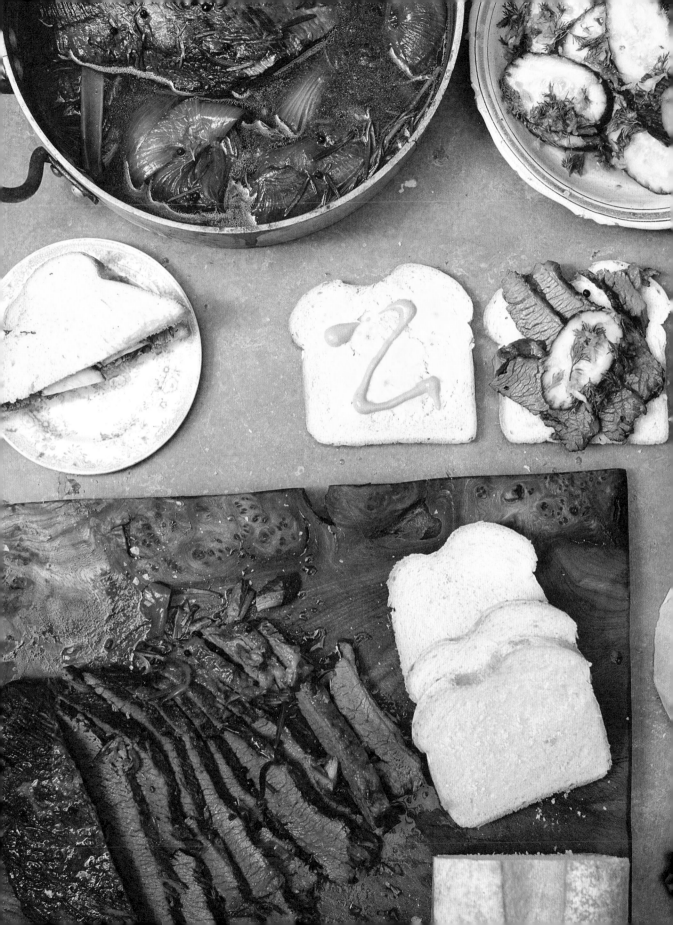

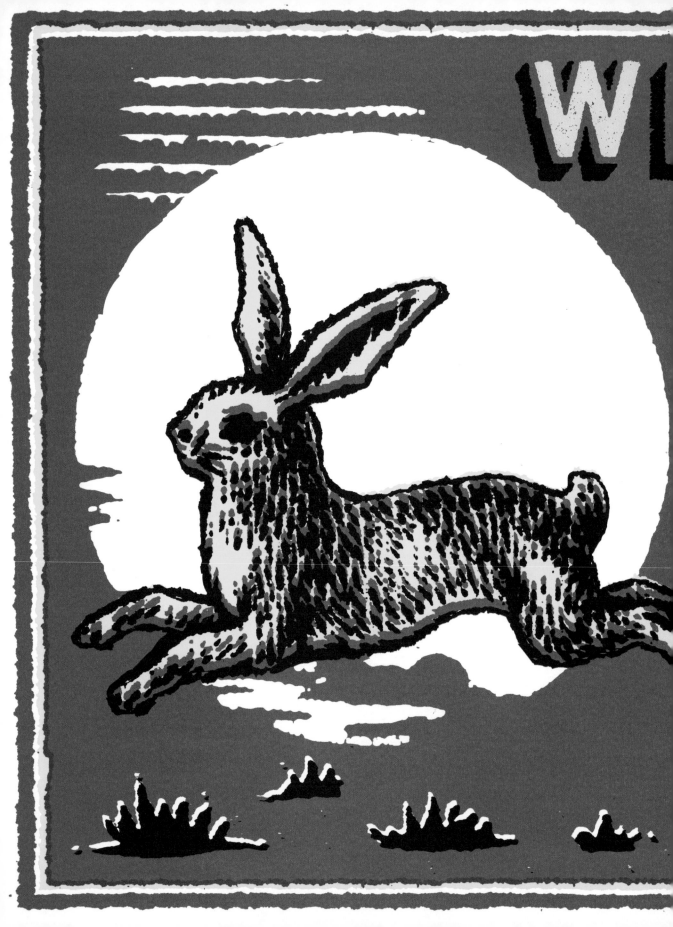

LD FOOD

I really wanted to put this chapter into the book because we are, and have always been, a nation of hunters and foragers. We have incredible wild food: pheasant, partridge, quail, pigeon, rabbit, venison, herbs, flowers, nuts, mushrooms ... But somewhere around the time of the industrial revolution, our ancestors didn't have the free time or inclination to pass on their skills for things like mushroom picking or hunting, which is such a shame. One thing's for sure, the Italian and Eastern European communities that live here still know what's what, and that's why they're out there picking mushrooms and selling them to gullible chefs who don't realize they're growing for free just down the road. There was a time when you would have gone hunting for snared rabbit, pigeon or other game birds, then done a swap with your mate for something he'd caught. And it wasn't that long ago - I remember locals bringing game birds into the pub and giving them to Dad in exchange for a few pints. But now that farmed meats are so easily available from supermarkets, this practice has become more of a leisure activity than common practice. There's a distinct and special flavour you get from wild food, whether it's wild garlic, mushrooms or a pigeon breast cooked just right. If you have a good butcher's shop or farmers' market in your area you'll be able to tap into this chapter really easily.

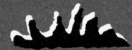

SEARED VENISON LOIN
SCOTTISH RISOTTO • GOLDEN PHEASANT HASH

SERVES 8 TO 10

For the pearl barley risotto
- 3 large leeks
- a few knobs of butter
- a few sprigs of fresh thyme, leaves picked
- olive oil
- sea salt and ground pepper
- 500g pearl barley
- 2 litres organic chicken stock
- 80g soft local cheese or Philadelphia cream cheese
- 80g good quality Cheddar cheese, grated
- a small handful of fresh flat-leaf parsley

For the hash
- 4 rashers of quality smoked streaky bacon
- 4 sprigs of fresh rosemary
- ½ a swede, peeled and halved
- 2 red onions, peeled and halved
- 1 large carrot, peeled
- 3 turnips (roughly 350g), peeled
- 4 pheasant breasts (roughly 400g), skin removed
- 200g chicken livers
- 2 heaped tablespoons bitter marmalade

For the venison
- 6 or 7 juniper berries
- red wine vinegar
- 700g venison loin in one fat piece, trimmed (ask your butcher to do this)

This recipe has three different elements to it, but you'll find there's a nice natural flow to the whole process and everything comes together around the same time. I've turned the pearl barley into a sort of Scottish risotto, to make a hero out of this incredible ingredient. The result is a silky, smooth dish that is just beautiful with game. I've used pheasant in the hash, but you can make it your own by embracing other kinds of game, or even pork, lamb or beef if you prefer.

Preheat the oven to 200°C/400°F/gas 6. Trim, wash and finely slice the leeks, then add them to a large deep pan on a medium heat with 2 knobs of butter, the thyme leaves and a drizzle of olive oil. Season, then cook gently for around 15 minutes, or until the leeks have softened. Stir in the pearl barley and half the stock, then put the lid on and cook for 20 minutes. After that time, add a splash of stock at a time, stirring and letting it absorb into the pearl barley before adding the next. Cook for a further 40 to 50 minutes, or until the pearl barley is a pleasure to eat.

While that's cooking, start the hash. Finely chop your bacon and the leaves from two of the rosemary sprigs. Add to a really large deep frying pan (at least 30cm wide) on a medium heat with a lug of olive oil. While that's crisping up, dice the swede, red onions, carrot and turnips into 1 to 2cm cubes, adding them to the pan as you go. Season well with salt and loads of pepper and keep moving everything around. Cook for around 30 minutes, or until the vegetables start to soften. Don't forget about the pearl barley. Pick the leaves from the two remaining rosemary sprigs into a pestle and mortar. Add the juniper berries and a good pinch of salt and pepper, then bash to a paste. Pour in a little olive oil and a swig of vinegar, then mix up and rub all over the venison loin and put it aside.

Season the pheasant breasts and chicken livers well, then chop into rough 1cm pieces and add to the pan of vegetables. Turn the temperature up to high, stir well and cook for another 5 to 10 minutes, or until the meat starts to brown. Taste and season the pearl barley if needed – if it's soft, turn the heat right down to low and add a knob of butter, the cheese and the chopped parsley, then pop the lid on. If it's not quite there, just stir in a little more stock and give it some time.

When you feel everything is about 20 minutes away from serving, add a little olive oil to a large frying pan on a high heat. Add the venison loin and cook for around 17 minutes, turning every 2 minutes until it's blushing and medium rare. Be brave! It's best blushing; if you overcook it, it will be tough and leathery. Place on a warmed plate and rub with a little butter to rest. The hash should be dark and lovely now, so stir in the marmalade to make it shiny. Thinly slice the venison and put the sizzling hash on a nice platter with the risotto. Lovely served with a green salad.

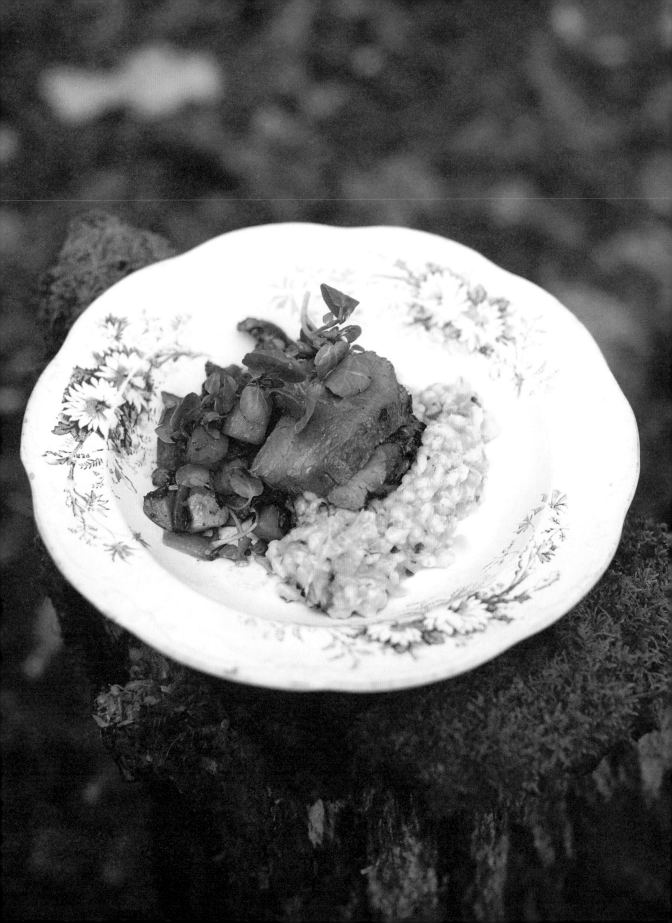

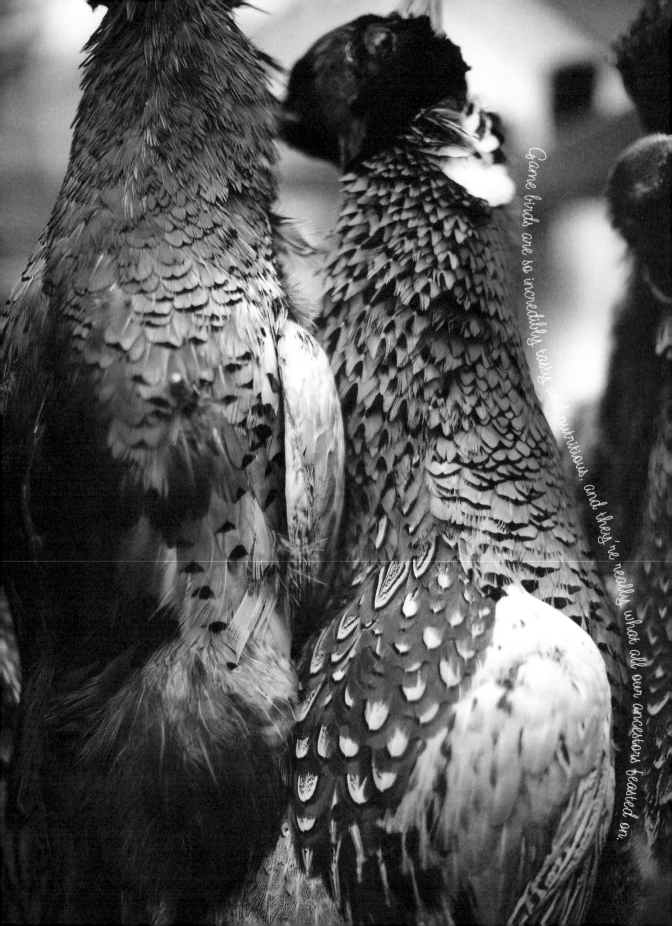

Game birds are so incredibly tasty and nutritious, and they're really what all our ancestors feasted on.

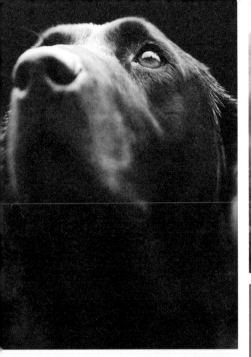

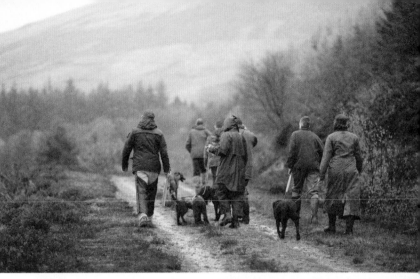

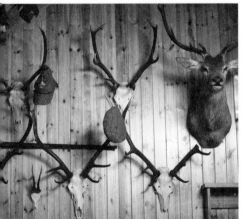

Game Shoots
Scotland has the most amazing wild game and stunning scenery. Being a 'beater' on a shoot there and driving the birds out of the undergrowth was great fun. The organization NOBS (I kid you not) can let you know all about shoots going on in your area. It's a great day out, you can earn a few quid and even take a brace of birds home at the end of it.
www.nobs.org.uk

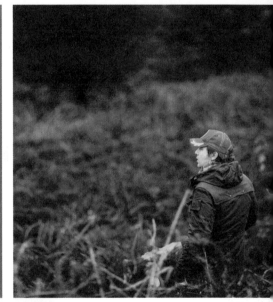

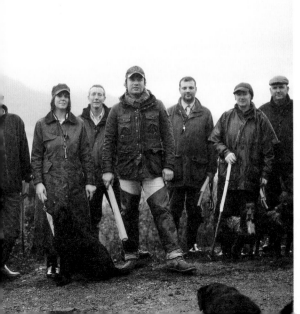

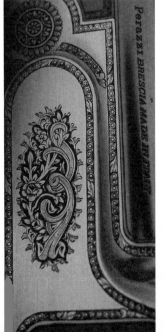

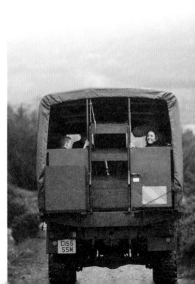

GORGEOUS PHEASANT
CREAMY FENNEL BAKE • APPLE MATCHSTICK SALAD

Any poultry or game would be lovely used in this recipe, but pheasant, guinea fowl or chicken work particularly well. It's definitely worth getting nice plump birds from a butcher if you can. The fennel and potato dish only really works if you cook a whole tray of it, so I suggest you eat half with the meal and save the rest for incredible leftovers for another day.

SERVES 6

For the pheasant
- olive or rapeseed oil
- 2 plump pheasants (roughly 800g each), cut into breasts, thighs and drumsticks (or ask your butcher to do this for you)
- sea salt and ground pepper
- 1 whole nutmeg, for grating
- 4 rashers of quality smoked streaky bacon, finely chopped
- a few small knobs of butter
- 2 cloves of garlic, peeled and crushed

- 4 sprigs of fresh rosemary, leaves picked
- 200ml good-quality apple juice
- 1 crunchy green apple
- 2 large handfuls of watercress, washed and spun dry
- 1 lemon
- 1 teaspoon runny honey

For the creamy fennel bake
- 600g Maris Piper potatoes, scrubbed
- 2 bulbs of fennel (roughly 400g), trimmed
- 1 white onion, peeled
- 4 cloves of garlic, peeled
- 2 fresh bay leaves
- 650ml organic chicken stock
- 250g fat-free thick natural yoghurt
- 1 tablespoon English mustard
- 100g Cheddar cheese, freshly grated

Preheat the oven to 180°C/350°F/gas 4. Put a large wide casserole-type pan (roughly 24cm wide) on a high heat and add a good lug of oil. Once hot, add the pheasant drumsticks and thighs, season well with salt and pepper and grate over a few scrapings of nutmeg. Fry for around 12 minutes, turning every minute or so until golden. Keep your eye on them.

Finely slice the potatoes (I like leaving the skins on), fennel and onion in a food processor using the slicer attachment, or by hand. Throw them into a high-sided roasting tray (roughly 28 x 35cm, and 4cm deep). Crush in the garlic, add the bay leaves, grate over half the nutmeg, then stir in the stock and season. Cover with tin foil, bring to the boil on a hob and simmer for around 20 minutes, or until the vegetables are tender.

By now the meat should be looking great, so pour away as much fat from the pan as you can, then add the chopped bacon and the pheasant breasts, skin side down. Stir and fry for 4 more minutes, then add a small knob of butter, crushed garlic and rosemary leaves. Pour in the apple juice and put into the oven to cook for around 25 minutes, but set the timer, because pheasant is not a forgiving meat.

When the vegetables are cooked, remove the foil, then quickly mix the yoghurt and mustard together in a small bowl, dollop and smear that all over the top and sprinkle over the grated cheese. Whack into the oven to cook for the same amount of time as the pheasant, or until golden and bubbling.

When everything is nearly done, slice the apple into matchsticks and toss in a bowl with the watercress, the juice of the lemon, about three times as much oil and a little seasoning. Slice the pheasant breast on a board with the thighs and drumsticks. Drizzle over the pan juices and a little honey from a height. Serve with the lovely creamy bake and enjoy.

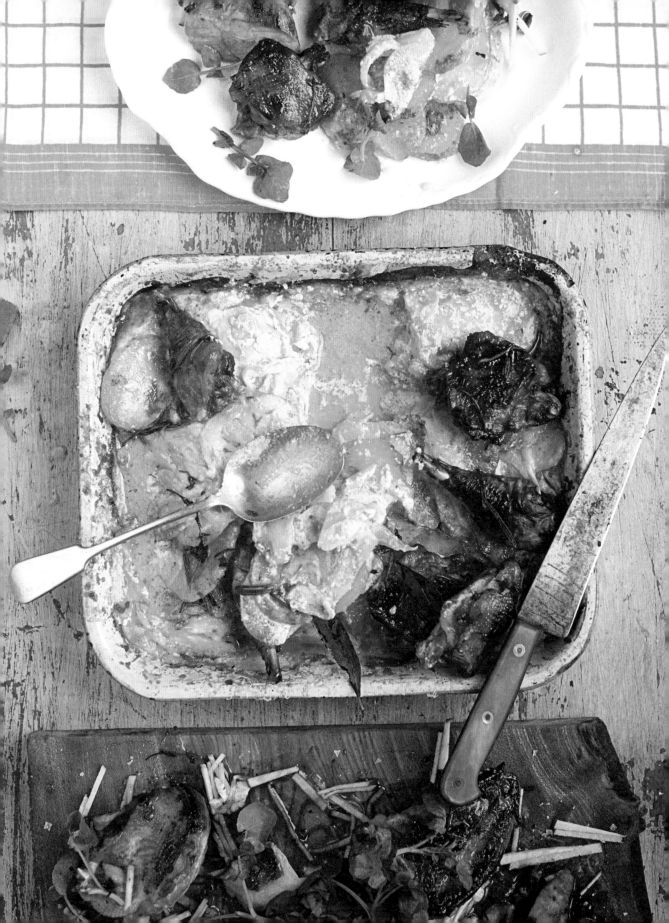

HONEY-ROASTED LEMON RABBIT
... WITH THE MOST BRILLIANT OFFAL SKEWERS

Whether farmed or wild, rabbit is wonderful, delicious meat. Because farmed rabbit can be slightly more tender than wild, I'm recommending you use it for this recipe. If you buy it from a proper butcher's, it should be very affordable indeed. Ask your butcher to put the offal aside for you, then joint the rabbit into two shoulders, two legs, four pieces of saddle and a couple of pieces of belly. It's really very simple, and if you want to see how it's done go to *www.jamieoliver.com/how-to* for a quick tutorial. Please give this a go – you'll love it.

SERVES 4

- 1 rabbit, skinned and jointed, including offal (ask your butcher to do this for you)
- 4 rashers of quality smoked streaky bacon
- olive oil
- sea salt and ground pepper

- 2 heaped tablespoons Colman's mustard powder
- ½-1 dried chilli, to taste
- 1 whole nutmeg, for grating
- 1 level teaspoon ground allspice
- 25g Cheddar cheese
- a bunch of fresh thyme

- 4 cloves of garlic, unpeeled
- 1 lemon, cut into wedges
- 1 tablespoon runny honey
- a knob of butter
- 2-3 tablespoons Worcestershire sauce
- a few pinches of cayenne pepper

Preheat the oven to 180°C/350°F/gas 4. Put the jointed rabbit pieces into a large bowl. Cut the bacon into chunky lardons and add them to the bowl. Drizzle over a few good lugs of olive oil and add a generous seasoning of salt and pepper. Sprinkle over the mustard powder, crumble in the dried chilli, finely grate over a third of the nutmeg and add the allspice. Give everything a really good toss to coat it in the flavours.

Pick out the pieces of rabbit belly from the bowl and spread them flat on a board. Grate over the cheese, pick over a few sprigs' worth of thyme tips, then roll up the meat and secure with cocktail sticks. Get a large non-stick frying pan (roughly 30cm wide), add a few good lugs of olive oil, then add everything from the bowl along with the rolled pieces of belly and the remaining thyme sprigs. Bash the cloves of garlic with the flat side of a knife and add these too, then cook for around 5 minutes on a high heat, turning every so often, until golden all over. Transfer everything to a snug-fitting tray (roughly 20 x 30cm), along with the lemon wedges and a good splash of water. Cover with foil and cook in the oven for 1 hour, or until the rabbit is tender. Once ready, use tongs to squeeze the lemon juice over the rabbit, discarding the skins. Drizzle over a tablespoon of honey from a height, then turn the oven up to 200°C/400°F/gas 6 and put the tray back into the oven for another 5 minutes to glaze and get beautiful.

Cut the rabbit livers, kidney, lungs and heart in half and thread them on to 1 or 2 metal or wooden skewers. Intersperse the offal (don't pack it on there too tightly), then put the original frying pan back on a high heat and add a knob of butter and a drizzle of olive oil. Put in the offal skewers – they will need only 2 minutes on each side – and when they're looking golden, hit them with 2 to 3 tablespoons of Worcestershire sauce and a few pinches of cayenne pepper. Take the skewers to the table with your roasted rabbit and some beautiful greens, and enjoy.

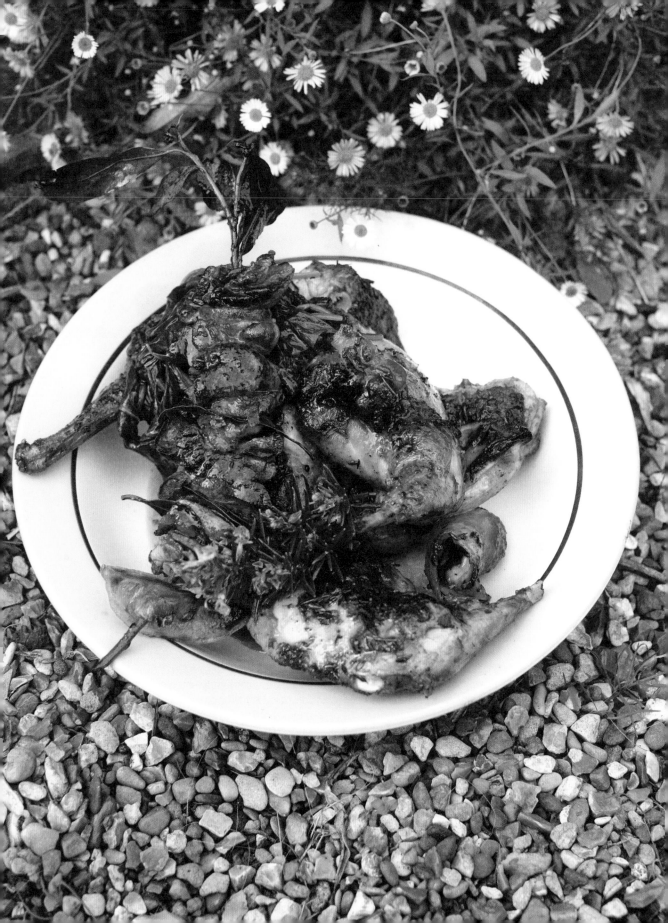

12-HOUR RABBIT BOLOGNESE

This is a wonderful evolution of that humble meat sauce we all love. You can create around fourteen incredible-tasting portions of bolognese out of one little rabbit, so it's beyond cheap to make. And most importantly, you can knock it together in around three minutes flat, then just allow the oven to turn it into a heavenly and delicious bolognese. Once it comes out of the oven you've got a rustic sauce that you can portion up and freeze for all sorts of beautiful meals in the days and weeks to come. If you aren't a lover of rabbit meat, I urge you to try this. It's cheap, it's tasty, and it's easy … Are you convinced yet?

MAKES ENOUGH SAUCE TO SERVE 14

- olive oil
- 3 rashers of quality smoked streaky bacon, roughly chopped
- 2 fresh bay leaves
- 2 sprigs of fresh rosemary
- 1 whole rabbit, skinned (ask your butcher to do this for you), including offal
- 1 bulb of garlic (left whole), white skin peeled away
- 2 leeks, washed, topped and tailed

- 2 carrots, washed, topped and tailed
- 2 sticks of celery, washed and trimmed
- 2 red onions, skin on, washed
- 20g dried porcini mushrooms
- 2 x 400g tins of chopped tomatoes
- 1 x 500ml can of light smooth beer/ale
- 2 tablespoons tomato purée
- sea salt and ground pepper

- 1 whole nutmeg, for grating
- ½ a lemon
- a few sprigs of fresh thyme

- *optional serving method: serves 6*
- 1 x 500g packet of dried pasta of your liking
- Parmesan or Cheddar cheese, for grating
- extra virgin olive oil
- a few sprigs of fresh thyme

Preheat the oven to 110°C/225°F/gas ¼. Put your largest casserole-type pan on a medium heat and add a lug of olive oil and the chopped bacon. Once it's lightly golden, add the bay leaves and rosemary sprigs and lay the whole rabbit and the offal on top. Drop in the whole garlic bulb, leeks, carrots, celery and onions, then add the dried mushrooms, tinned tomatoes, beer, tomato purée, and just enough water to cover everything (roughly 1 litre). Bring to the boil, and season generously with loads of black pepper and a few pinches of salt. Finely grate in half the nutmeg, put the lid on, then pop the casserole into the oven and leave to cook for 12 hours.

Once cooked, let the stew cool down a little, then get yourself a big pair of clean Marigold gloves and another large pan. This is where you make it a pleasure to eat, so pick through small handfuls of stew at a time, taking out any bones or vegetable skins. Discard the herbs, and flake the beautiful meat off the bones and into the clean pan. Scrunch the vegetables and offal in your hands as you go and break them into smaller pieces. Pour any juices left behind into the new pan, then go back in and have another rummage to make sure you haven't missed anything. Have a taste and correct the seasoning. Finely grate in the zest of half the lemon and pick in a few thyme tips to brighten up the sauce. Divvy the sauce up between sandwich bags and either freeze them, or keep in the fridge.

When you want to make your rabbit bolognese, simply reheat a small ladle of sauce per person in a pan over a medium heat and cook around 80 grams of pasta per person. Spaghetti and penne are favourites of mine for this. Boil according to packet instructions in salted water, then drain, reserving some of the starchy cooking water. Toss with your sauce and a little splash of the cooking water to make it silky then add a nice handful of cheese. Taste and check the seasoning then serve immediately with another good sprinkling of cheese, a drizzle of extra virgin olive oil and some fresh thyme tips.

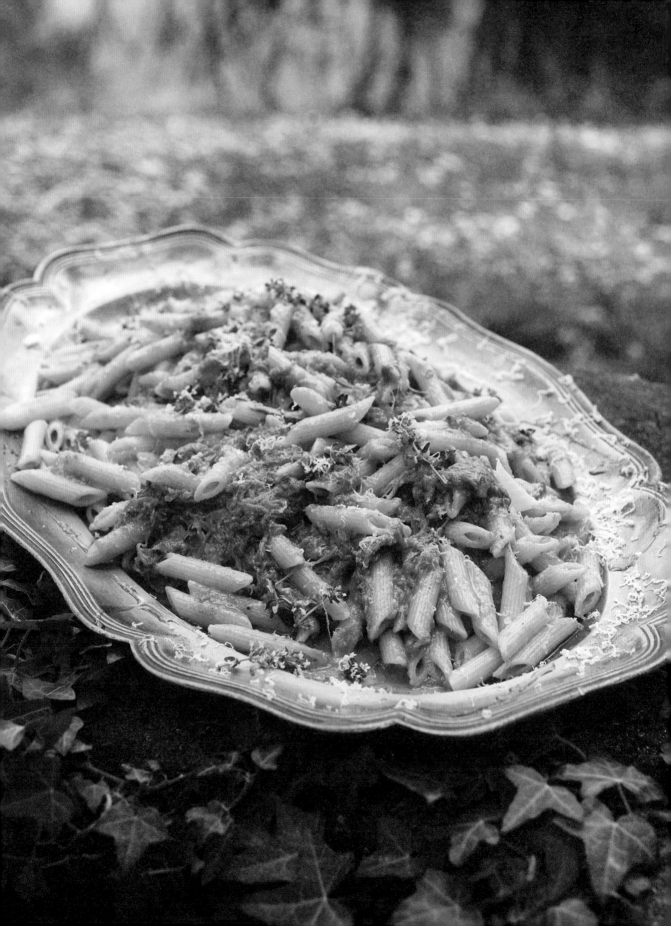

The Cowal Peninsula has to be one of the most beautiful, quiet, tranquil places.

SEARED PEPPERED STEAK
MIXED WILD MUSHROOMS • WATERCRESS

Because of Britain's amazingly lush pastures (thanks to all the rain), we have access to some of the best beef in the world, and this simple recipe is a great way of celebrating that, alongside another beautiful ingredient we have in abundance in woods and fields all over the country: wild mushrooms. Without question, the combination of steak, wild foraged mushrooms, little pinches of herbs and watercress will have been served together in many ways over the years – it's simplicity itself. For me, this really is the perfect Friday night dinner. If you're cooking a medium rare steak you can knock the whole thing out in 10 minutes, no problem. In this recipe, I'm cooking one large steak from a butcher's and slicing it into two portions, which is the nicest way to make this, but you could also cook two smaller steaks, if you like.

SERVES 2 STRAPPING LADS

- 1 x 400g sirloin or rib-eye steak
- sea salt and ground pepper
- olive oil
- 2 tablespoons nice port
- a small knob of butter

- 3 good handfuls (roughly 250g) of mixed mushrooms, such as mini Portobello, ceps, chestnuts, oysters, trimmed, cleaned and thickly sliced
- 1 clove of garlic, peeled and finely sliced

- a few sprigs of fresh thyme
- 2 tablespoons single cream
- 1 lemon
- 1 generous handful of watercress
- English mustard, to serve

Preheat a large, thick-bottomed pan or griddle pan on a high heat until screaming hot. Season the steak with salt, pepper and a drizzle of olive oil, then rub all over with the seasonings. Place the steak in the pan with a little olive oil and turn every minute until cooked to your liking. You need to use your instincts, but for a steak that's about 2.5cm thick, around 2 to 3 minutes on each side will give you medium rare. Cook it a little longer if you like it more well done, or for less time if you prefer rare steak. Once you're happy with how it's cooked, add the port to the pan – don't worry if it flames – and as soon as it subsides, add a small knob of butter, shake the pan around, then remove the steak and the juices to a plate.

Quickly wipe the pan out with a ball of kitchen paper, then put back on a high heat with a drizzle of olive oil. Add the mushrooms. Toss and cook them for about 2 minutes, then add the sliced garlic and pick in the thyme leaves. Keep tossing and cooking for another 2 minutes, or until the mushrooms start to turn golden, then add the cream. Jiggle the pan a little to coat the mushrooms, then season to taste, add a little squeeze of lemon juice and remove from the heat.

Cut the steak into 0.5cm slices, removing any unwanted fatty bits, then quickly dress those slices of meat in the incredible resting juices and divide between your plates along with the lovely mushrooms. Dress the watercress quickly with the juice of half the lemon to make it fresh and zingy, and put a big pinch of it on each plate. Serve with some nice English mustard for dolloping on the side and a hunk of crusty bread to mop up all the juices, if you like.

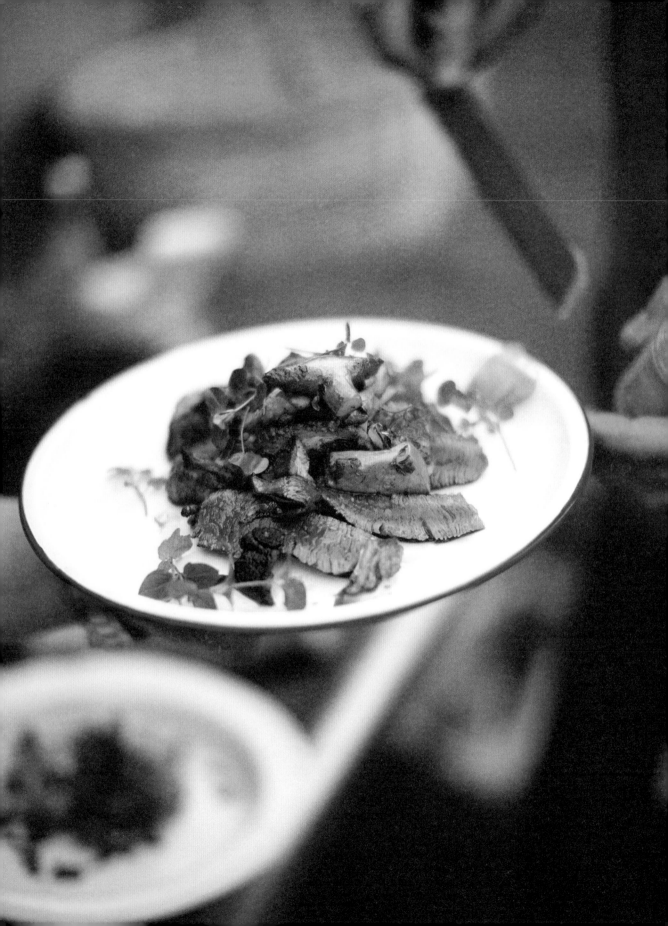

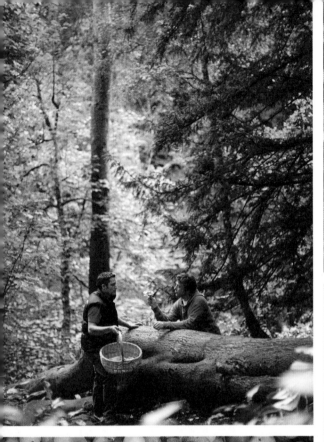
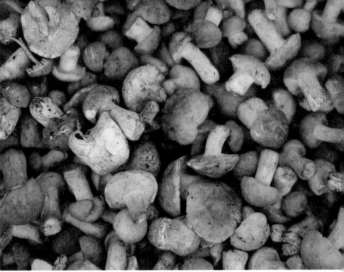
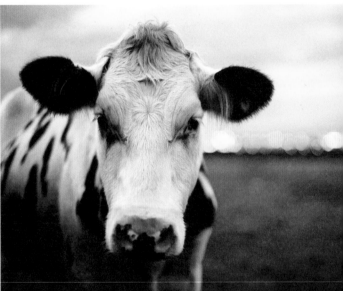
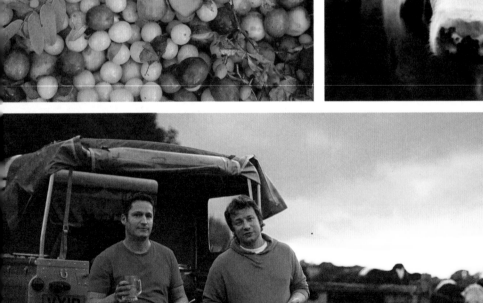

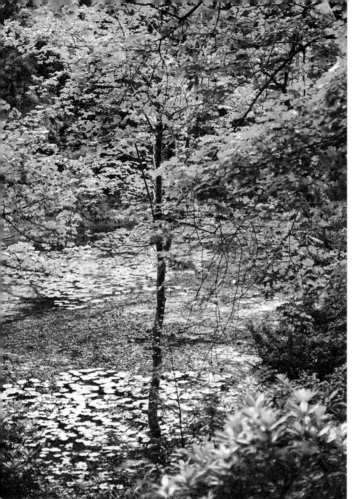

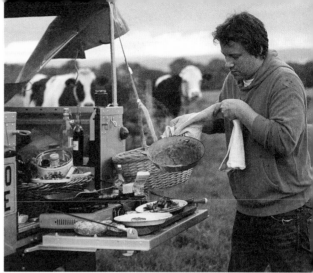

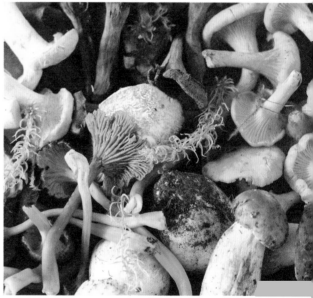

Wild Mushroom Foraging

I went out foraging with Toby Gritten, the chef and owner of The Pump House pub in Bristol. He showed me how plentiful the wild mushrooms, fruits, nettles, flowers and sorrel were in the local woods. Toby incorporates lots of the food he forages into the dishes he makes for his pub's restaurant. To me, that's such an exciting and clever way to cook - he's obviously a proper chef, and I admire his approach to using local ingredients, not to mention some of our older, more traditional recipes. If you get a chance to visit his place, you must check out the Bath chaps on his menu. It's one of his signature dishes. We cooked some of the mushrooms as the sun set. Great food.

www.the-pumphouse.com

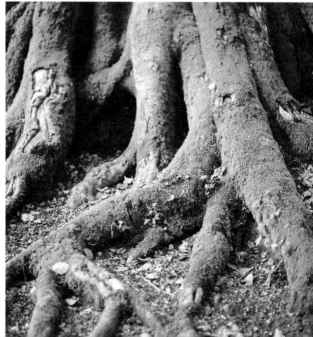

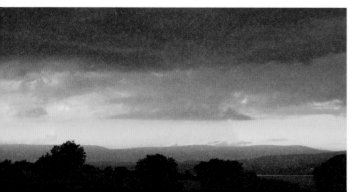

FLYING STEAK SANDWICH
STICKY ONIONS • MUSTARD • COTTAGE CHEESE

Pigeon gets a bad rap, but good wild country birds (not the mangy kind you see wandering around cities!) produce one of the most delicious and underrated meats in the world (as long as it's cooked medium rare). In the past, I've seared pigeon breast, put it inside some lovely bread and had people tell me it's the best steak sandwich they've ever had! So here's how it's done … This makes a brilliant casual lunch, dinner or snack with a nice salad.

SERVES 4

- 2 red onions, peeled and finely sliced
- olive oil
- sea salt and white pepper
- 1 teaspoon soft brown sugar
- 2 sprigs of fresh thyme, leaves picked
- 4 tablespoons red wine vinegar
- 1 ciabatta loaf
- 2 sprigs of fresh rosemary, leaves picked
- 4 pigeon breasts, skin on
- 1 whole nutmeg, for grating
- 2 fresh bay leaves
- Worcestershire sauce
- English mustard, to serve
- a large handful of watercress, to serve
- cottage cheese, to serve

Turn the oven to 180°C/350°F/gas 4. Put the onions into a large pan on a medium low heat and add a lug of olive oil, a pinch of salt and white pepper, the sugar and the thyme leaves. Put the lid on and cook for 30 minutes, stirring occasionally. After this time, remove the lid, turn the heat up to high and give the onions a good stir, then add the vinegar and stir again. Leave the lid off and continue to cook down until the onions are really sticky and slightly golden. Keep your eye on them.

Put the ciabatta into the hot oven. Heat a large non-stick pan on a high heat. Finely chop the rosemary leaves and put them into a mixing bowl. Add the pigeon breasts, drizzle over some olive oil, season with salt and pepper and grate over a few scrapings of nutmeg. Toss the pigeon until coated. Once the pan is really hot, add a lug of olive oil and the bay leaves and put in the breasts, skin side down so they crisp up nicely. Cook for around 2½ minutes on the skin side and 1 minute on the other side for tender and blushing medium-rare meat, which trust me is what you want - anything over that and it will be tough and boring. As you remove the pan from the heat, shake in a few good drizzles of Worcestershire sauce, then toss the meat in the juices. Move to a board and slice thinly at an angle.

Get the warm bread out of the oven, open it out with a serrated knife, put it on a nice board and spread as much mustard as you dare on one side (be confident - you can spread a little butter on if you want, but I don't because the meat juices are enough). Put big pinches of watercress and those sticky onions down one side. Arrange the slices of pigeon around the sandwich, then dollop small amounts of cottage cheese in and around the meat. Push the top of the sandwich down and hold it for a couple of seconds so it sucks up all those juices. I always stab a knife through the sandwich to hold it together and make it look manly when you take it to the table. Serve next to a pint of good British ale.

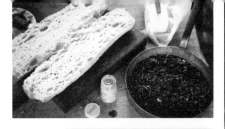
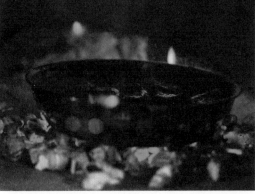
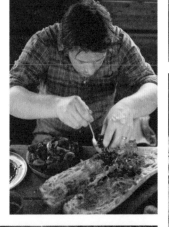
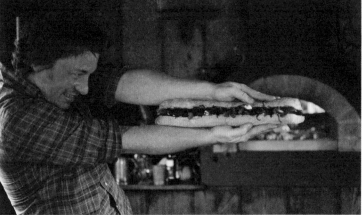
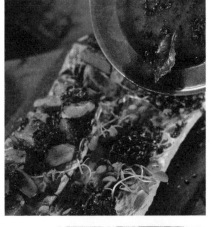
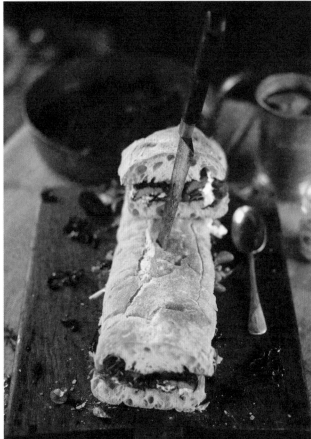
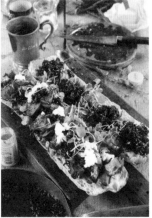

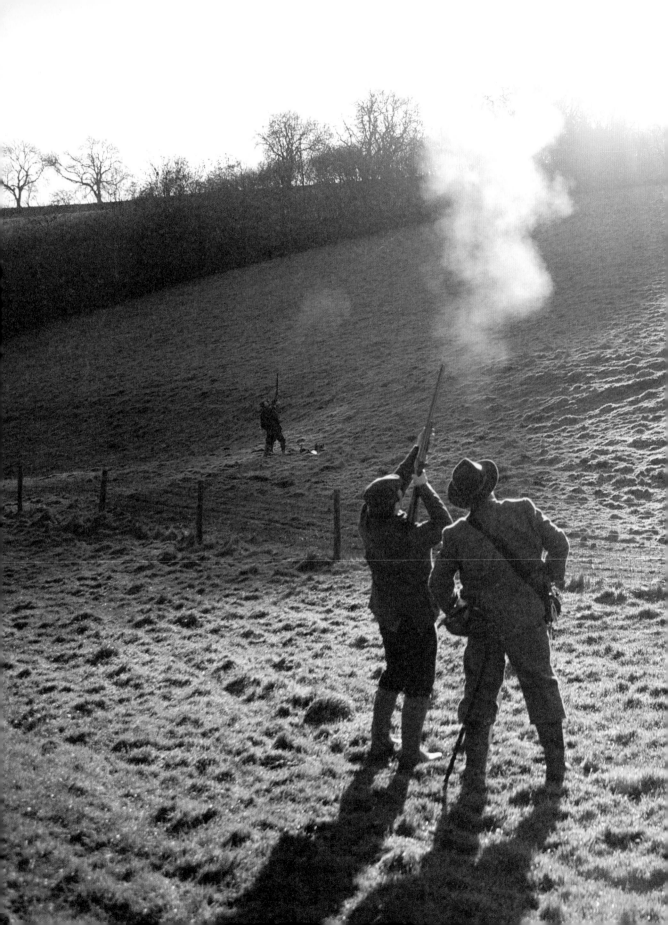

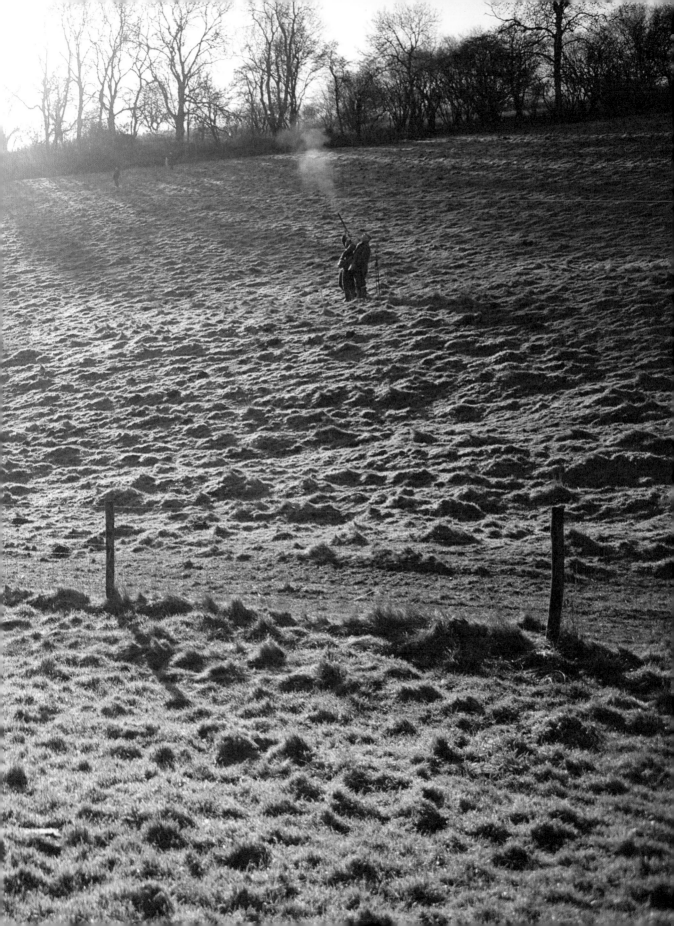

GOLDEN-GLAZED PARTRIDGE
STUFFING BALLS • DELICIOUS LENTILS

All good butchers have seasonal game at certain times of the year. You've probably seen those little birds in the butcher's shop window and wondered what to do with them. All I'll say is that you never know until you try, so here's a recipe that will guarantee you a really tasty dinner. Partridge isn't ultra gamey, so it's a great place for game virgins to start; it has a delicious mild flavour with attitude. I hope this recipe convinces you that it's something special.

SERVES 4

- 1 red onion, peeled and finely chopped
- olive oil
- red wine vinegar
- sea salt and ground pepper
- 4 partridges
- a few sprigs of fresh thyme and rosemary

- 12 very thin rashers of quality smoked streaky bacon or pancetta
- 4 quality sage and onion Cumberland sausages
- 250g puy lentils
- *optional:* 1.3 litres organic chicken stock

- 2 or 3 cloves of garlic, unpeeled
- a few fresh bay leaves
- good-quality blueberry jam
- good extra virgin olive oil
- 200g washed baby spinach
- natural yoghurt, to serve

Preheat the oven to 200°C/400°F/gas 6. Put the onion into a medium-sized pan with a lug of olive oil, a swig of red wine vinegar and a pinch of salt and pepper. Cook over a medium heat for 10 to 15 minutes to sweeten the flavours, stirring occasionally, while you prep your partridges. Rub them all over with olive oil, salt and pepper, then stuff them with the thyme and rosemary and drape 3 rashers of bacon over the breasts of each bird. Tie the bacon on with a piece of string – use the picture to guide you or have a look at the video on *www.jamieoliver.com/how-to* for guidance – but don't worry, it doesn't have to be perfect. Put the partridges into a snug-fitting roasting tray.

Pinch the sausage meat out of the skins, then roll each sausage into 3 little balls and place them all around the partridges. Cook in the oven for about 30 minutes, or until golden. As soon as the birds go in the oven, stir the lentils into the pan of onions and pour in enough stock or water to cover by about 2.5cm (roughly 1.3 litres). Bash the garlic and add to the lentils along with the bay leaves. Bring to the boil, then turn down the heat to medium and simmer for about the same time as it takes to cook the birds, or until the lentils are soft but still holding their shape. Add a splash more stock or water if needed.

When the birds are ready, take them out of the oven. Put a heaped tablespoon of the blueberry jam in the corner of the tray and push it around so it melts. As it becomes syrupy, spoon or brush the melted jam over the partridges and stuffing balls and return them to the oven for just a few minutes to glaze. Check your lentils – this requires you to really pay attention and taste, season, taste, season until you've got them just right. They should be cooked to a nice loose consistency by now, so season generously to taste with salt and pepper and a swig of vinegar and extra virgin olive oil until they taste delicious.

Put the spinach on to a platter, spoon over the hot lentils, then place the partridges and the balls of sausage meat on top of the lentils and drizzle over any juices from the roasting tray. Dollop some yoghurt over the lentils and dive in.

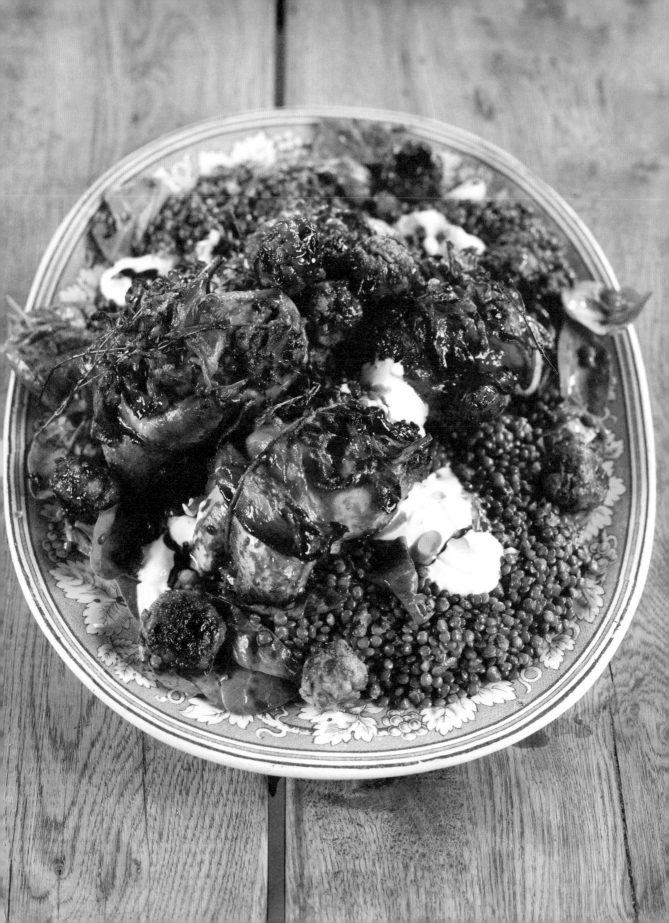

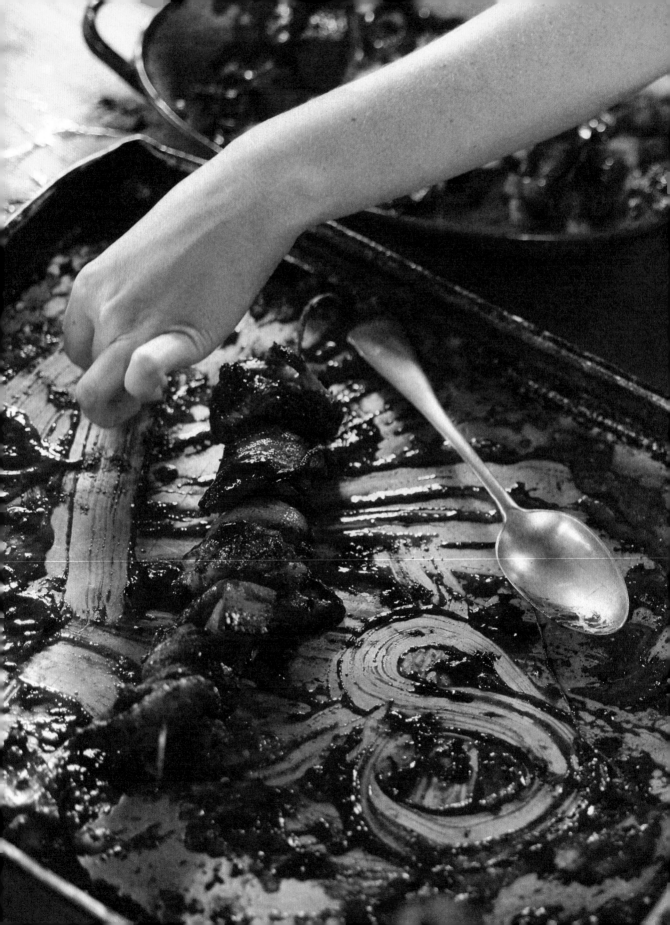

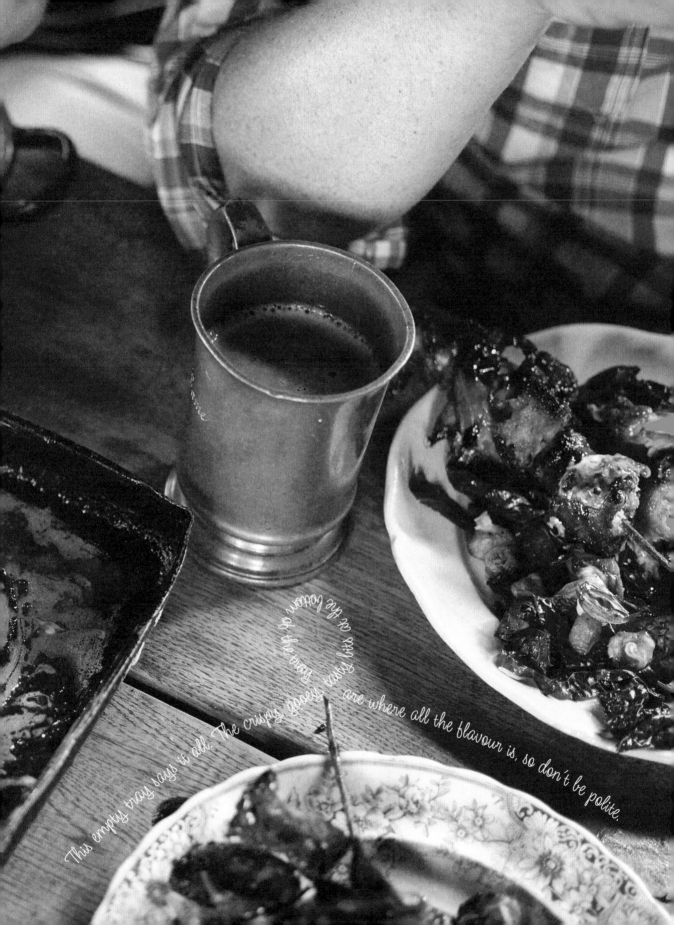

This empty tray says it all. The crispy, gooey, tasty bits from the tray or at the bottom of the tray are where all the flavour is, so don't be polite.

ROAST QUAIL SKEWERS
DELICIOUS SMASHED CELERIAC & FENNEL

The quail may be a small bird, but when it's served like this, a little goes a long way. These skewers can be as humble, or as exciting and surprising, as you like. Take a bit of pride in putting them together and use common sense when you're assembling them, so that things that need more heat, like the legs and thighs, go on the ends and the delicate breasts that need a bit more protection go in the middle of the skewer. Don't jam things on there so tightly that the heat can't circulate and crisp things up. The point of these skewers is that they are good fun to make and even more fun to eat. Get your butcher to divide each quail into two legs and two breasts, through the bone. Tasty and finger-lickin' good.

SERVES 4

- 1 celeriac, trimmed, peeled and cut into 2cm dice
- 1 bulb of fennel, trimmed, peeled and cut into 2cm dice
- a knob of butter
- 2 sprigs of fresh thyme, leaves picked
- olive oil
- sea salt and ground pepper

- 4 quality Cumberland sausages
- 4 rashers of quality thick-cut smoked streaky bacon
- ½ a loaf of sourdough bread
- 1 large pear, or 2 small ones
- 4 quails, jointed
- 8 fresh bay leaves
- 8 cloves of garlic, slightly crushed

- 4 sprigs of fresh rosemary, leaves picked and finely chopped
- 1 whole nutmeg, for grating
- 4 tablespoons runny honey, for drizzling
- cider vinegar
- natural yoghurt, to serve
- 4 long skewers

Preheat the oven to full whack (about 240°C/475°F/gas 9). Put the diced celeriac and fennel into a casserole-type pan with the butter, thyme leaves, a lug of olive oil, a good pinch of salt and pepper and 200ml of water. Leave the lid askew and cook slowly over a medium heat for 1 hour, stirring every 10 minutes and smashing them up a little as you go.

Slice each sausage and bacon rasher into three and put into a mixing bowl. Cut the bread into 2.5cm cubes and add to the bowl. Cut each pear into quarters lengthways, then cut each quarter in half widthways to make 8 chunks. Add the pears to the bowl of meat along with the jointed quails, bay leaves, lightly crushed garlic cloves, chopped rosemary and a good pinch of salt and pepper. Drizzle a few good lugs of olive oil over everything, add a few gratings of nutmeg, then toss to coat everything nicely.

Start and finish each skewer with a quail leg, and basically skewer and alternate and intermingle all those lovely ingredients together (bread, bay leaves, breasts, sausages, pear … you get the idea) so they flavour each other as they cook. Put the skewers on a tray and bang it on the top shelf of the oven (after your smash has had just over 30 minutes) to roast for 20 minutes, turning as needed. When the time is up, take the skewers out of the oven, drizzle the honey and a touch of cider vinegar all over them, then return them to the oven and cook for a few more minutes, or until dark, sticky, beautiful and glazed.

Move the skewers to a serving platter and add a little swig of water to the tray they were cooked in. Quickly scrape and stir all the goodness off the bottom of the pan to make a thickish sauce, then add 3 tablespoons of yoghurt and marble the two together. Drizzle those sticky, lovely pan juices all over and around the skewers. Smash up your celeriac and fennel and serve with some fresh seasonal greens such as spinach, runner beans or broad beans.

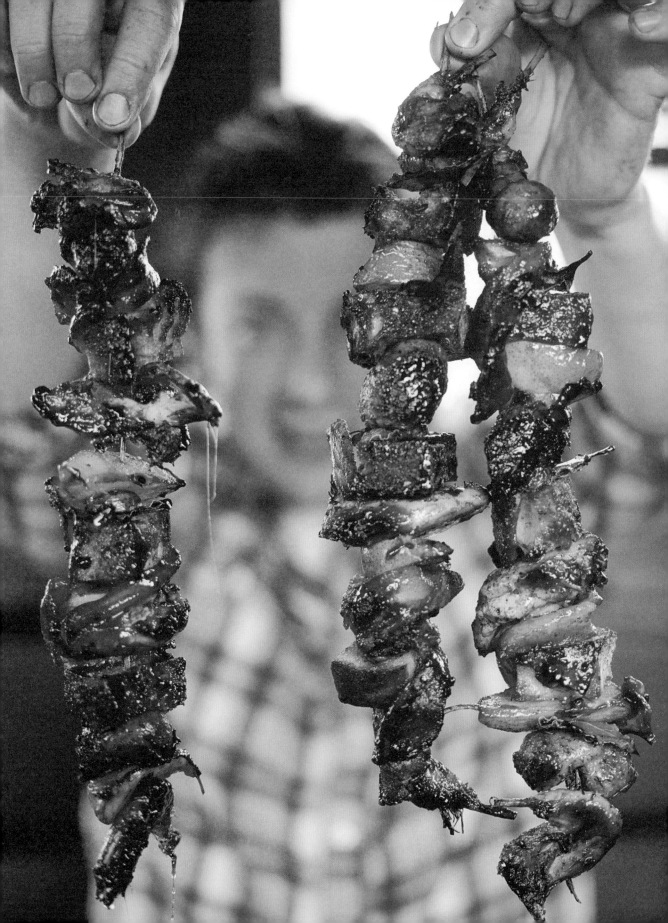

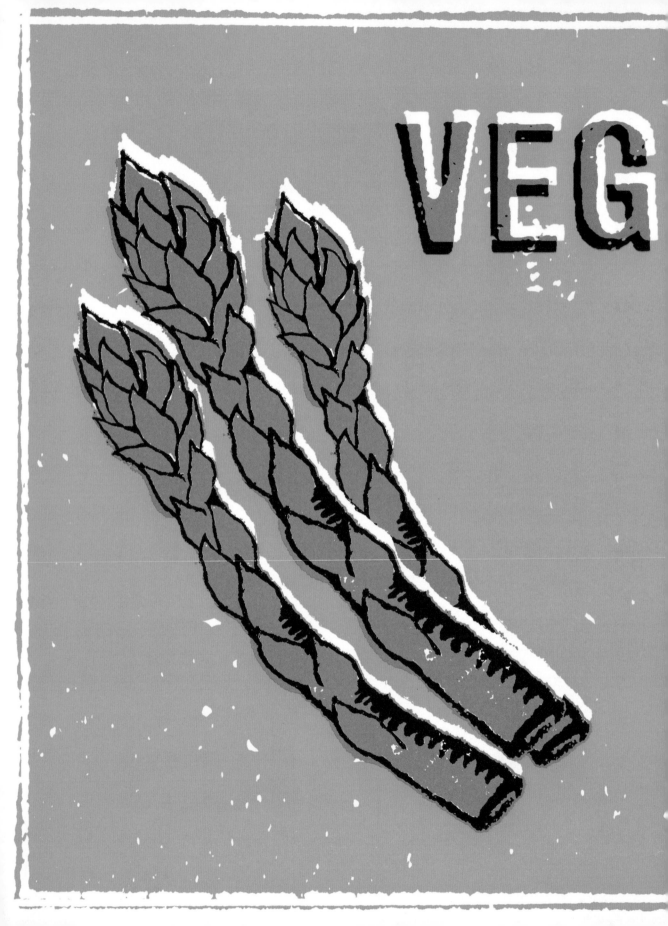

ETABLES

ecause we have four very distinct seasons and spring is often slow in coming, our vegetables have plenty of time to develop their flavours. And when they do come into season, they're an absolute joy to eat. So with this bundle of recipes I'm giving you the things I enjoy cooking and feeding my family over the course of the year. This is all about bigging up great vegetables, making them even more beautiful to eat, and giving you really quick recipes for lovely things like British asparagus, green runner beans, exciting mashes and comforting gratinated sweet leeks or creamed spinach. You can serve these dishes with food from other chapters, but in actual fact some of these recipes are so good you could easily eat them on their own.

RED CABBAGE & CRISPY BACON

What an absolute hero of a cabbage recipe this is. It's dead simple, and by using a food processor to slice the cabbage you create a more delicate vegetable dish. This cooked cabbage is brilliant for cold autumn or winter days, and I actually make a very similar version of this every Christmas. Any leftovers are always great reheated in the two or three days afterwards to pad out all sorts of quick dinners.

SERVES 6 AS A SIDE

- ½ a red cabbage (roughly 800g)
- olive oil
- 6 rashers of quality smoked streaky bacon, finely sliced
- 2 sprigs of fresh rosemary, plus a few extra to serve
- sea salt and ground pepper
- 2 tablespoons golden caster sugar
- red wine vinegar
- a large knob of butter
- runny honey

Get rid of the tatty outer leaves from your cabbage. Trim the base and cut the cabbage into wedges. Run them through the slicing attachment on your food processor, or finely slice them.

Put a large roasting tray on a high heat. Add a good lug of olive oil and the sliced bacon. Strip in the leaves from the rosemary, and add a pinch of salt and a good pinch of pepper. Cook and stir for 5 to 10 minutes, until crisp and lightly golden, then spoon the bacon into a bowl, leaving the fat behind in the tray. Turn the heat down to low, then add the sugar to the tray and keep stirring until it starts to caramelize. Add a couple of good lugs of red wine vinegar, followed by the shredded red cabbage (if the mixture seems to tighten up when you add the vinegar, don't panic, it will sort itself out). Add the crispy bacon, then toss and stir everything together.

At this point, add another splash of red wine vinegar and a generous splash of water to the tray and cover it with tin foil. Leave to tick away over a medium heat for 30 to 40 minutes, stirring every few minutes, until the cabbage is soft and delicious. Add a splash of water now and then, if you think it needs it. Stir in the butter and a few generous drizzles of runny honey, have a taste to check the balance of flavours, season to taste, then serve.

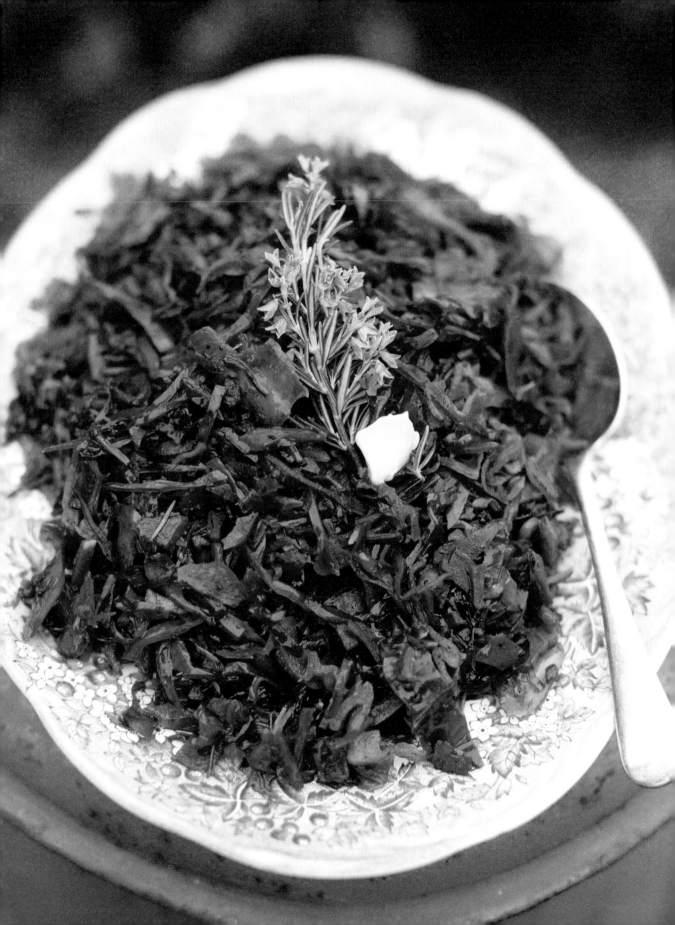

TASTY SHREDDED BRUSSELS

So many people, especially kids, whinge and whine when faced with a plate full of Brussels sprouts, but as far as I'm concerned these humble vegetables have had a bad rap, thanks to too many people cooking the hell out of them and making them sad and soggy. I love and adore them, and for me, this is one of the nicest ways to cook them. It's all about developing an intense flavour base, then cooking the Brussels right at the end so they retain their flavour and stay light, fresh and soft. This is such a simple dish to make, and it goes with literally anything, from fish to white or dark meat. You can even serve any leftovers the next day as a cold and exciting salad. Give it a go. If you're one of the haters, I hope this converts you.

SERVES 6

- olive oil
- 2 quality Cumberland sausages
- 1 white onion, peeled
- a few sprigs of fresh thyme, leaves picked

- 1 heaped teaspoon fennel seeds
- 500g Brussels sprouts, tatty outer leaves removed
- 2 heaped teaspoons runny honey

- 2-3 tablespoons cider vinegar or white wine vinegar
- sea salt and ground pepper

Put a large frying pan on a medium heat and add a splash of olive oil. Once it's hot, squeeze the sausages out of their skins straight into the pan and use a wooden spoon to break up the meat as it fries. Run the peeled onion through the thin slicing attachment of your food processor, or slice it as finely as you can, then add it to the pan with the thyme leaves and fennel seeds. Cook, stir and take care of everything for about 10 minutes, or until you have lovely, golden caramelized onions and small pieces of sausage meat.

Meanwhile, quickly run the sprouts through the same slicing attachment of your food processor (or slice them finely by hand if you absolutely have to). Put aside while you stir the honey and cider vinegar into the pan with a pinch of salt and pepper. Cook for a few more minutes until really golden and sticky (you're in control, you want it golden, not burnt), then sprinkle the sliced sprouts all over the top with a pinch of salt and pepper. Pour in 150ml of water, then cover with a lid or tin foil and leave to simmer on a medium heat for 10 minutes, or until the Brussels are tender and a pleasure to eat. Remove the lid and take the pan to the table, then gently fold the steamed sprouts through the lovely base flavours and serve.

PS: At Christmas time, some dried sour cranberries and chestnuts thrown in is epic!

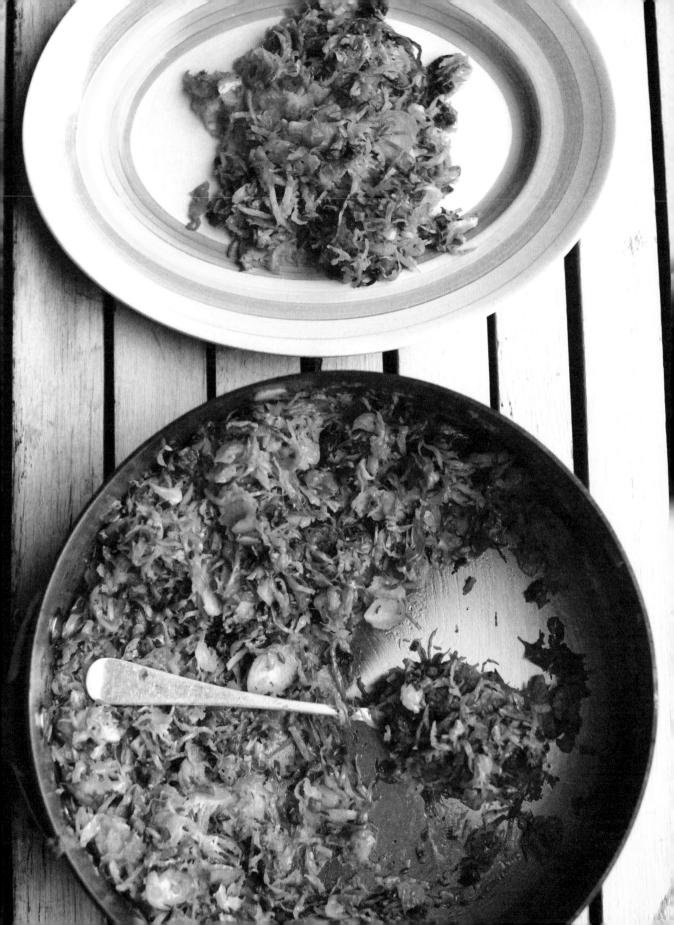

KING OF MASH: IRISH CHAMP

This is possibly one of the best potato recipes in the world. It's completely easy to make, but it's not as simple as just mashing any random flavour into the potatoes. Thanks to our Irish brothers and sisters, we get an infusion of leeks or spring onions simmered in milk with seasoning and herby greens, like wild lovage (which is very similar to yellow celery leaves) or watercress. That, with some good seasoning and a few knobs of butter, and we're talking about an epic cousin of mashed potato. It seems to go with everything, and can be used as a base for cool starters with lovely things like steamed asparagus and soft poached eggs, creamy wild mushrooms, or a few slices of delicate smoked salmon. Basically it's a great veg dish to have up your sleeve.

SERVES 6

- 1kg Maris Piper potatoes
- sea salt and ground pepper
- 2 spring onions
- 1 leek
- 150ml milk
- 1 fresh bay leaf
- 50g butter
- a small handful of watercress
- a small bunch of fresh flat-leaf parsley, leaves picked and roughly chopped
- a small handful of yellow celery leaves or lovage, roughly chopped

Peel the potatoes while you bring a large pan of salted water to the boil. Cut the potatoes into 2.5cm chunks, then add them to the pan and boil them fast for around 12 to 15 minutes, or until tender when poked through with a knife.

While the potatoes are boiling, wash and trim both ends of the spring onions and the leek, then slice them as finely as you can. Pop them into a pan with the milk, bay leaf, a good pinch of salt and pepper and the butter. Bring everything to the boil, then turn down to a gentle simmer and leave to poach and infuse for 7 or 8 minutes.

Once the potatoes are cooked, drain them and leave to steam dry in a colander for a few minutes. Put them back into the pan and use a potato masher to smash them up a bit, mashing in ladlefuls of the incredible infused milk mixture as you go. Once you've added it all, and it's at the consistency you like, have a taste and season again if need be. Roughly chop the watercress, discarding any thick stalks and keeping back a few nice leaves for serving. Stir the chopped leaves through the mash.

Just before you serve, gently bring the champ up to heat with a lid on and stir in the parsley and most of the celery leaves. Sprinkle over the reserved watercress and the rest of the celery leaves and welcome to the land of champ!

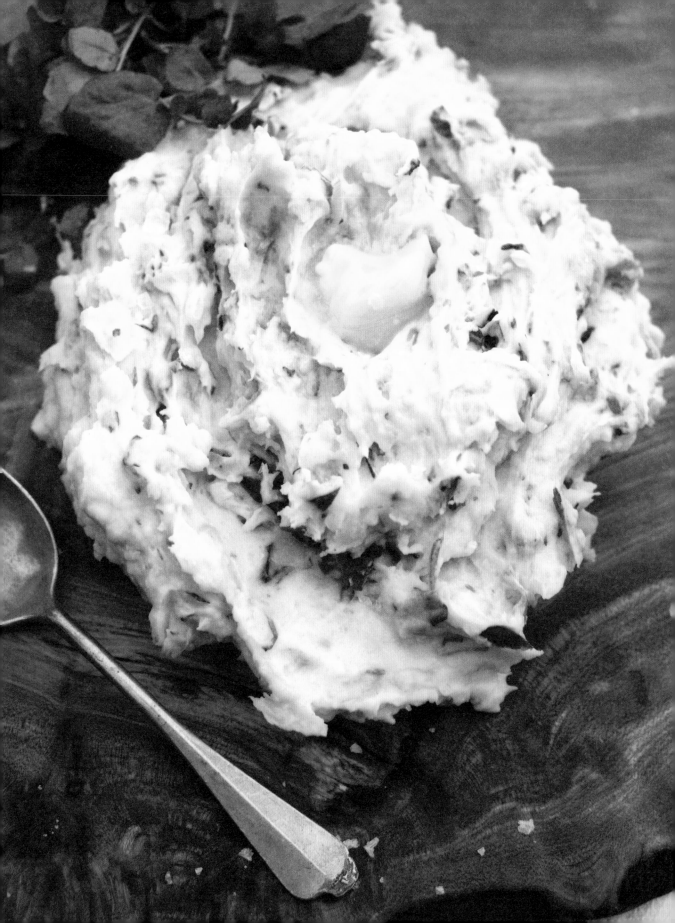

BLANCHED ASPARAGUS
POACHED EGG • FRESH SMOKED SALMON

Believe it or not, for many years poached eggs were just getting me every time. They were busting, or just generally not great … It was really only once I started looking after chickens that I started to get the hang of making them. I think even as a chef I'd been taught to create a vortex in the water then pop the egg into the middle, but if you're cooking for lots of people, that's a pain. So this new way guarantees a perfectly poached pouch of egg every time. The exciting thing is that by simply tying the egg up in clingfilm with a few herbs you can flavour the eggs and have confidence they're going to cook all right.

SERVES 4

- sea salt and ground pepper
- 2 knobs of butter
- 2 lemons
- olive oil
- dried chilli flakes

- inner yellow leaves from 1 head of celery
- a few sprigs of fresh tarragon
- 4 large free-range eggs

- 500g asparagus, woody ends snapped off
- 8 slices of smoked salmon (roughly 240g)

Half-fill a medium-large saucepan with water, season generously with salt and bring to the boil. Instead of putting a lid on, put a large bowl on top but don't let it touch the water. Put the butter, a pinch of salt and pepper and the juice of 1 lemon into the bowl.

This is going to sound cheffy, but it's simple, so bear with me … Tear off 8 sheets of good-quality clingfilm, each roughly 40cm square. Get yourself 4 teacups or small bowls and rub the rims with olive oil. Place a double layer of clingfilm on top of each one and carefully push it in so that it snugly lines the cups. Use your finger to lightly oil the inside – this will help your egg come out easily at the end. Put a tiny pinch of salt, pepper and chilli flakes into each cup then pick the celery and tarragon leaves and divide them between the cups too – try to help these flavours to spread up the sides, if you can.

Carefully crack the egg into the clingfilm, then gently push the yolk down so the egg white surrounds it (without it breaking). Bring the clingfilm up into a bundle, then tie it in a knot and try to squeeze the knot down so it creates a perfect pouch and seals it (imagine a goldfish in a fairground plastic bag). Once the water is boiling, remove the bowl (the butter should be melted now) and place your eggs in the water along with the asparagus. It takes between 5 and 6 minutes at a gentle simmer for a large egg. Place the bowl or a lid back on top and after 3 or 4 minutes remove the asparagus to the bowl of lemony butter and quickly toss.

Meanwhile, arrange 2 pieces of smoked salmon on each plate. Pull out one of your eggs after 5 minutes and have a little feel (it should have a similar texture to fresh mozzarella). If it still seems undercooked, pop it back in for another minute or so.

Neatly divide the asparagus between your plates. Cut off the clingfilm knots with a pair of scissors, peel away the rest, then carefully lift the eggs with a tablespoon and serve them right on top of your asparagus. If you've done a good job, not only will you have perfect poached eggs, but the herbs and seasonings will have cooked into the egg and become one, like a stained glass window, which is really cute. Poke a knife into the egg to let the yolk run, and serve with wedges of lemon on the side.

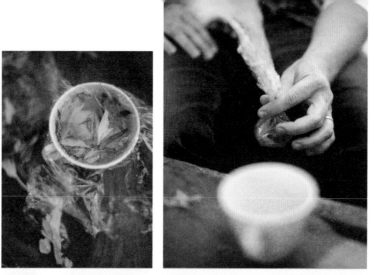

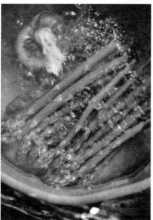

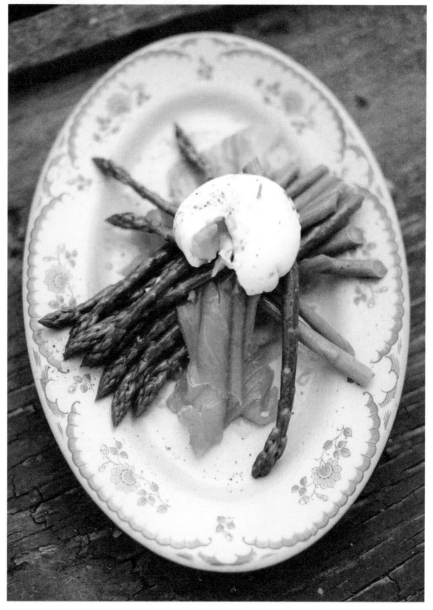

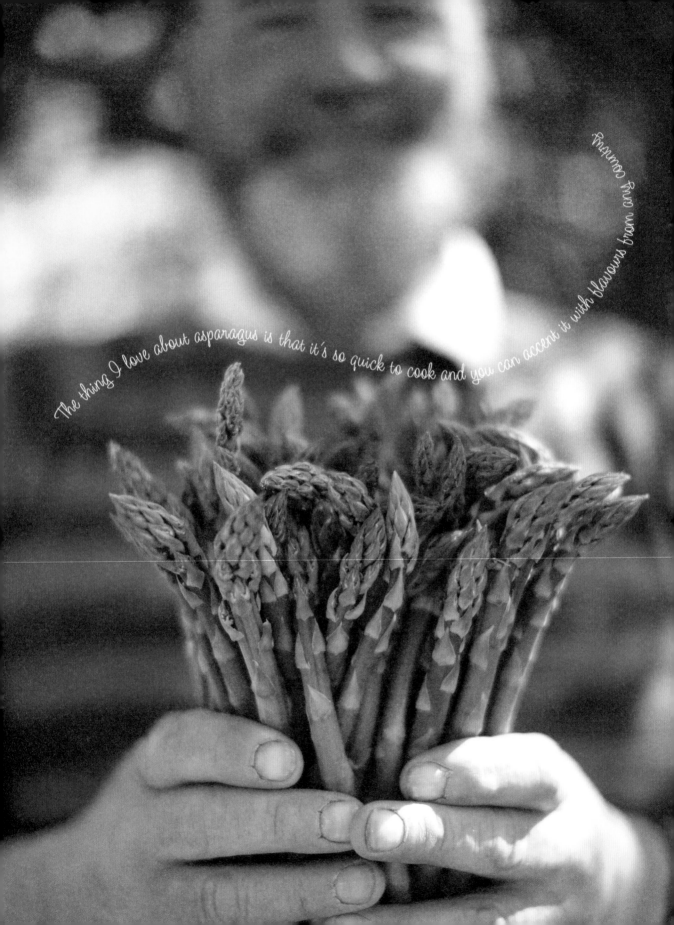

The thing I love about asparagus is that it's so quick to cook and you can accent it with flavours from any country.

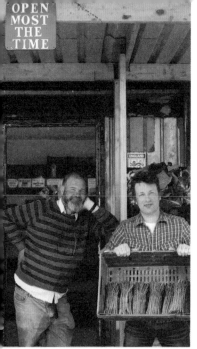

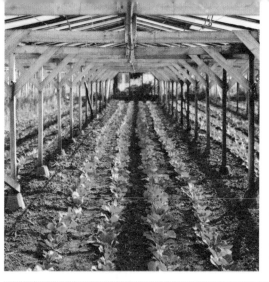

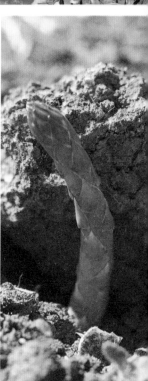

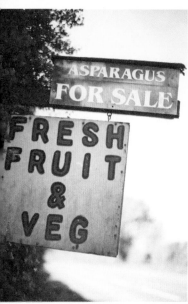

ASPARAGUS
FOR SALE

FRESH
FRUIT
&
VEG

Incredible Asparagus

Billy Byrd is an asparagus farmer, or grass farmer as he calls it, in Evesham, Worcestershire. He grades his beautiful asparagus into sprue, standard and best bunches for competitions. Despite a really dry year, you can see in the pictures how powerful asparagus is as it literally bursts through the ground, lifting up clods of mud in its relentless efforts to get to the sunlight.

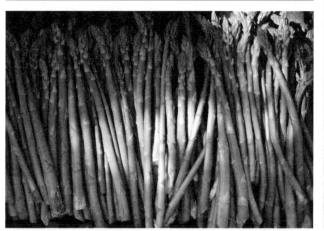

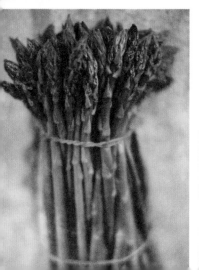

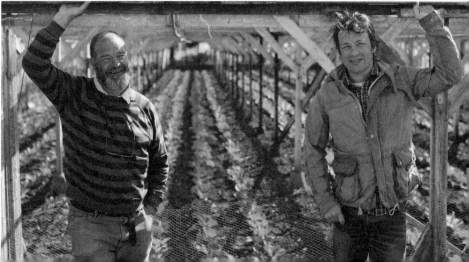

AMAZING ASPARAGUS FOUR WAYS

Asparagus is the first vegetable of spring, and an absolute joy to eat. These quick little recipes are some of my favourite ways to prepare it. Make sure you try them all – they're equally good.

THESE SERVE 4 AS A SIDE OR STARTER

Steamed Asparagus and Quick Tomato Sauce

Bring 2.5cm of water to the boil in a large pan. Meanwhile, pick the leaves from 4 sprigs of **fresh rosemary**, slice 4 rashers of **quality smoked streaky bacon** into matchsticks, and halve 4 **large ripe tomatoes**. Grate the tomato halves cut side down on a fine grater, discarding the skins. Put 500g of washed **asparagus** (woody ends snapped off) into a colander and place over the pan of boiling water. Cover with a lid or tin foil and cook for 3 to 4 minutes, or until just tender. Meanwhile, put a large frying pan on a high heat. Add a lug of **olive oil** and the sliced bacon. Once the bacon is crispy, add the rosemary leaves and cook for about 40 seconds, then remove both to a plate. Add a knob of **butter** to the same pan, then add the tomato, bring to the boil and season well. Move the asparagus to a serving platter, pour over the hot tomato sauce, scatter over the crispy bacon and rosemary and serve.

Worcestershire Asparagus and Mushrooms on Toast

Peel and finely slice 4 cloves of **garlic**. Put a large frying pan on a high heat and add a good lug of **olive oil**. Whack 4 slices of **nice bread** into the toaster. Slice 2 handfuls of **mushrooms** (brushed clean) and 500g of washed **asparagus** (woody ends snapped off) into bite-sized chunks. Add them to the hot pan with the sliced garlic and toss and fry for around 4 minutes. Finely chop a small handful of **fresh flat-leaf parsley** and add most of it to the pan, along with 8 tablespoons of **Worcestershire sauce** and a knob or two of **butter**. Take the pan off the heat and shake and stir around for 30 seconds, or until the sauce has reduced down. Season to taste, then spoon over the slices of hot toast and top with the rest of the parsley.

Lemon Buttered Grilled Asparagus and Shaved Lancashire Cheese

Put your griddle pan on a high heat. Place 500g of washed **asparagus** (woody ends snapped off) on the dry griddle pan. Turn and lightly char on both sides until just tender (roughly 2 to 3 minutes on each side), then toss in a large bowl with a knob of **butter**, a good squeeze of **lemon juice** and a pinch of **salt and pepper**. Divide between plates or serve on a big platter. Toss 2 large handfuls of **salad leaves** with a little **extra virgin olive oil**, a pinch of **salt and pepper** and a good squeeze of **lemon juice**. Use a speed-peeler to shave over a nice crumbly **British cheese like Lancashire or Ticklemore**, and serve.

Minted Raw Asparagus Salad with Baby Spinach and Fresh Garden Peas

Put 2 large handfuls of washed **baby spinach leaves** and 2 large handfuls of freshly podded **spring peas** into a salad bowl. Finely slice a handful of **fresh mint leaves** and add to the bowl, then use a speed-peeler to shave 8 large spears of raw washed **asparagus** (woody ends snapped off) into ribbons. Season with a good pinch of **salt and pepper**. Squeeze in the juice of 1 **lemon**, and drizzle over three times as much **extra virgin olive oil**. Crumble over a small handful of **soft goat's cheese**, then toss and serve on a platter. The peas always fall to the bottom of the bowl, so pick them up, scatter them over the top and serve.

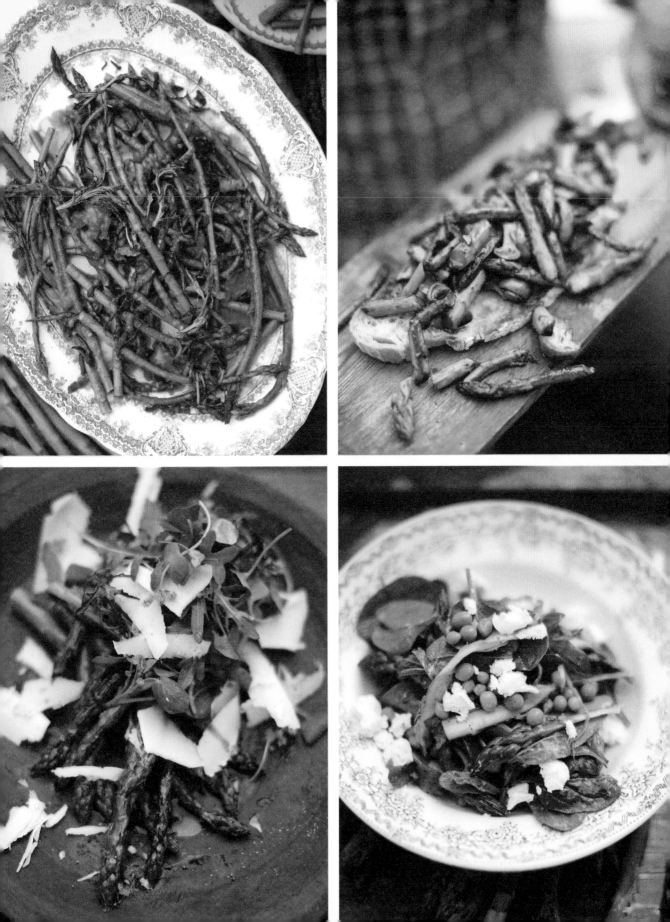

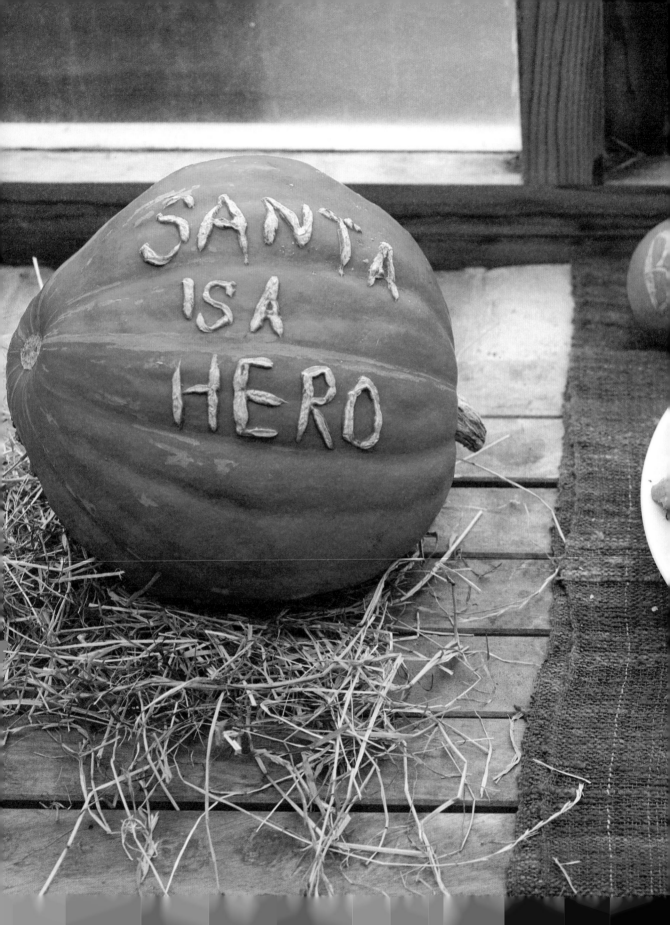

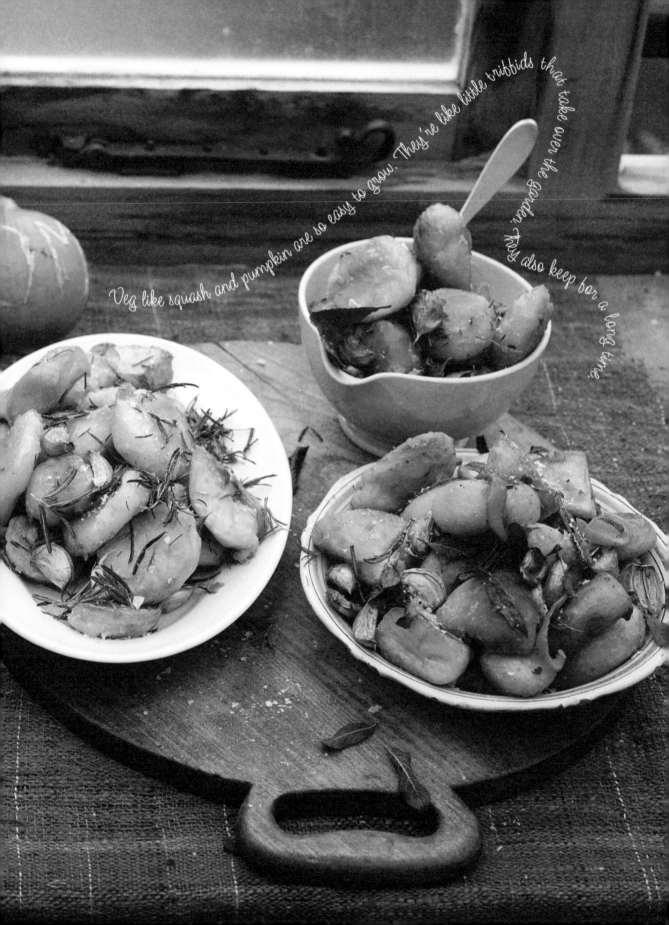

Veg like squash and pumpkin are so easy to grow. They're like little triffids that take over the garden. They also keep for a long time

CREAMY CRUNCHY LEEKS

If you're looking for a straightforward way to make a gratin, this is a goodie and a great vehicle for bigging up all sorts of veg, from thinly sliced fennel or celeriac to baby turnips, shallots and even spring onions. Every family feast should include a few really good vegetable side dishes, and if one of those side dishes happens to be crispy, rich, bubbling and lovely like this one, that can only be a good thing.

SERVES 4 AS A SIDE

- 1 rasher of quality smoked streaky bacon, finely sliced
- 2 tablespoons rapeseed or olive oil
- 1 fresh bay leaf
- 350g baby leeks

- sea salt and ground pepper
- 250ml organic chicken stock
- 5 tablespoons single cream
- 50g Caerphilly, Cheddar or any delicious cheese, crumbled
- 1 clove of garlic, peeled

- 3 thick slices of stale white bread, crusts removed
- a small bunch of fresh thyme, leaves picked

Preheat the oven to 200°C/400°F/gas 6. Put a medium-sized pan on a medium heat. Put the bacon, the oil and the bay leaf into the pan, and fry for a few minutes until lightly golden.

While that's happening, top and tail the leeks, trim and pull back any tough leaves, split the leeks lengthways in half, then wash well. Slice them into 2cm pieces and add them to the pan. Stir together, season generously with salt and pepper, then pour in the stock and cream, bring to the boil, and simmer for around 10 minutes. At that point, turn the heat off and stir in most of the cheese (remove any rind first). The mixture will still be quite runny at this point, but don't worry, it will thicken up in the oven. Meanwhile, put the garlic and bread into a food processor with the thyme leaves and pulse until you have nice coarse flavoured breadcrumbs.

If your pan is ovenproof you can simply pop it straight into the oven; if not, decant the creamy leeks into a shallow earthenware dish (roughly 20 x 25cm). Sprinkle over the incredible breadcrumbs and crumble over the remaining cheese, and cook on the top shelf of the oven for around 30 to 40 minutes, or until golden and crispy. Serve with absolutely anything you like.

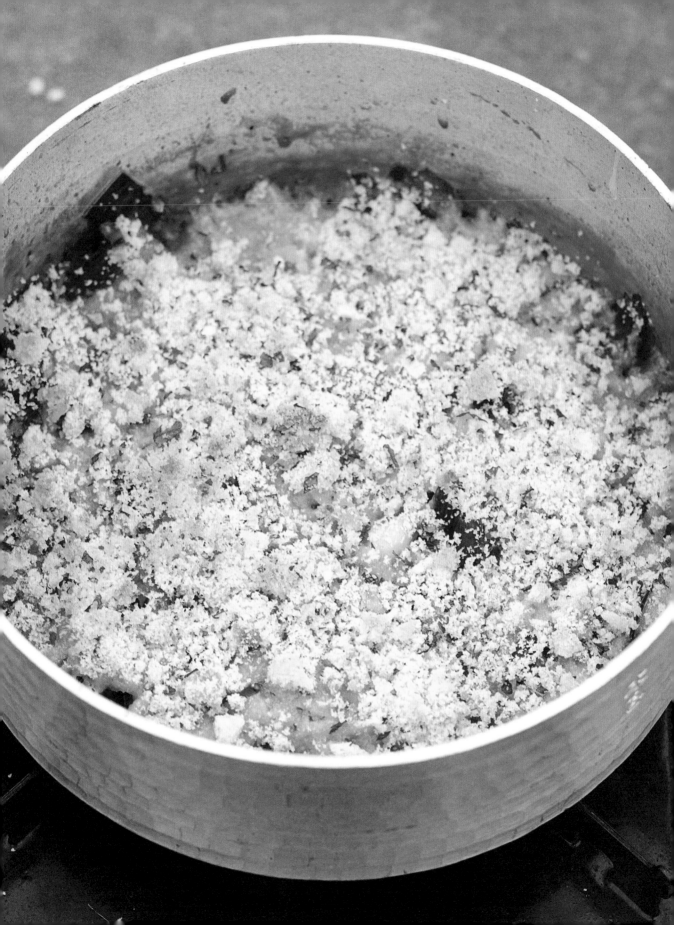

KILLER GREEN BEANS
... ON AN AWESOME SPICY TOMATO SAUCE

For some reason, I'm completely besotted with runner beans. The gardener of King Charles I brought them to Britain in the 1600s from Central America. They were actually grown as a pretty plant before we started tucking into them, but now we love them. They're only really available for a couple of months each year, so they're definitely worth making a fuss over, and to be honest, I think they're fairly underrated. There's no doubt that they're delicious served simply with a knob of butter and a pinch of salt, but it's really nice to do other things with them too. I've gone for a saucy base to toss the just-cooked beans through, but you could also braise them in butter, garlic and chilli with a load of other beautiful greens.

SERVES 4 TO 6

- 6 medium-sized ripe tomatoes
- 3 spring onions, trimmed
- 3 anchovy fillets in oil
- a knob of butter
- olive oil
- sea salt and ground pepper
- 450g runner beans
- extra virgin olive oil

Halve your tomatoes, then carefully grate them, cut side down, on a box grater so you get a kind of bruised tomato slurry. Discard the skin left behind. Finely slice the spring onions and anchovies. Put them into a hot frying pan with the butter, a lug of olive oil and a pinch of salt and pepper. Jiggle the pan about for a bit, then add the grated tomato. As it comes to the boil, season to taste, then turn the heat down to a simmer and cook for 5 to 8 minutes, until it starts to thicken a little, then turn off the heat. (Feel free to liven things up with a swig of Worcestershire sauce or Tabasco at this point if you like.)

While your sauce is cooking, put a large pan of salted water on to boil and push the runner beans through a bean slicer (they only cost a quid or two and are worth having if you don't already). Boil them hard and fast for about 4 minutes, or until tender and a pleasure to eat. Drain them, and quickly bring the tomato sauce back up to the boil. Pour the sauce on to a platter and use tongs to place the beans right on top. Drizzle over a little extra virgin olive oil and serve right away. Let your guests toss everything together at the table.

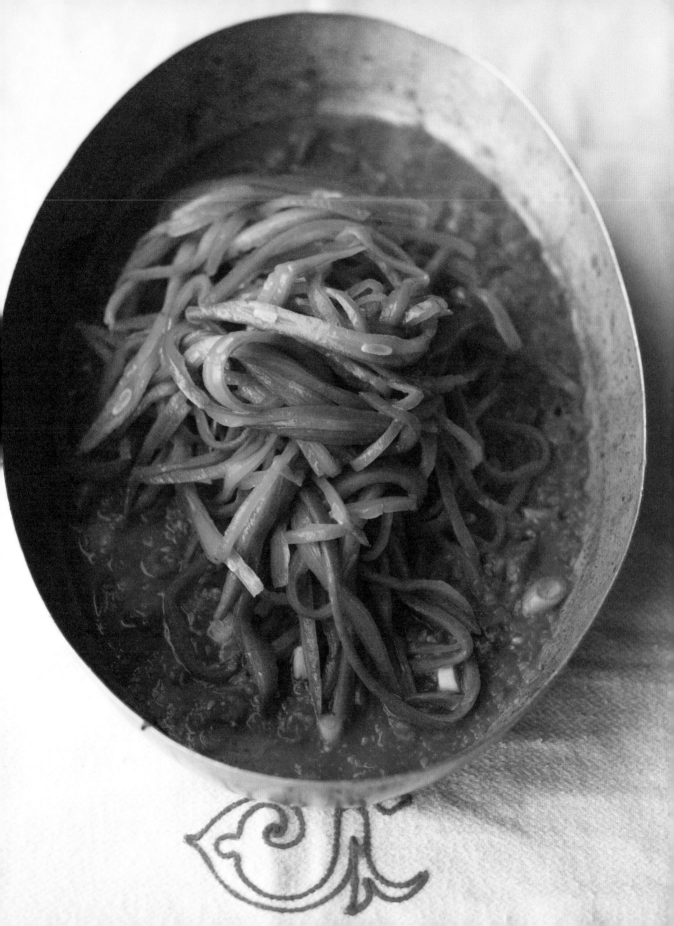

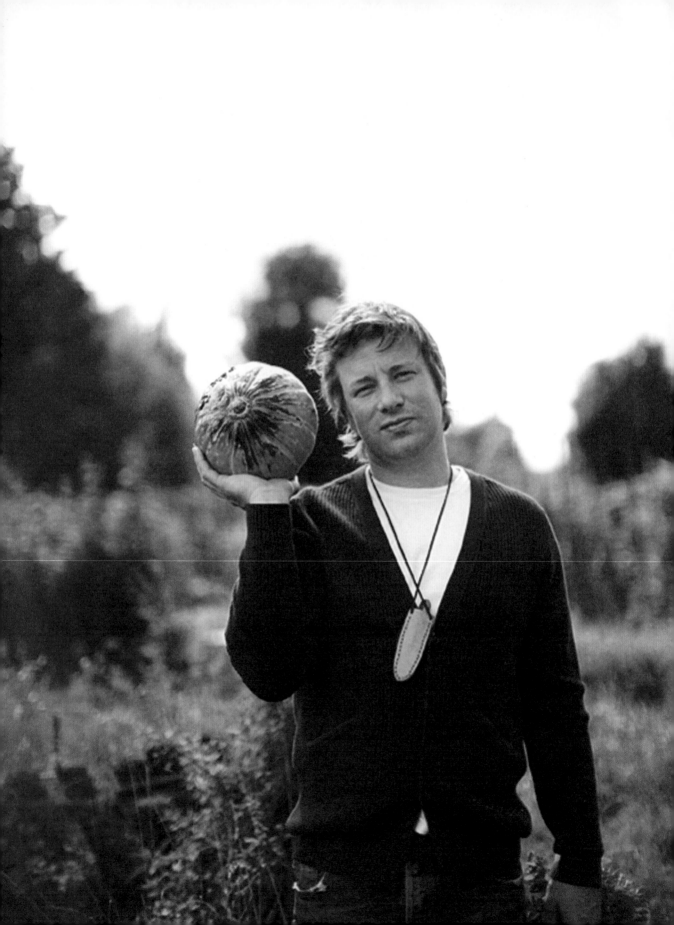

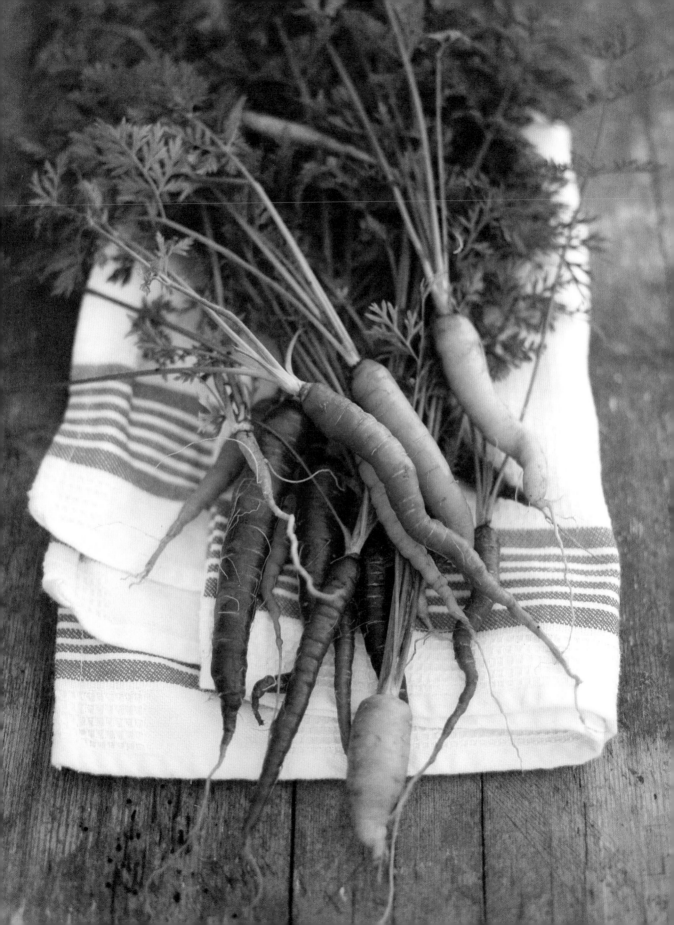

SPEEDY BUTTER BEANS

This is a really simple, convenient bean dish to knock out if you ever get caught for time but want something delicious to serve next to grilled meats or chicken. It can pretty much embrace any greens or soft herbs, whether it's chard, kale, cabbage, or even chopped rocket, parsley or basil, so feel free to switch it up depending on what you have.

SERVES 6 TO 8 AS A SIDE

- 2 x 540g jars of butter beans
- sea salt and ground pepper
- 12 cherry tomatoes, quartered
- a knob of butter
- white wine vinegar
- 1 tablespoon sun-dried tomato paste
- Tabasco sauce
- 100g baby spinach, chard or shredded cabbage

Tip the beans and their juices into a pan on a medium high heat. Add a good pinch of salt, bring to the boil, then turn the heat down and simmer for a few minutes. Add the tomatoes to the pan with a knob of butter, a swig of white wine vinegar, the tomato paste and a splash or two of Tabasco. Mash a few of the beans with a potato masher or a hand blender and stir them back into the rest, to give the whole dish a lovely creaminess. Bring back to the boil, then lower the heat and simmer for 10 minutes, or until the sauce has thickened and is tasty and delicious.

Just before you're ready to serve, throw in the greens and let them wilt down. Spinach only needs 1 minute, but if you're using chard give it 2 minutes, and shredded cabbage will need around 5 minutes. Just use your instincts, then check the seasoning and serve.

PS: Another great thing to do with this dish is to add the greens, then decant everything into a nice ovenproof dish, sprinkle over some breadcrumbs and a tiny bit of freshly grated cheese, and gratinate in the oven at 180°C/350°F/gas 4 until golden and bubbling.

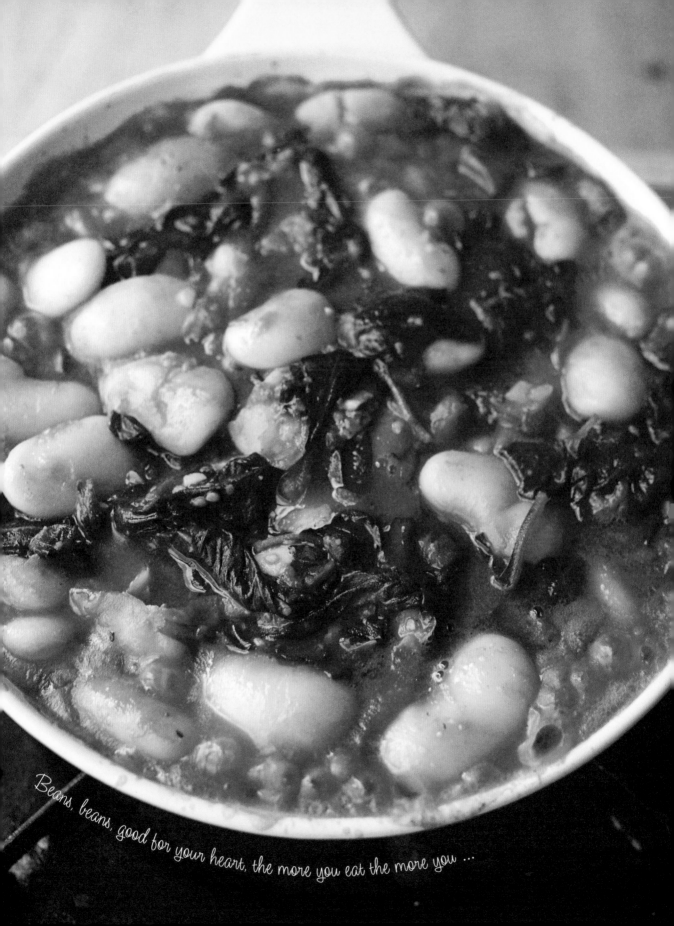

Beans, beans, good for your heart, the more you eat the more you ...

MASHED POTATO FOUR WAYS

Neeps and Tatties

Fill a large pan with cold water, add a good pinch of **sea salt** and put it on a high heat. Peel 1 large **swede** (roughly 1kg), and cut it into 2cm chunks. Once the water is boiling, add the swede and cook for 15 minutes. Meanwhile, peel 1kg of **potatoes** and cut them into 2.5cm chunks. When the 15 minutes is up, add the potatoes and cook for a further 10 to 15 minutes, or until everything is soft and cooked through. Drain, leave to steam dry for a minute, then mash with a good pinch of salt and **white pepper** and a knob of **butter**.

Potato and Smashed Fennel with Crispy Thyme Breadcrumbs

Fill a large pan with cold water, add a good pinch of **sea salt** and put it on a high heat. Pick the herby tops off 5 **fennel bulbs** and put aside. Trim off the base of each bulb, as well as any stalks or woody bits, and cut each one into 10 wedges. Peel 1kg of **potatoes** and cut them into 2.5cm chunks. Once the water is boiling, add the fennel and potatoes and cook for 15 to 20 minutes, or until tender. Meanwhile, fry a handful of **breadcrumbs** with a little **olive oil** in a non-stick pan on a high heat for 3 to 5 minutes. As they crisp up, throw in a small handful of picked **thyme leaves** and remove from the heat. Drain the veg and let them steam dry for a minute, then mash up with a good pinch of salt and pepper and a few knobs of **butter**. Scatter over the crispy breadcrumbs, and fennel tops and drizzle over a little **extra virgin olive oil**.

Potato and Celeriac Smash

Fill a large pan with cold water, add a good pinch of **sea salt** and put it on a high heat. You need to buy roughly a 1.4kg **celeriac** to get 1kg for the smash. Trim and peel the celeriac and peel 1kg of **potatoes**, then cut everything into 2.5cm chunks. Once the water is boiling, add the celeriac and potatoes and cook for 15 to 20 minutes, or until everything is soft and cooked through. Drain in a colander, leave to steam dry for a minute, then return the veg to the empty pan and have a good old mash up. Add a little swig of **single cream**, a knob of **butter**, and a good pinch of salt and **pepper**. Have a taste and correct the seasoning, then pop the lid on to keep it warm. If you like your mash really smooth, pop it into a food processor and pulse until smooth, but don't blitz it too much, otherwise it will go gluey and wet.

Potato and Rustic Jerusalem Artichoke with Bay Oil

Fill a large pan with cold water, add a good pinch of **sea salt** and put it on a high heat. Peel 1kg of **potatoes** and cut them into 2.5cm chunks. Chop the top and bottom off 1kg of **Jerusalem artichokes**, then peel and chop them into 2cm chunks - adding them to the water as you go. Cook for 5 minutes, then add the potatoes and cook for around 15 to 20 minutes, or until tender. Drain, and leave to steam dry. Meanwhile, bash 2 **bay leaves** and a pinch of salt to a pulp in a pestle and mortar. Remove the stalks, then muddle in 4 tablespoons of **olive oil** and a swig of **white wine vinegar**. Mix together, taste and season, and put aside. Put the drained veg back into the pan, then crudely smash up with a few good knobs of **butter** and a good pinch of salt and **pepper**. Serve with the bay oil drizzled all over.

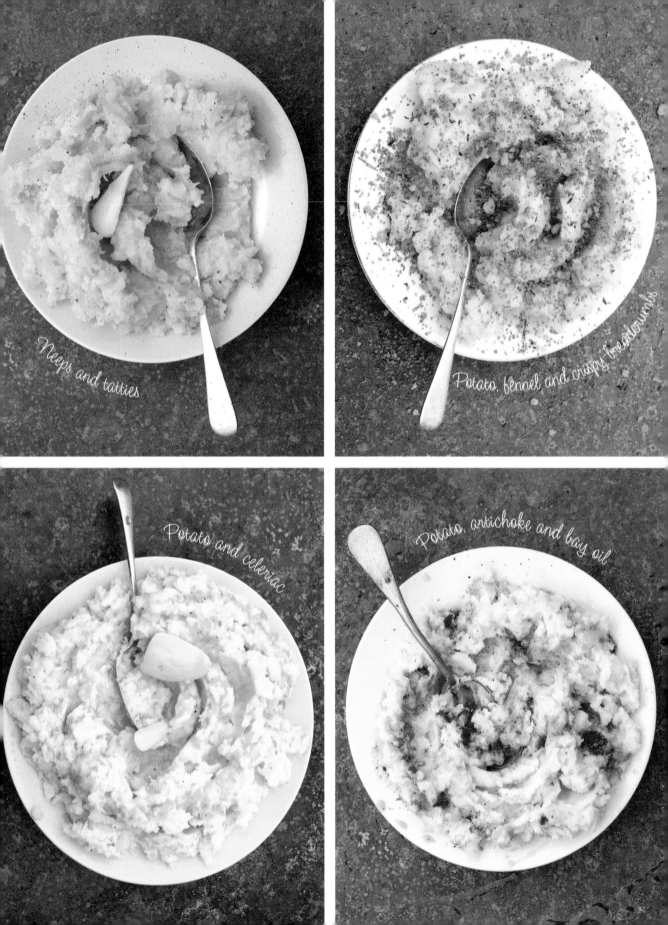

Neeps and tatties

Potato, fennel and crispy breadcrumbs

Potato and celeriac

Potato, artichoke and bay oil

BAKED CREAMED SPINACH

This is a win-win dish – it's not hard in the slightest to make, but the results are golden, bubbling and delicious. It's especially nice with grilled meat or chicken. You can make it with cabbage, Swiss chard, peas, broad beans and, believe it or not, even escarole or iceberg lettuce … basically anything green! Although I love spinach when it's fresh, many chefs will tell you that the best creamed spinach is made with frozen spinach, and I won't disagree. It's dehydrated and dense already, so you get a really nice, super-intense creaminess. Enjoy.

SERVES 6 AS A SIDE

- olive oil
- a large knob of butter
- 4 cloves of garlic
- 1 red onion
- 1 medium-sized tomato

- 1 whole nutmeg, for grating
- 450g frozen spinach, or 3 x 200g bags of washed baby spinach
- 150ml single cream

- 50g breadcrumbs
- 50g Cheddar cheese
- sea salt and ground pepper

Turn the oven grill to high. Put a drizzle of olive oil into a large saucepan on a medium heat and add the butter. Peel and slice the garlic and onion as finely as you can. Add the sliced garlic and onion to the pan and cook for around 5 minutes, or until softened but not coloured. Finely chop and add the tomato, then finely grate over a quarter of the nutmeg.

Cook everything over a medium heat for a further 5 minutes, or until soft and beautiful, then add the spinach, a small splash of water and the cream, if you're using fresh spinach you'll need to add it in batches, letting each one wilt down a bit before adding more. Place a lid on the pan and simmer slowly for 5 minutes, stirring occasionally. When everything looks thick and lovely, pour it into a snug-fitting ovenproof dish or pan (about 22cm x 15cm, and 6cm deep).

Sprinkle over the breadcrumbs and grate over the cheese, then put the dish under the grill and let it bubble away for 5 to 8 minutes, or until just golden and gorgeous.

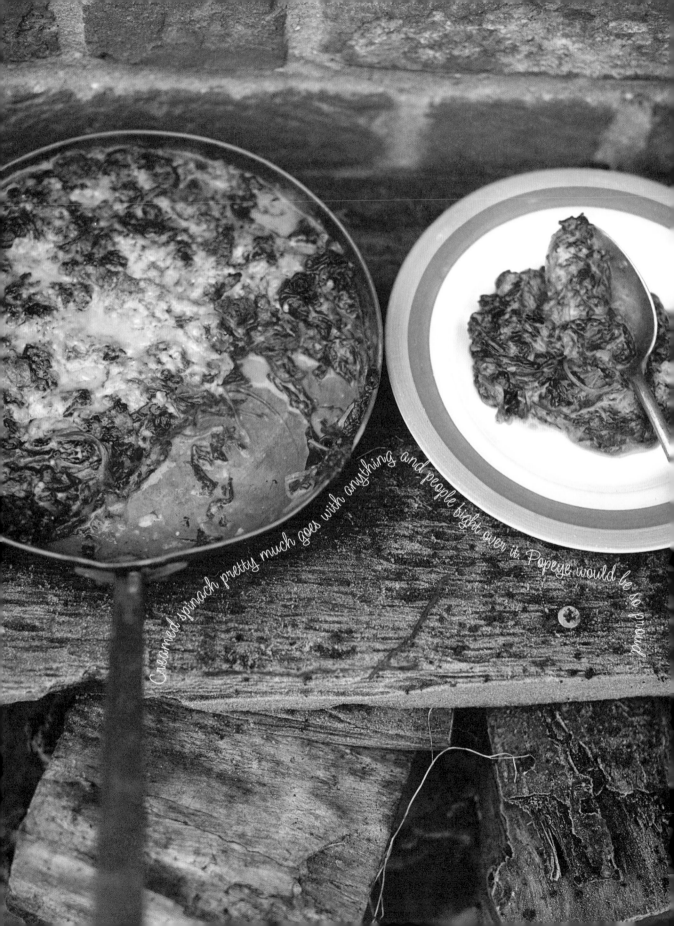

Creamed spinach pretty much goes with anything and people fight over it. Popeye would be so proud.

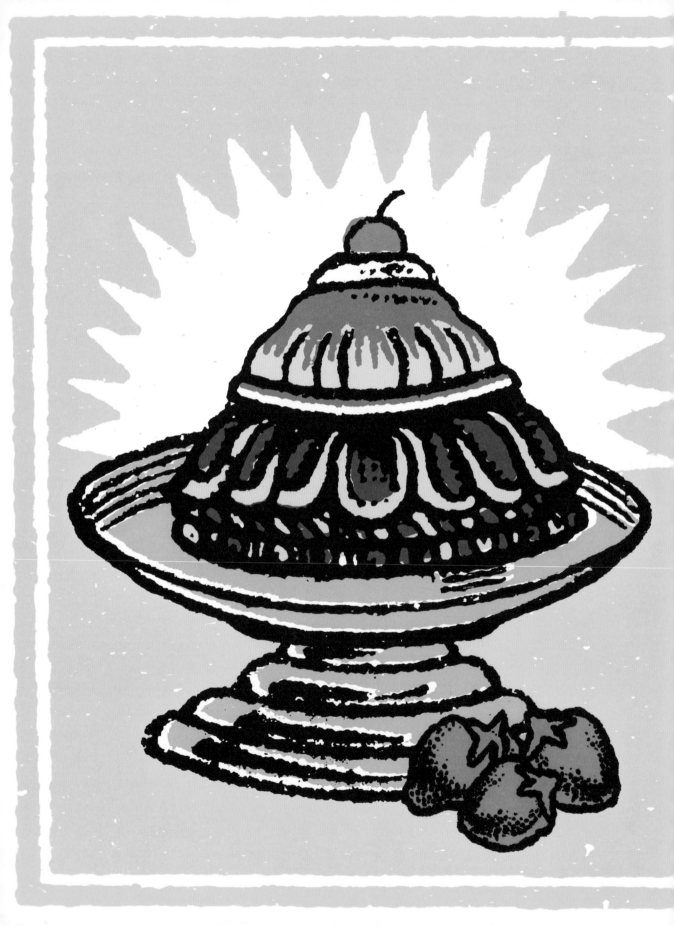

Puddings

For me, British puddings are some of the most informal, yet luxurious desserts in the world. There's something joyful, gregarious and in your face about them. I think their flavours are the best in the world, though admittedly many of the spices we love to use in our puddings have come to us from other countries. One of the things I love most about our desserts is that they're not particularly hard to make, and not so accurate or precise that you feel you have to be on your best behaviour when you tuck into them. The word 'pudding' is now a sort of generic word for dessert, but the true definition of a pudding is something large, wobbly, heroic and wonderful! There are a few of those things in this chapter (my mum's retro trifle is definitely one of them) – but I've also included a few other beauties that will make everyone cheer when you put them on the table. It goes without saying that these are treats – but every once in a while, a spoonful or two of something beautiful won't do you any harm.

ELDERFLOWER SUMMER PUDDING
... A CRACKING DESSERT FOR TOM, ALICE & THIBAULT AEDY

Tom, Alice and Thibault (or 'Thibs') have very cool parents who made a lovely donation at an event benefiting the Ecology Trust, The Aspinall Foundation and The Rainforest Foundation this year. Because I happen to know their whole family are fans of another berry dessert of mine, I've dedicated this recipe to them. The British summer is something we all look forward to, and if this pudding is made during a month when all the fruit is at its best it will be a total joy. If you want to add blackcurrants, mulberries or little wild strawberries to the mix, feel free. You don't want to cook the fruit completely, you just want to encourage the juices out of the berries so they bleed through the white bread. It's totally easy to assemble this type of pudding once you've seen it done, so go and watch a quick tutorial at *www.jamieoliver.com/how-to* before you get started.

SERVES 8 TO 10

- olive oil
- a loaf of nice white bread
- 4 tablespoons seedless blackcurrant jelly or jam
- 1kg mixture of fresh strawberries, raspberries and blackberries
- 4 ripe peaches
- 1 bay leaf
- 100g caster sugar
- 1 vanilla pod, halved lengthways, seeds scraped out
- 2 oranges
- 1 lemon
- elderflower cordial
- *optional:* clotted cream or ice cream, to serve

Rub a 1.5 litre pudding bowl with a little olive oil, then line it with 2 long sheets of clingfilm, crisscrossed so there are no gaps inside the bowl and there is quite a bit of overhang. Cut 12 slices of bread, each about 1cm thick, and remove the crusts. Smear one side of each slice with a thick layer of jelly or jam, then press 10 slices into the pudding bowl, jam side up, overlapping them as you go, so there are no gaps. Save 2 slices for the top.

Put a small handful of the prettiest-looking berries into the fridge for garnishing the pudding the next day. Hull the strawberries, cut any larger ones in half, then put them into a medium-large saucepan with the rest of your berries. Halve and stone the peaches, then tear them into little pieces and add to the pan with the bay leaf, the sugar and the vanilla pod and seeds. Squeeze in the juice of the oranges and lemon and stir over a medium heat for around 5 minutes.

Once the fruit has softened a little, discard the bay leaf and vanilla pod and use a slotted spoon to transfer the fruit to the lined pudding bowl. After each spoonful, drizzle in 1 tablespoon of elderflower cordial (you want about 4 tablespoons in total). Push everything down firmly with the back of the spoon to really compact it, then put the saucepan with the cooking juices aside. Lay the remaining 2 slices of bread, jam side down, on top of the pudding, and plug any gaps with more bread, if needed. Gently press down on the top, and pull the overhanging clingfilm over to cover. Place a small plate that fits within the diameter of the bowl on top of the pudding and put something heavy, like a mortar or a few tins of something, on top. Put it into the fridge overnight to set and firm up. Pour the leftover juices from the pan through a sieve into a small pan and simmer gently for around 8 to 10 minutes, or until you have a glossy syrup. Pour it into a little jug, leave to cool, then cover and put into the fridge.

The next day, peel the clingfilm off the top and turn the pudding out on to a serving plate. Gently coax it out of the bowl using the clingfilm, but have patience - it will all be worth it. Peel away the clingfilm, drizzle over some of the cold syrup from the jug, and sprinkle over the reserved fresh berries. Serve with some clotted cream or ice cream and enjoy!

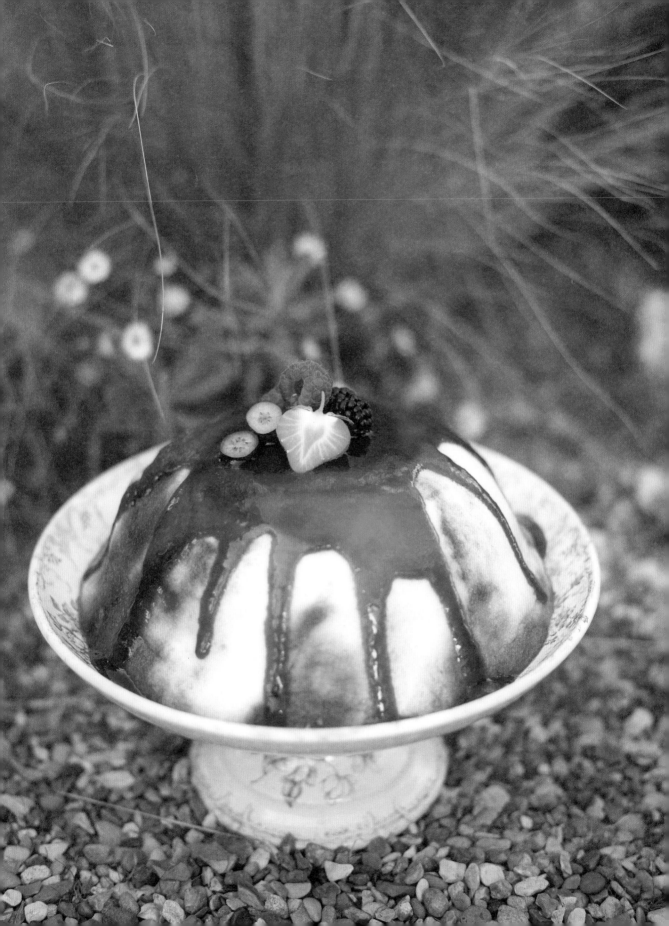

PERFECT POACHED PEARS
BRAMBLE SAUCE • THICK CLOTTED CREAM

Some people say it's hard for fruit-based desserts to hit that pleasure spot in the same way a cake or pudding can, but honestly these poached pears with this syrupy brambley sauce are really heavenly, and actually very convenient for something like a dinner party. The brambles (raspberries or blackberries, as they are also known) add a richness and gentle acidity that works so well with the sweet pears, but you can also use mulberries or bilberries. Plus, they look like little jewels on the platter, so you'll earn points for presentation, which is never a bad thing. At the beginning of spring, brambles start popping up all over country roads and hedgerows, and picking your own when the fruit ripens in autumn is awesome. So keep your eyes open and use wild-picked ones if you can. A little tip for you if you're picking your own fruit is to add just a few bramble leaves to the syrup – this somehow seems to unleash even more of their flavour. Try it.

SERVES 8

- 1 litre good-quality apple juice or apple cider
- 200g demerara sugar
- 3 or 4 fresh bay leaves
- 1 vanilla pod, halved lengthways, seeds scraped out
- 2 cloves
- 1 small lemon or orange
- 8 firm pears (the blush varieties are lovely)
- 150g brambles
- *optional:* clotted cream, whipped cream, ice cream or custard, to serve

In a deep-sided pan, heat the apple juice or apple cider and the sugar together on a high heat with the bay leaves, the vanilla pod and seeds, the cloves and a few strips of peel cut from the lemon or orange. Cook for 5 minutes, or until the sugar has dissolved into a light, thin syrup.

While that's happening, carefully peel the pears so they look beautiful, leaving their stalks on if you can. Take the pan off the heat and sit the pears inside, taking care not to splash the hot syrup but making sure the pears get covered. Scrunch and wet a piece of greaseproof paper and place it on top of the pears, forming a sort of lid, so they are completely covered. Turn the heat down to low and simmer slowly for about 20 minutes, or until the pears are lovely and soft but still holding their shape nicely. To test whether they're done, just poke one with a small knife until you hit the core – if the knife slides in easily, they're good to go.

Carefully move the pears to the middle of a cute serving platter using a slotted spoon, and just pop in the oven at the lowest temperature to keep warm. Turn the heat under the pan up to high and reduce the syrup down for 30 minutes, or until it's just thick enough to coat the back of a spoon. Stir it occasionally to make sure it isn't catching. At this point, add the brambles and cook for 5 minutes, or until the syrup turns an amazing colour. To serve, take the platter out of the oven and carefully pour the bramble syrup all over the top of the pears. Blob some clotted cream, whipped cream or ice cream on the side, then put right in the middle of the table.

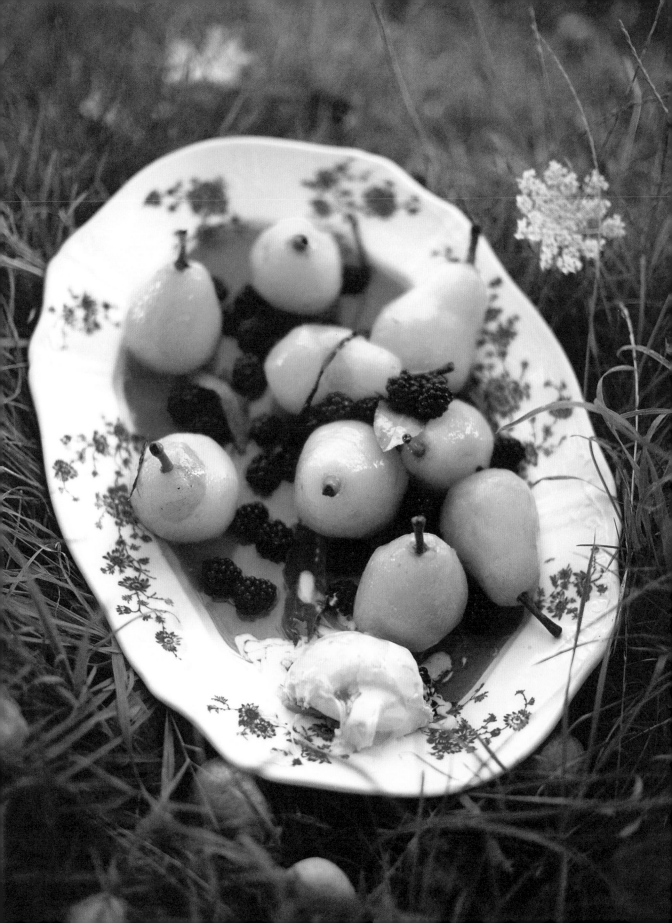

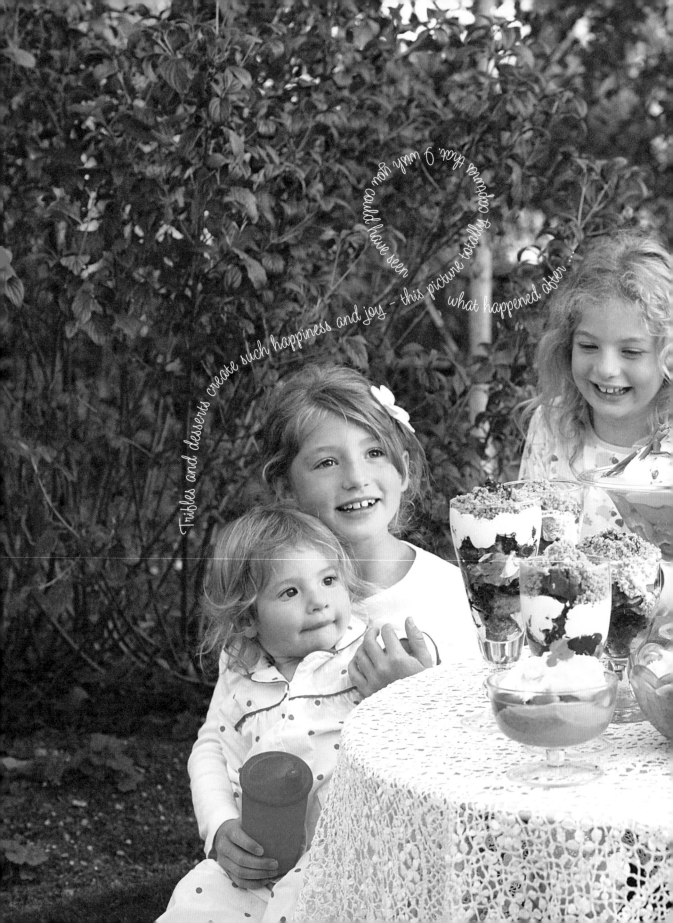

Trifles and desserts create such happiness and joy – this picture totally captured that. I wish you could have seen what happened after...

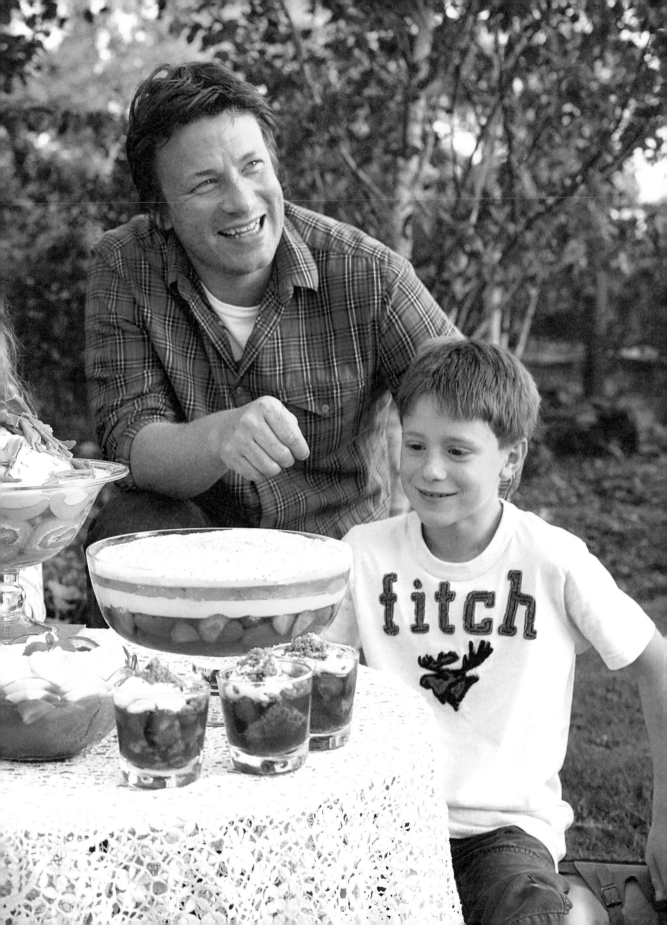

JOYFUL TRIFLES

Both of these trifles are an absolute joy. My mum's retro trifle is a blast from my past. It uses some iconic products from my childhood and just looking at it makes me feel like a kid again. The Wimbledon trifle is my fun homage to one of our great sporting institutions.

My Mum's Retro Trifle

SERVES 14

- 1 x 440g vanilla Swiss roll, sliced 2cm thick
- 500g strawberries, hulled and sliced
- 125ml Cointreau
- 1 x 135g packet of strawberry jelly

- 630ml full-fat milk
- 4 teaspoons golden caster sugar
- 1 x 35g sachet of strawberry blancmange
- 3 x 298g tins of mandarin segments, drained
- 1 x 135g packet of orange jelly

- 500ml ready-made Bird's Custard
- 300ml double cream
- 1 teaspoon vanilla extract

To serve
- cute sprinkles

Lay the slices of Swiss roll all over the bottom of a glass trifle dish (roughly 30cm wide), overlapping them. Scatter over the strawberries, then drizzle over the Cointreau. Dissolve the strawberry jelly in 300ml of boiling water, then add 300ml of cold water and mix. Once cool, SLOWLY pour the jelly all over the sponge and leave in the fridge for 3 hours to set. When it's set, put 30ml of milk into a bowl and stir in 2 teaspoons of the sugar and the blancmange. Pour 600ml of milk into a medium saucepan and bring to a gentle boil. Add the milk to the blancmange mixture, whisking as you bring it back to the boil. Pour it back into the bowl and leave to cool, then SLOWLY pour that over the strawberry jelly, and put into the fridge for 3 hours.

Make the orange jelly the same way as the strawberry jelly. As it cools, scatter your mandarin segments over the set blancmange. SLOWLY pour over the orange jelly and leave to set for another 3 hours. At this point, GENTLY spread the custard all over the orange jelly. Whip the double cream with the vanilla extract until you have soft peaks, and CAREFULLY spread that over the custard. Leave overnight before serving with sprinkles on top.

Wimbledon Trifle

SERVES 12

- 250g sticky ginger loaf, cut into 1cm slices
- 500g ripe strawberries, hulled
- 3 sprigs of fresh mint

- 9 leaves of gelatine
- 200ml Pimm's
- 550ml good-quality fizzy lemonade, chilled in the fridge

- 6 teaspoons caster sugar
- a splash of vanilla extract
- zest of 1 lemon
- 300ml double cream

Divide the slices of ginger loaf between 12 small glass tumblers, overlapping them. Halve the strawberries and divide between the tumblers. Tear over a few mint leaves, then put the glasses in the fridge for an hour. Soak the gelatine in a little water for 3 minutes. Place a saucepan on a low heat and add the Pimm's. As soon as it's hot, drain the gelatine leaves and place in the pan. Whisk until dissolved. Pour the chilled lemonade into the pan of Pimm's, stir, then SLOWLY divide between the tumblers, so the jelly comes just above the strawberries. Return to the fridge for about 2 hours.

Once set, bash up the remaining mint leaves in a pestle and mortar with the of sugar and put aside. Add a splash of vanilla extract and the lemon zest to your cream and whisk until just soft and peaky. Blob the lemony cream over each little trifle and top with the mint sugar.

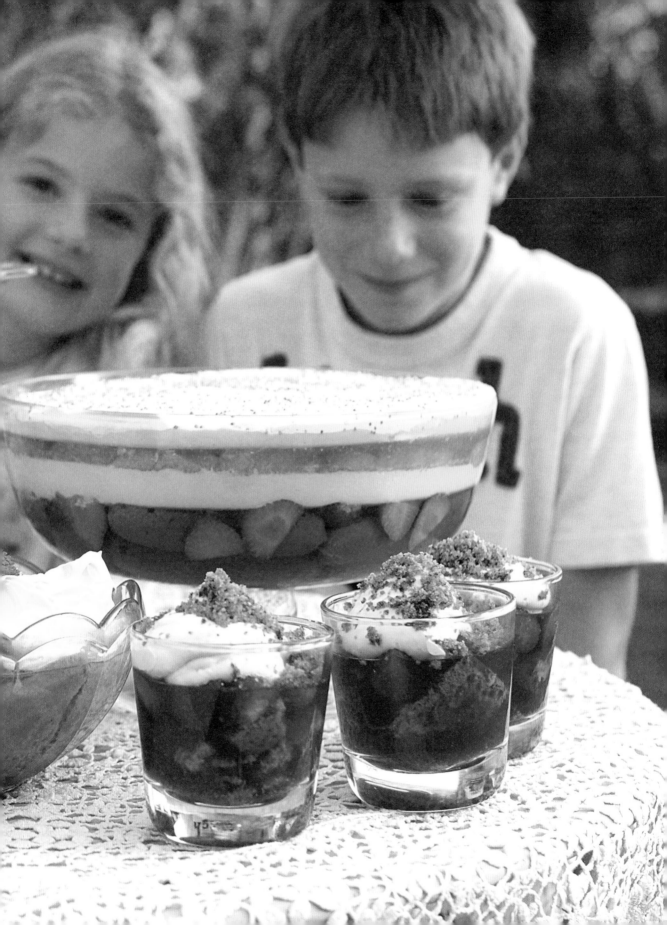

CHOCOLATE ORANGE STEAMED PUD

If my mum ever asked me as a kid what dessert I wanted for special occasions, I would always say I wanted this. It's one of my all-time favourites. It's got lightness, chocolate, orange and a silky dark sauce that oozes out of it. It's my pleasure to pass this recipe from my mumma to you lovely people. I've adjusted it slightly, because that's what sons do, but I've got a feeling you'll love it.

SERVES 8 TO 10

For the dark chocolate sauce
- 100g unsalted butter
- 100g golden syrup
- 100g good-quality dark chocolate (preferably 70% cocoa solids), bashed up
- 2 tablespoons milk

For the sponge
- 50g dark chocolate (preferably 70% cocoa solids), chilled
- 100g unsalted butter, softened, plus extra for greasing
- 85g golden caster sugar
- 200g self-raising flour

- zest and juice of 1 orange
- 1 large free-range egg
- 3 level tablespoons cocoa powder
- 8 tablespoons milk
- *optional:* seasonal soft fruit and double cream

Your first job is to make your chocolate sauce, so get yourself a 1.5 litre pudding bowl and put in all the sauce ingredients. Find a large pan with a lid that you can comfortably sit the pudding bowl inside, then pop the bowl in and pour a few inches of hot water into the pan. Simmer over a medium heat and gently stir every so often until you have a dark smooth chocolate sauce. Turn the heat off, then carefully remove the bowl from the pan and gently angle and tilt it so the chocolate sauce covers the inside of the bowl. Put aside while you make the sponge.

Smash or roughly chop the cold chocolate into little pieces and put it into a large mixing bowl with the rest of the sponge ingredients. Stir together until well mixed, then carefully spoon into the pudding bowl containing the chocolate sauce. Grease a small sheet of greaseproof paper and loosely cover the top of the bowl, with the greased side facing down. Put a sheet of tin foil on top, stretch it down over the rim of the pudding basin and scrunch it all around. Wrap about 2 metres of string twice around the rim of the bowl, tie it in a double knot, then attach the other end to the opposite side with a double knot to make a handle – this will make pulling the bowl out at the end much easier. Go to *www.jamieoliver.com/how-to* for a quick tutorial if you like.

Place the pudding bowl in the pan you used earlier. Top the pan up with enough hot water to come halfway up the bowl, and put the lid on. Bring to the boil, then turn down the heat and leave to simmer for 2 hours. Set a timer, and top up with water every now and then to keep a fairly constant level.

When the time is up, carefully pull out the bowl, cut away the string and remove the foil and greaseproof. Put a nice serving platter or plate on top of the bowl, then carefully and confidently flip the bowl over so it's upside down on the platter. Gently remove the bowl and use a spatula to encourage any sauce left behind to drizzle out. Lovely served with seasonal soft fruit and a dollop of lightly whipped cream.

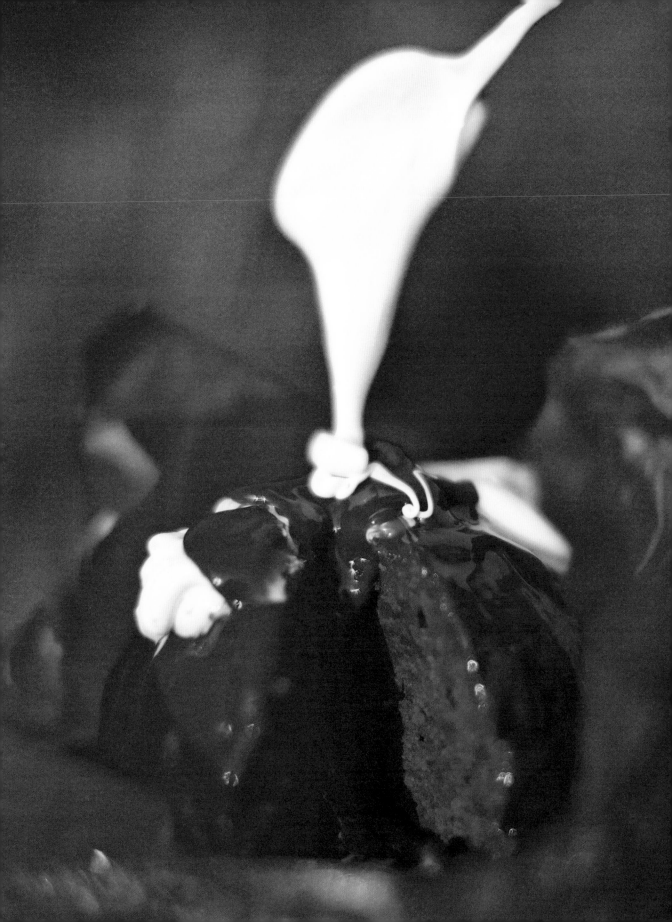

RHUBARB & RICE PUDDING

In Yorkshire, there's a fairly small area known as the rhubarb triangle. Loads of the amazing British rhubarb that is loved and eaten all over Europe, including forced rhubarb, is grown there. Forced rhubarb is denied light as it grows. Weirdly, the result is the most incredibly pink, tender and naturally sweet rhubarb around. It's to die for. This recipe works with either regular or forced rhubarb – just make sure to taste your stewed fruit towards the end so you get the right level of sweetness. I've kept the quantity of sugar fairly low, so you get a good balance between the sweet, creamy rice pudding and the sweet and sour fruit. If you like, you can add a little more creaminess to your rice pudding by stirring in a tablespoon of clotted cream just before serving. It makes it that little bit more heavenly.

SERVES 6 TO 8

For the rice pudding
- 200g pudding rice
- 1.2 litres semi-skimmed milk
- 2 vanilla pods
- 4 tablespoons golden caster sugar

For the Pimm's stewed fruit
- 3 tablespoons golden caster sugar
- 1 orange
- 1 lemon
- 2 fresh bay leaves

- 60ml Pimm's
- 500g rhubarb, trimmed and cut into 2cm chunks
- 400g strawberries, hulled and quartered

Put the rice and milk in a large non-stick saucepan (roughly 25cm in diameter). Halve the vanilla pods lengthways, then scrape out the seeds and add the pods and the seeds to the pan, along with the golden caster sugar. Bring everything to a gentle simmer over a medium heat, and stir regularly as it cooks for around 20 to 30 minutes. Once the rice is lovely and soft, pour on to your largest serving platter. Don't forget to pull out the vanilla pod halves.

While your rice pudding is ticking away, put the sugar for the stewed fruit in a large pan on a medium heat and add strips of peel from your orange and lemon. Squeeze in the juice from the orange and add the bay leaves and Pimm's. It might flame but that's OK – just let it subside then add the chopped up rhubarb and leave to stew away for 5 minutes with the lid on, or until tender. (It's your call whether you want tender chunks, a rhubarb compote, or a mixture of soft and chunky – so stew it down to whatever consistency you like.) Stir the strawberries into the rhubarb and cook for another 3 to 4 minutes with the lid off, or until the strawberries are soft but still holding their shape. Discard the bay leaves and orange and lemon peel, then spoon and ripple that hot fruit over the rice pudding, dragging your spoon slowly in a figure of 8 so it looks pretty.

PS: If by some slim chance you have any leftovers, you can either reheat them in the oven the next day, or what I like to do is put them in a dish, cover with clingfilm and pop in the freezer. Take out about 30 minutes before you need to serve for a sort of rice pudding ice cream.

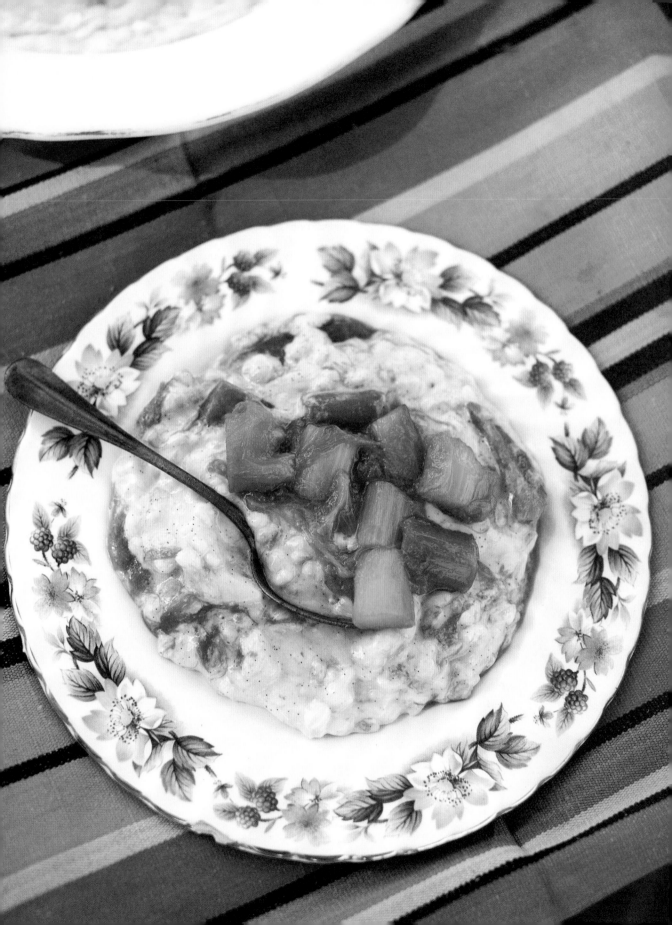

SWEET SMASHED HONEYCOMB
WARM CHOCOLATE SAUCE • SWEET SUMMER BERRIES

Honeycomb is one of those beautiful things you've either forgotten you knew how to make, or never realized you could. The process of making it is a bit like magic: one minute you've got a hot caramel, then within a few seconds of adding the bicarb you've got a sprawling frothy concoction rising up the sides of the pan. It's great fun, but it's well worth having a sugar thermometer so you get the caramel bang on 150°C. Once it cools, you can crack that hardened honeycomb into chunks and serve it with a bowl of melted chocolate to make your very own version of a Crunchie bar. Put this out at a party and watch it go like the clappers, or smash it into fine pieces and sprinkle it over ice cream to add a sweet crunch.

MAKES A TRAY FOR 10

- 1 heaped teaspoon bicarbonate of soda (roughly 8g)
- 250g golden caster sugar
- 2 heaped tablespoons runny honey
- *optional:* 100g good-quality dark chocolate (70% cocoa solids), melted, to serve
- *optional:* 150g punnet of fresh raspberries, to serve

Line a shallow baking tray (roughly 25 x 35cm) with a sheet of greaseproof paper. Measure out your bicarb so that it's ready to go - you'll need to work quickly once the sugar reaches the right temperature. Put the sugar, honey and 50ml of water into a medium-sized, deep, heavy-bottomed pan. Stir together and heat to 150°C on a sugar thermometer. Whatever you do, do NOT touch or taste the caramel, as it will burn. It's best to keep kids and pets out of the room while you make this.

As soon as the caramel reaches the right temperature, turn the heat off and add the bicarb, whisking quickly and carefully to combine it. It will froth right up, but that's normal. Carefully pour the mixture out on to your lined tray right away, then gently tilt the tray a little from side to side to get the mixture to spread out into a fairly even layer (again, being careful to make sure you don't come into contact with the hot caramel). Leave to one side to cool, then crack it into bite-sized pieces. Serve with melted chocolate for dunking and fresh berries on the side.

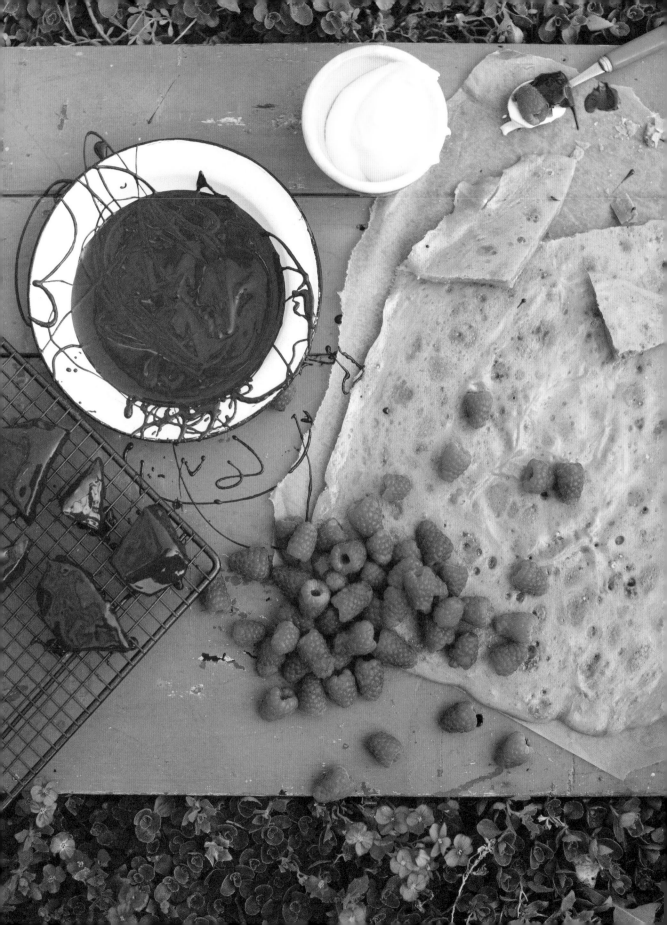

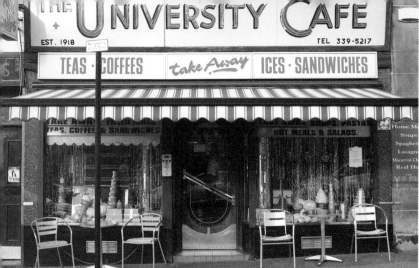

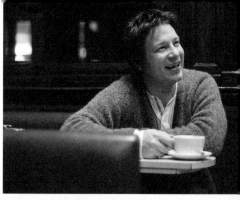

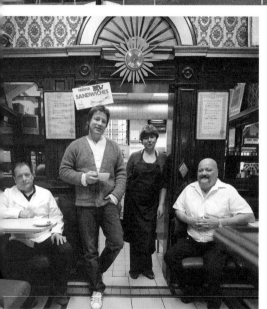

The University Café

I love the University Café. It's a welcoming old-school place on Glasgow's Byres Road run by a lovely family of Italian descent. The art director on all my books, John Hamilton, used to come here all the time as a kid with his grandma, and I bet it hasn't changed much since then. That's why everyone loves it. Great ice cream, proper coffee and big beautiful jars of boiled sweets.

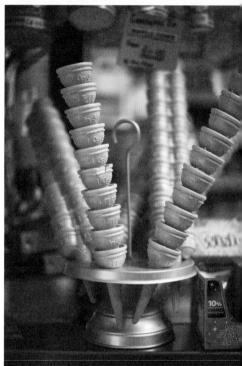

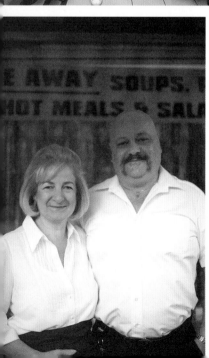

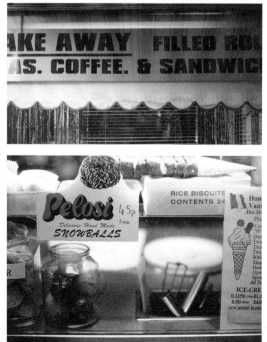

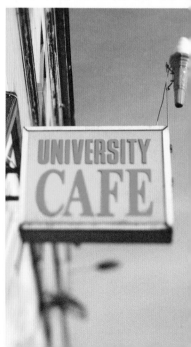

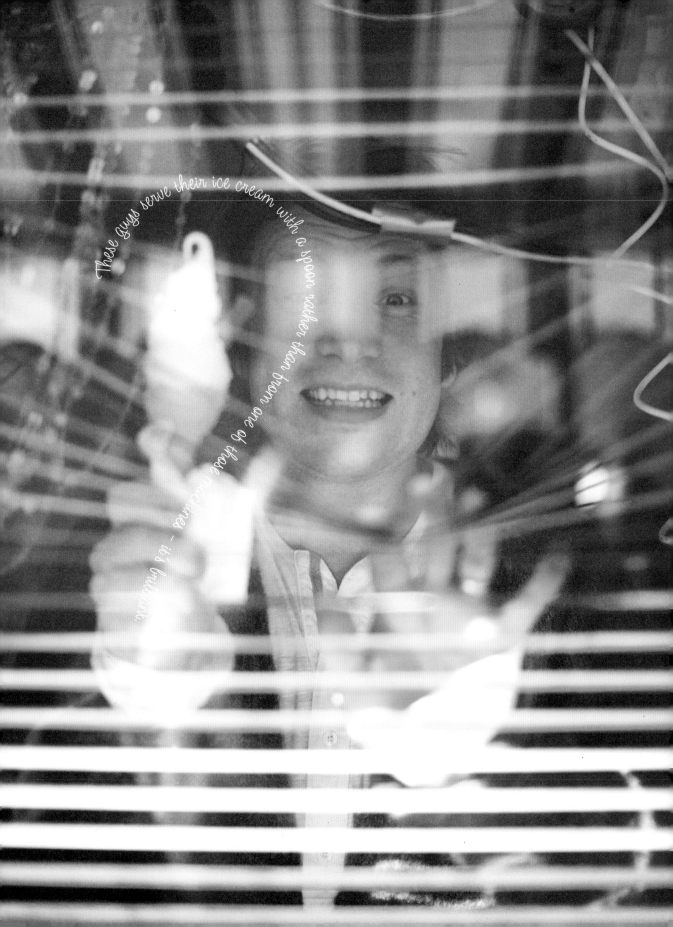

These guys serve their ice cream with a spoon rather than from one of those machines – it's brilliant.

RETRO ARCTIC ROLL

In the 60s and 70s, having a frozen dessert you could serve at a moment's notice was the posh thing to do. The simple but glorious arctic roll started popping up everywhere, from restaurants to school and hospital menus. Eventually it became seen as something a bit naff and tacky, but I think smearing a homemade sponge with quality jam, good ice cream and a little bashed-up honeycomb is easy, fun, and just a bit silly. Roll it up, freeze it for a few hours, and you'll get sweet and sour, crunch and softness, all in one mouthful. Heaven.

SERVES 14

For the sponge
- 3 large free-range eggs
- 100g golden caster sugar, plus extra for sprinkling
- 75g plain flour
- a few knobs of butter, for greasing
- 1 heaped teaspoon cocoa powder

For the filling
- 2 x 500ml tubs of good-quality ice cream, vanilla and chocolate
- 300g good-quality strawberry or raspberry jam
- 1 Crunchie or Dime bar or a bag of Maltesers, bashed up

To serve
- 200g fresh berries
- juice of ½ a lemon
- *optional:* edible flowers

Preheat the oven to 180°C/350°F/gas 4. Move the ice cream to the fridge so it starts to soften. Crack the eggs into a mixing bowl, add the sugar, and whisk until pale, fluffy and at least doubled in size. You can do this with an electric mixer, or by hand if you've got the muscle. Once it's looking good, sift in the flour and slowly fold it through with a spatula. Grease a baking tray (roughly 26 x 36cm) with butter, then line it with greaseproof paper and grease that too. Spoon half your sponge batter on to the tray, blobbing it about in different places, then sift the cocoa powder into the remaining batter and fold it in. Spoon the chocolatey sponge into the gaps on the tray, and use the spoon to drag it through the white sponge in S-shapes and circles until it looks beautiful and marbled. Make sure there are no gaps. Place the tray on the middle shelf of the oven and bake for 12 to 15 minutes, or until cooked through.

Grease another large sheet of greaseproof paper with butter and sprinkle over a few good pinches of sugar. Take the sponge out of the oven and confidently flip it over on to the paper. This is all really simple, but if you need a bit more help, go to *www.jamieoliver.com/how-to* where you'll find a video to guide you through it. Peel and discard the top piece of paper, then, while the sponge is still warm and flexible, loosely roll it up into a long sausage, including the paper, and leave it to cool for around 20 minutes.

Once cooled, gently unroll the sponge and spread over half of the jam. Take big dessertspoons of your soft ice cream and randomly distribute them over the sponge, leaving the last 5 or 6cm at one end free of filling so that it creates a seal when you roll it up. Put whatever you don't use back in the fridge. Dollop over teaspoons of the remaining jam, then sprinkle your bashed-up chocolate bar all over. Use a spatula to smear everything into a fairly smooth dense layer.

Confidently, start rolling the sponge up again, making sure there's no paper inside it. If the filling starts to slip out, just push it back in. Twisting the ends and squeezing it into a long, fairly even ice-cream sausage. Pop it into the freezer for 3 hours, and take it out around 5 to 10 minutes before you want to use it so it thaws enough to slice. Unwrap your arctic roll, take a slice out of each end to expose the frozen insides, and serve with fresh summer fruits tossed in lemon juice and a pinch of sugar, or any edible flowers if you have them.

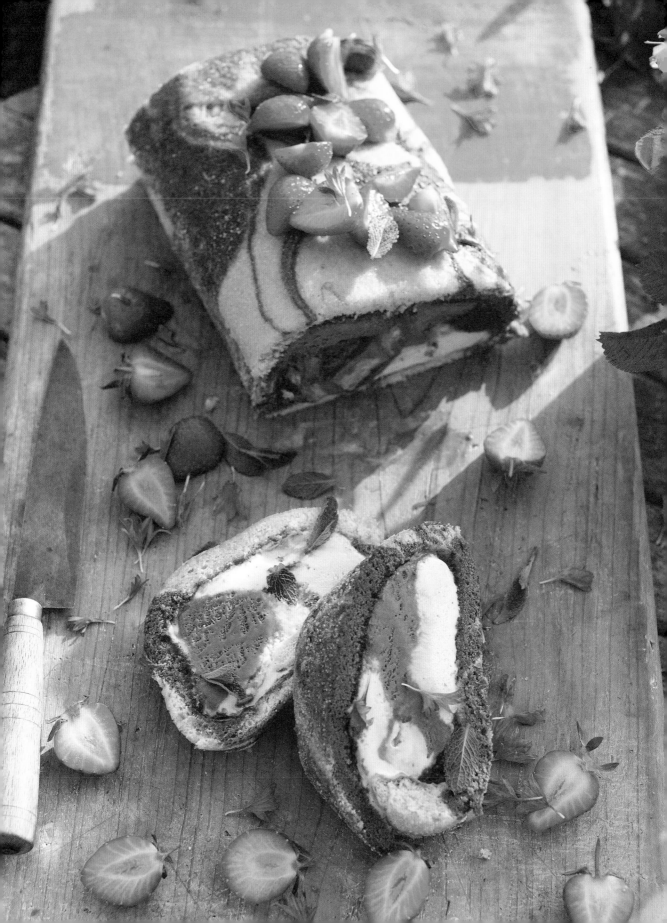

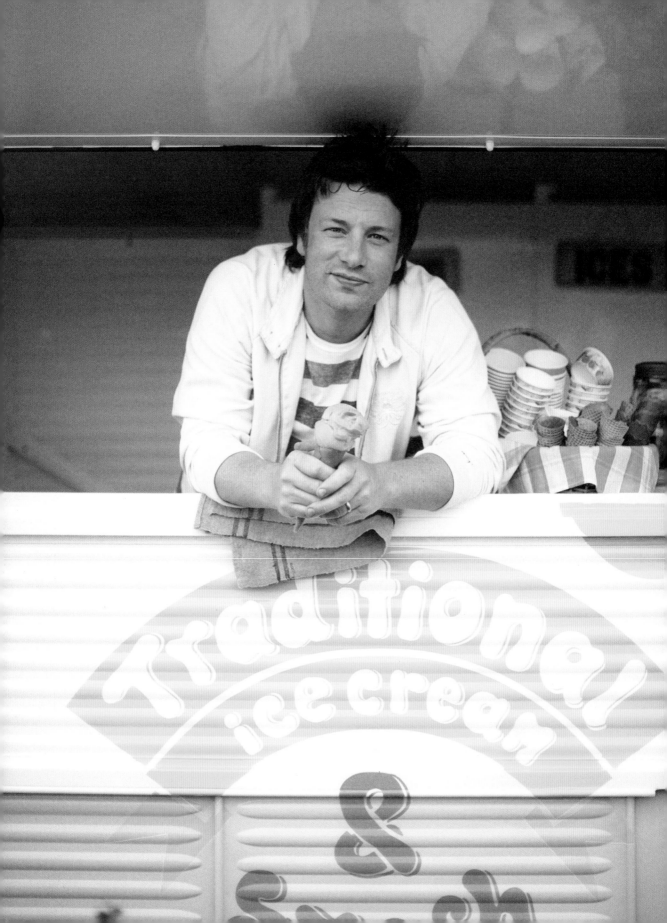

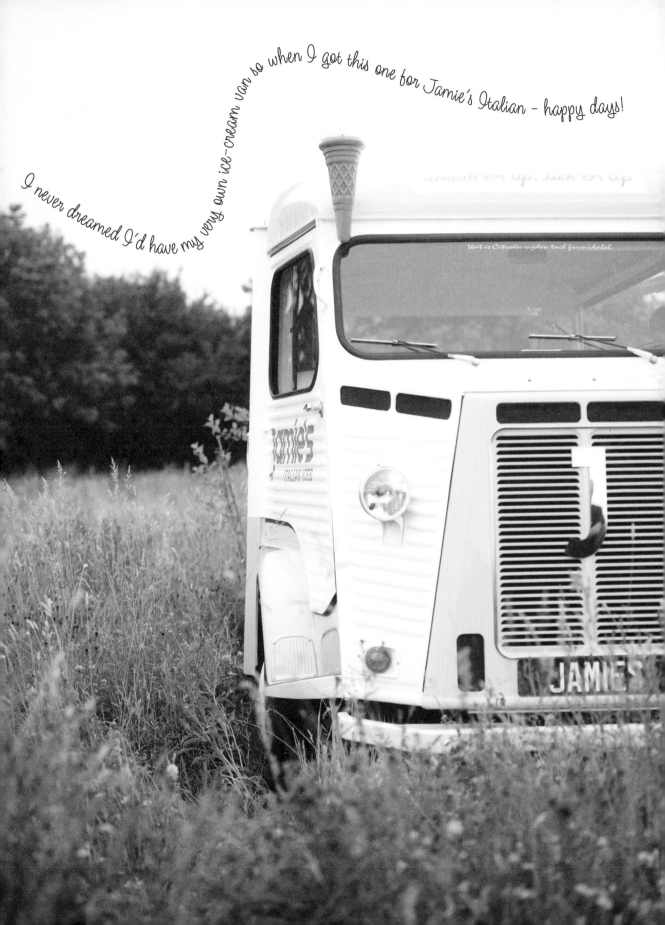

I never dreamed I'd have my very own ice-cream van so when I got this one for Jamie's Italian – happy days!

CITRUS CHEESECAKE POSSETS
LEMON • CLEMENTINE • ORANGE • GRAPEFRUIT

You'll get four or five of the most heavenly spoonfuls from one of these little pots. I was inspired by the quintessential British lemon posset when I made them. Historically, possets were hot drinks made with milk or cream, and they date right back to medieval times. They eventually became creamy cold desserts, like syllabubs, which are lovely but can be quite rich. Sometimes, all you need to satisfy a dessert craving is a few mouthfuls of something zingy and delicious, so I've made these into tiny little pots and used a cheesecake base to add crunch and contrast to that creamy filling. I'm using digestive biscuits, but if you're partial to a ginger biscuit, shortbread or similar, feel free to use those instead.

Whether serving these in glasses or espresso cups, they really look gorgeous, cute and have a simplicity and classiness to them that I love. Once you've got this recipe down, you could make half a batch using one juice, and half with another, so you end up with different coloured layers in each pot, or you could try a blend of citrus juices like lime and lemon, or pink grapefruit and orange. Get as creative as you like.

MAKES 8 TO 10 LITTLE POTS

For the biscuit base
- 50g blanched almonds
- 5 digestive biscuits
- 30g unsalted butter, melted

For the creamy filling
- 200ml freshly squeezed juice (8-10 lemons or 3-4 oranges)
- 100g golden caster sugar

- 1 vanilla pod, halved lengthways, seeds scraped out
- 600ml double cream

Toast the almonds in a non-stick pan until golden brown and allow to cool. Bash up the biscuits and almonds in a bowl using the end of a rolling pin, then stir in the melted butter. Mix together really well, then divide between little pots, glasses or espresso cups. Use the back of a spoon or your thumb to pack the mixtures down, then pop them into the fridge to firm up.

Wash your chosen fruit, then carefully peel delicious thin strips of zest with a good speed-peeler, making sure you avoid the bitter white pith (this is very important). Squeeze 200ml of the juice into a measuring jug, with a sieve balanced on top to catch any pips, and put aside.

Put your sugar, strips of zest, citrus juice and the vanilla pod and seeds into a pan on a medium heat and bring to a simmer. Stir gently until the sugar dissolves and you have a thick syrup – this will take roughly 14 to 16 minutes on a medium low heat. Remove from the heat and pour in the cream. Place back on the heat, but turn it down to low, and simmer gently for around 10 minutes, gently whisking as you go so you get good flavour infusion, with a pastelly hint of the colour of the fruit you've chosen, and the mixture becomes thick and glossy.

Take your chilled pots out of the fridge. Pass the flavoured cream through a sieve to remove the peel and vanilla pod, then divide the mixture between the little pots. Cover with clingfilm and put into the fridge to set for roughly 2 hours before serving.

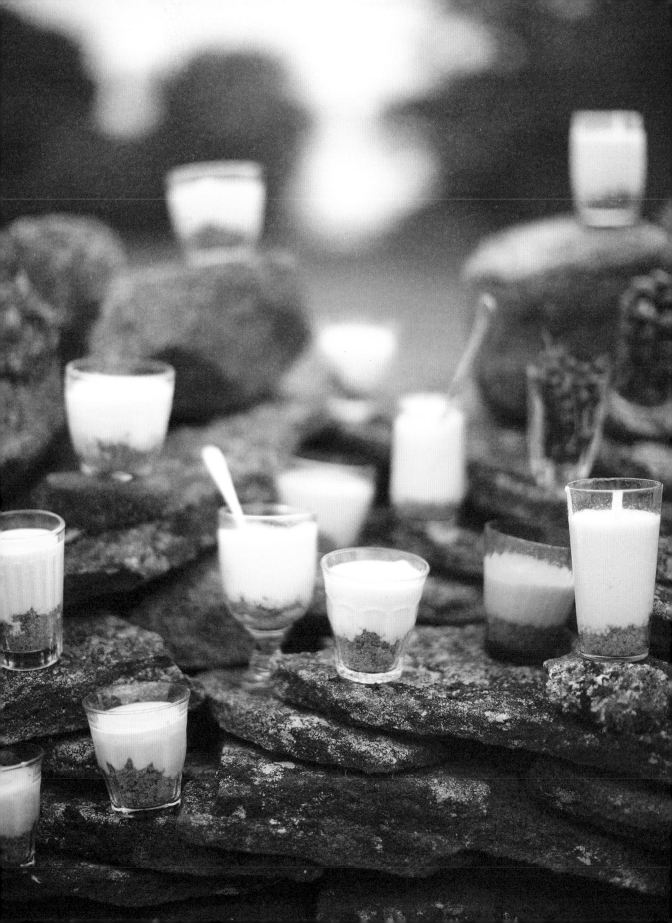

ECCLEFECHAN TART
DOLLOP OF WHISKY • GINGER CREAM

Tarts and cakes burn beautiful memories in people's minds and this one is no exception. It's definitely a treat and an indulgence, but I think you're going to 'fechan' love it. The filling is absolutely gorgeous and the pastry is so damn light it snaps into shards when you eat it, which is only ever a good thing. This is my version of the original tart, which is named after a lovely little village in the south of Scotland. The filling is rich and tasty because of the dried fruit – and supermarkets these days have such a phenomenal choice of dried fruits, so let's make the most of them.

SERVES 12

For the pastry
- 250g plain flour, plus extra for dusting
- 125g unsalted butter, cubed
- sea salt
- 50ml/large shot of whisky

For the filling
- 150g unsalted butter, at room temperature

- 150g light brown sugar
- 3 large free-range eggs
- 150ml double cream
- 1 heaped tablespoon black treacle
- 300g mixed dried fruit, such as raisins, cranberries, cherries or blueberries
- 1 teaspoon finely chopped stem ginger

- 1 lemon
- 1 orange

To serve
- 150ml double cream
- 1 tablespoon stem ginger syrup
- 25ml/small shot of whisky
- black treacle for rippling through

Preheat the oven to 180°C/350°F/gas 4. Put the flour into a mixing bowl with the cubes of butter and a pinch of salt. Use your fingertips to pinch the butter into the flour, but don't overwork it. Add the whisky and push, pat and bring it together without kneading it. Cover it with clingfilm and pop it into the fridge until needed, or just give it 15 minutes to relax.

Dust a clean surface and a rolling pin with flour and roll the pastry out until it's about the thickness of a £1 coin and large enough to cover a 25cm loose-bottomed tart tin. Roll the pastry up around your rolling pin then unroll it over the tin. Gently encourage the pastry into the tin, using your thumb and forefinger to mould it in as you go. Don't worry if there are holes, you can always patch them. Prick the pastry all over with a fork. Scrunch up and wet some greaseproof paper under a tap, then line the tart case with it. Fill nearly to the top with uncooked rice, then pop it into the bottom of the oven and cook for 10 minutes to stop the pastry shrinking. After the time is up, get the pastry case out of the oven, remove the greaseproof paper and rice, then return it to the oven for another 5 minutes, or until lightly golden. You can keep the rice to use for blind baking another time.

Meanwhile, cream the butter and sugar for the filling together in a bowl or food processor. Beat the eggs into the mixture one by one until smooth. Mix in the cream. Take the pastry case out of the oven and spoon the black treacle all around the base. Scatter over all your dried fruit and stem ginger, then add a few sweeps of lemon zest and the zest of half an orange. Pour and spoon over the filling mixture, then jiggle the tart case gently to help everything settle. Put it back into the oven and cook for about 30 to 35 minutes, or until golden and still slightly wobbly.

Let the tart cool for about 30 minutes. To serve, whip the cream with a tablespoon of the syrup from the stem ginger and a thimble of whisky. Ripple a tiny drizzle of treacle through at the very end, then dollop a spoonful over a slice of your tart.

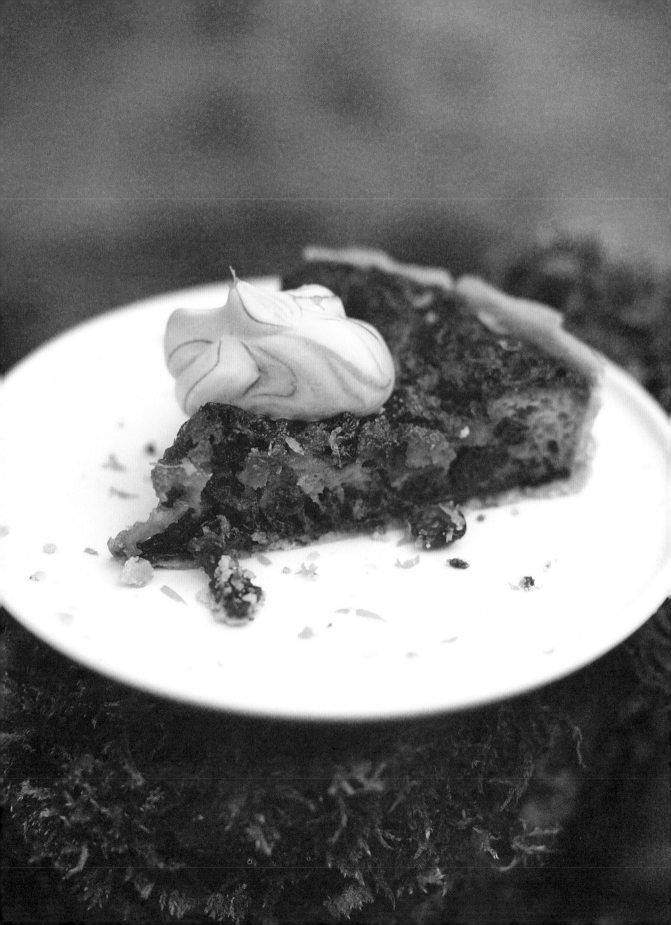

FLAPJACK CRUMBLE

The logic behind the invention of this wonderful dessert is very simple: you take two things in life that make you really happy and you find a way of incorporating them into one beautiful thing, thus giving you the gigantic double whammy that is the mighty flapjack crumble. As much as I make, and honour, traditional crumbles, every now and then it's nice to give people something unexpected – something that makes them sit up, ask questions and get excited about the fact that a delicious flapjacky base has found its way into their favourite dessert. I love it.

SERVES 10 TO 12

For the flapjack base
- 50g mixed nuts, such as hazelnuts or shelled walnuts
- 1 ball of stem ginger
- 125g unsalted butter, plus extra for greasing
- 3 tablespoons golden syrup
- 175g jumbo rolled oats
- 75g mixed dried fruit, like apricots, sour cherries, raisins or blueberries, chopped

For the apple filling
- 1 cooking apple, peeled and cored
- 6 medium-sized good eating apples, peeled and cored
- 100g dark brown sugar
- a good pinch of ground cinnamon
- 1 whole nutmeg, for grating
- a swig of brandy or sloe gin
- 300g blackberries

For the crumble topping
- 75g unsalted butter, chilled and cut into 1cm cubes
- 100g plain flour
- 100g demerara sugar
- 1 orange
- quality ice cream, custard or natural yoghurt, to serve
- grated orange zest, to serve

Preheat the oven to 180°C/350°C/gas 4. Bash the nuts for your flapjack base in a pestle and mortar or in a metal bowl with a rolling pin, and roughly chop the stem ginger. Melt the butter and golden syrup in a saucepan on a low heat. Put the oats, bashed-up nuts, stem ginger and dried fruits into a big bowl, then pour over the melted buttery syrup and mix together so all the oats end up shiny and coated. Spoon this mixture into a greased ovenproof dish or tin, roughly 24cm wide x 6cm deep. Use the back of a spoon to press the mixture down into the bottom and up the sides of the dish, so it's an even 0.5cm thickness all over, then bake in the oven for 20 minutes, or until golden and lovely. Don't panic if it shrinks down slightly, as you can use the back of a spoon to push it back into place while it is hot.

Meanwhile cut each apple into 12 and put the pieces into a large heavy-bottomed pan on a medium heat. Add the brown sugar and cinnamon, grate over some nutmeg and add a good swig of brandy or sloe gin. Cover with a lid and stew for 5 minutes, or until the fruit has started to soften. Remove the lid and cook for another 5 minutes or so, until the sauce has thickened up a bit. When it's good, simply stir in the blackberries and take off the heat.

In a clean bowl, quickly make your crumble topping by rubbing the butter into the flour and sugar until you have fine crumbs – you can also do this in a food processor. Grate over the zest from the orange, give the mixture a quick stir and put aside.

Pour the stewed fruit into the dish containing the flapjack base, filling it right to the top. Sprinkle over the crumble topping, then put in the hot oven for 50 minutes, or until the fruit is bubbling up around the edges and the top is golden and biscuity. Serve warm, with a scoop of good ice cream, some custard or a dollop of natural yoghurt and a grating of orange zest.

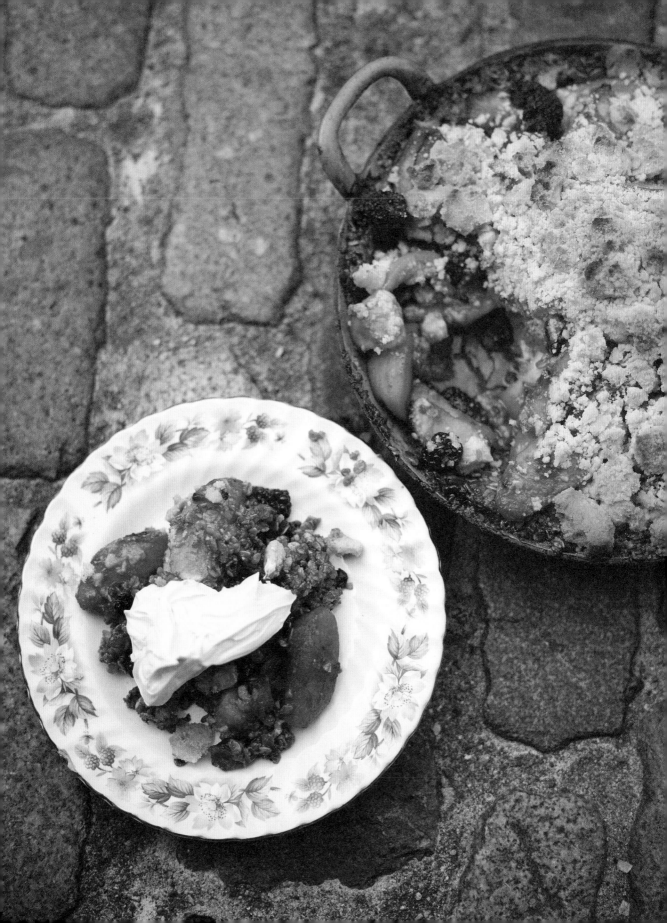

APPLE PEPPER POT CAKE

This sticky, spongy, gorgeous pudding is my homage to Bristol. I perfected it there by taking most of the spices that the lovely Guyanese family I met put into their incredible pepper pot meat stew, and using them to add mega flavour to this otherwise classic apple sponge. These spices would have been introduced during the colonial era via Bristol's ports, and now they're in so many of the foods we love. Feel free to use pears, quinces or peaches in this sponge. It's a flexible recipe. And if you don't have any molasses handy, a tablespoon of black treacle plus a tablespoon of golden syrup will do the same job.

SERVES UP TO 14

For the caramelly sauce
- 200g unsalted butter, cubed, at room temperature, plus extra for greasing
- 200g golden caster sugar
- 2 tablespoons molasses
- 1 level teaspoon ground cinnamon
- 1 level teaspoon ground ginger
- a pinch of ground cloves
- 3 tablespoons clotted cream or single cream

For the sponge
- 6 or 7 small/medium eating apples, such as Cox or Braeburn quartered and cored
- 125g unsalted butter, at room temperature
- 125g golden caster sugar
- 2 large free-range eggs
- 225g self-raising flour, sifted
- ½ a level teaspoon bicarbonate of soda
- 200ml good-quality dry cider
- 2 oranges

Grease the bottom and sides of a 24cm circular cake tin and line with greaseproof paper. Preheat your oven to 180°C/350°F/gas 4. Put the cubed butter for your sauce into a saucepan large enough to hold all your apple quarters in one layer. Add the caster sugar, molasses and ground spices then gently bring everything to the boil. Turn down the heat and simmer, stirring occasionally, until the sauce starts to thicken. Be careful because caramel is very hot and can burn badly. At this point, add the quartered apples and cook for a few minutes while you make the sponge, but keep a close eye on them and stir occasionally so they don't catch.

Cream together the butter and sugar for the sponge, then add the eggs, one at a time, mixing them in as you go. Fold in half the flour, the bicarbonate of soda and the cider. The mixture might look like it's splitting, but don't worry. Mix well, then fold in the remaining flour and the zest from the oranges, and stir again.

Put the prepared cake tin on to a baking tray lined with greaseproof paper (just in case any hot caramel seeps out during cooking). Spoon the sticky apples into the bottom of the tin in a fairly even layer, along with any of the caramel that happens to come with them. Put the pan with the remaining caramel aside for later, then pour the sponge batter over the apples and give it a jiggle to spread the mixture out a bit. Put the cake tin and baking tray into the hot oven on the middle shelf to cook for around 35 to 40 minutes. Insert a skewer into the middle of the cake after 35 minutes - if it comes out clean the cake's ready, if not, just bake for a further 5 minutes.

Once cooked, let the cake cool for 10 minutes (no longer or you won't be able to turn it out). Warm the reserved caramel on a low heat and gently stir in the cream. Go back to your cake and spoon away any escaped caramel so it can't burn you, then pop a serving plate on top of the cake and quickly and confidently flip it over. Ease the tin off the overturned cake, then cut into wedges and serve with the remaining sticky, creamy caramel sauce drizzled on top.

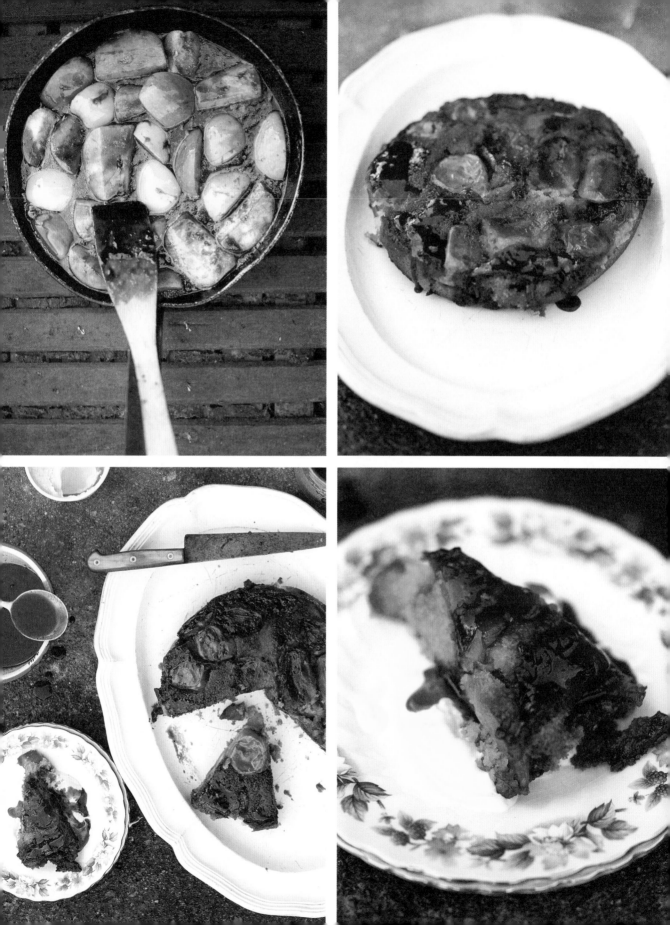

CHOCOLATE PUDDING BOMBE

Puddings you can make ahead of time and leave in the freezer until you need them are great. Especially around the holidays, which is when I tend to make this one. I see this dessert as a sort of cross between a summer pudding and an arctic roll, so it hits a lot of those retro buttons. Because it's an assembly job, anybody at all can make this – so if you've got someone at your house who won't muck in because they say they can't cook, put them to work on this!

SERVES 10

- 2 x 500ml tubs of good-quality vanilla ice cream
- 1 x 1kg panettone
- 125ml sweet sherry
- 3 heaped tablespoons good-quality raspberry jam
- 25g shelled pistachios
- 75g tinned cherries, drained
- 40g glacé clementines (or other glacé fruit), thinly sliced
- 2 clementines, 1 peeled and sliced into rounds, the other left whole
- 200g good-quality dark chocolate (70% cocoa solids), bashed up

Get your ice cream out of the freezer so it can soften a little while you get things ready. Line a 2-litre pudding bowl with three layers of clingfilm. Use a serrated knife to slice four 2cm-thick rounds of your panettone, then cut them in half. You'll have some panettone left over, so keep this for another time (I love it sliced and toasted). Arrange six of the slices in a single layer around the bowl and push them down if they overlap. Drizzle some sweet sherry around the sponge so it soaks in, then use the back of a spoon to smear the jam over the sponge.

Add 1 tub of ice cream to the bowl and use the spoon to spread it around in a thick layer. Sprinkle in the pistachios, cherries and glacé fruit, then layer the clementine slices on top. Add the other tub of ice cream. Spread it out, working quickly so the ice cream doesn't completely melt. Put the rest of the panettone slices on top of the ice cream, make sure there are no gaps, then drizzle over some more sweet sherry and cover the bowl tightly with clingfilm. Put a plate on top and press everything down, then freeze overnight, or longer.

When you're ready to serve it, put the bashed-up chocolate into a bowl and get it over a pan of simmering water on a really low heat. Leave the chocolate to melt while you unwrap your amazing winter bombe and carefully turn it on to a beautiful serving dish. Add a few gratings of clementine zest to the chocolate, and when it's nicely melted, pour it over the top so it oozes down the sides and looks delicious – from this point, you've got around 10 minutes before the chocolate freezes and gets hard, so get serving.

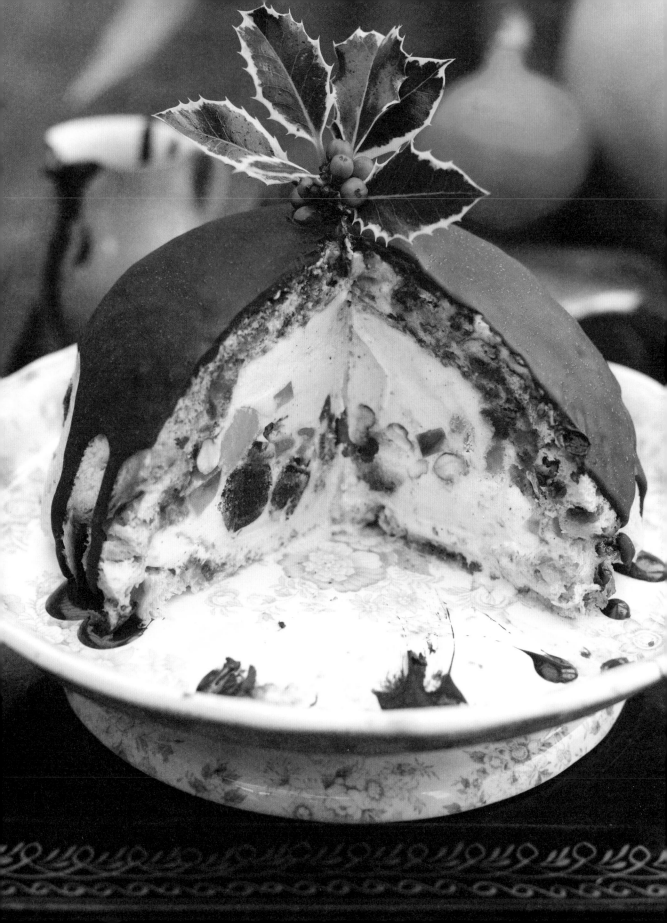

VELVETY CHOCOLATE POTS
A THIMBLE OF BRANDY • BEAUTIFUL RIPE CHERRIES

Putting a really straightforward, easy-to-make chocolate recipe in this book felt like the right thing to do, because first, who doesn't love a light and creamy chocolate treat? And second, my Fifteen students happened to be having a chocolate seminar on the day I was shooting some recipes for the book. When they came upstairs with a tray of very simple mousse I thought there was something wonderfully humble about the fact that they were using milk chocolate rather than the posher dark variety. So I made this version, using brandy and some lovely fresh cherries, though rum and stem ginger in syrup would also be delicious, as would whisky and orange. Basically, chocolate is a wonderful carrier of flavours, so good luck. Just don't over whip it!

SERVES 12

For the mousse	To serve
• 250g good-quality milk chocolate	• 200g cherries, raspberries or strawberries
• 500ml double cream	• 50g good-quality milk chocolate (kept in the fridge)
• 50g caster sugar	
• 25ml/shot of brandy	

Smash the chocolate for the mousse and place it in a large heatproof glass bowl. Sit the bowl over a pan of gently simmering water, making sure the water doesn't touch the base of the bowl, and leave it there until the chocolate has melted. Once silky and smooth, immediately remove from the heat and put aside to cool for around 5 minutes.

Whip the cream and sugar together with a balloon whisk until you have very soft peaks, then use the whisk to stir in the brandy. Gradually pour the cooled melted chocolate into the cream and gently fold it in with the whisk until just combined. Please don't over whisk it.

Pour the chocolate mixture into cute little cups, glasses or dishes, or spoon it into disposable plastic piping bags so that you can pipe it into any receptacle you like. It sounds a bit cheffy, but piping bags are available online and in cook shops, or you can create the same effect by using a sandwich bag with the corner snipped off. Either way, make sure the chocolate chills in the fridge for a couple of hours before you serve it.

Just before serving, scrape the chilled chocolate with a knife, or grate it, and sprinkle some on top of each chocolate pot. These are lovely served with soft, sweet and sour seasonal fruit like cherries, strawberries or raspberries, and if you're feeling extra naughty you can finish them off with a small blob of whipped cream on the top.

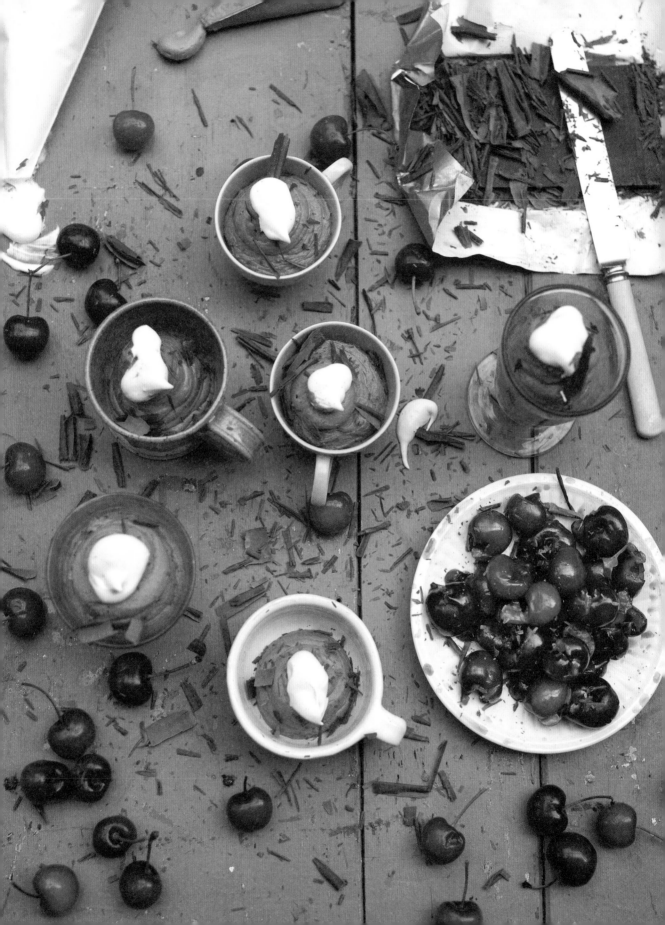

BONNIE CRANACHAN

When the Scots have something to celebrate, like the legendary Burns Night when they toast the poet Robbie Burns over a haggis feast and copious amounts of whisky, the elements for this dessert are often put out on the table, just waiting to be assembled. I love cranachan, partly because it's delicious and exciting, like a sort of Scottish sundae, but also because the whisky and cream are so good together, and somehow seem to make the fresh raspberries and crunchy oats taste even better. Although traditionally this dessert is made with cream, or a blend of cream and a Scottish soft cheese called crowdie, I've cut the cream with yoghurt to make my version rich, but also a little bit lighter on the tummy.

SERVES 6

- 500g frozen raspberries or strawberries, or a mixture
- a sprig of fresh rosemary
- 3 tablespoons runny honey
- 1 orange
- 100g pinhead or rolled oats
- 100g flaked almonds
- 1 vanilla pod
- 150ml double cream
- 2 tablespoons caster sugar or treacle
- 150ml low-fat yoghurt
- a splash of whisky
- 150g fresh raspberries or other summer fruit

Put the frozen berries, rosemary sprig and 1 tablespoon of honey into a small saucepan and grate over the zest and squeeze in the juice from the orange. Bring everything to the boil, then turn down the heat and simmer for roughly 10 minutes, or until it's thick and syrupy. Get rid of the rosemary sprig, then pour the mixture into a serving bowl and leave to cool.

While the fruit is bubbling away, put the pinhead or rolled oats in a dry medium non-stick frying pan on a medium heat. Stir and gently toast them for around 5 minutes, or until they are golden (making sure they don't catch), then tip them into a second serving bowl and put it on a table with a spoon. Put that same frying pan back on the heat and add the remaining 2 tablespoons of honey and the flaked almonds. Toss around for a few minutes, until the almonds are lightly golden and sticky, then remove to another serving bowl and put that on the table with a spoon too.

Cut the vanilla pod in half lengthways and scrape out the seeds. Put the double cream and caster sugar or treacle into a bowl, add the vanilla pod seeds and whisk until you get soft peaks, then fold in the yoghurt and whisky. Spoon into a nice serving bowl, cover with clingfilm and pop into the fridge, along with the stewed berries, while you enjoy your dinner.

When you're ready to serve, simply take all of the elements - the stewed berries, toasted oats, sticky almonds and flavoured cream - to the table with a bowl of fresh raspberries or other fruit, a handful of spoons and some tumblers or bowls. The joy is letting everyone build their own cranachan, either by layering up the ingredients and eating it like a sundae, or simply lobbing what they like into their bowl and mixing it all up.

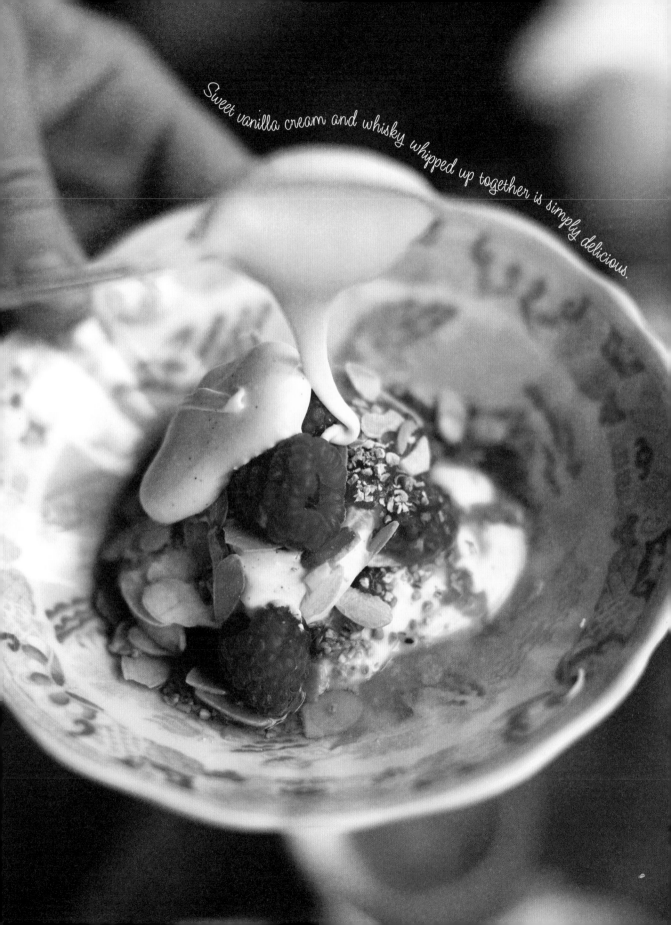

Sweet vanilla cream and whisky whipped up together is simply delicious.

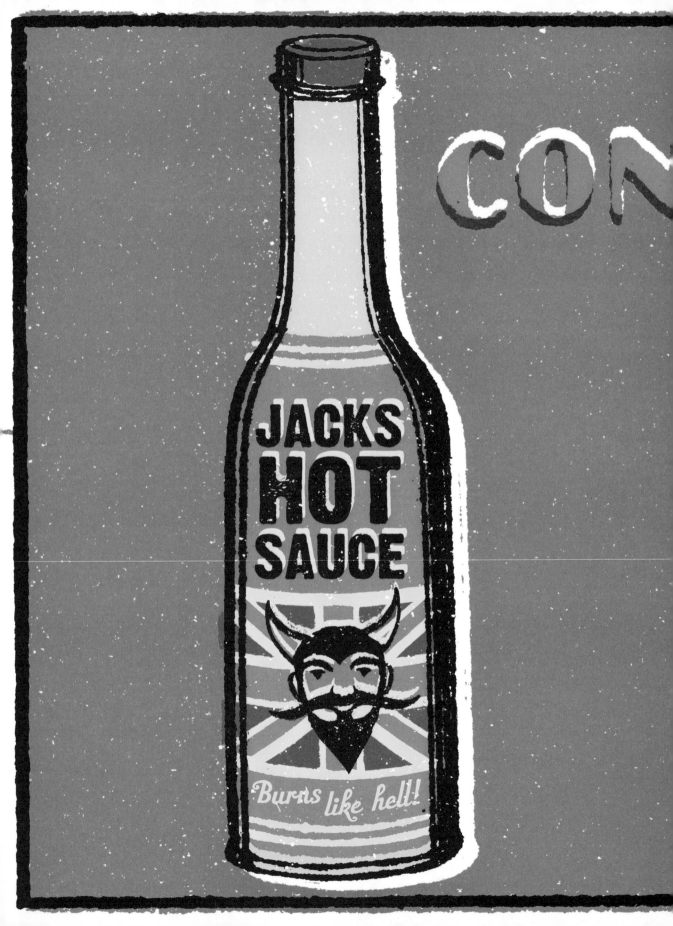

CON
DIMENTS

This chapter is really important to me because at the heart of nearly every recipe in this book is a condiment. Where would a salad be without a swig of good vinegar? Where would lamb be without mint sauce? What roast beef dinner would be complete without a smear of horseradish sauce? And this love of condiments is nothing new. Preserving fruits and vegetables in chutneys and jams was common practice in the days long before there were freezers and fridges. Mustard is actually ancient, and our medieval ancestors went mad for their mint and horseradish. It's quite funny to see how similar our tastes still are! So please have a look at this chapter and really think about how simple this stuff is to make. This is about giving you the power to make your food rock the party and be truly unique. I hope the ideas here inspire you to make your own.

THE BEST PICCALILLI

This wonderful pickle transforms ordinary garden veg into something vibrant and exciting, thanks to the gorgeous Indian flavours that are added to the base ingredients. As a nation, Britain has fallen in love with this pickle, and there are recipes for it dating as far back as the mid-1700s! Without meaning to brag, I think this is by far the best piccalilli I've ever had. It's brilliant with so many things – from a wedge of pork pie, to a ploughman's lunch, or even a ham sandwich. I know everyone seems to want quick meals these days, but I think setting aside two hours once a year to make this is a great thing to do. Believe me, your own piccalilli always blows the stuff you find in the stores away. Keep a few jars in your larder and give the rest away to your favourite people – everyone who tries it will absolutely love it.

MAKES ROUGHLY 3 LITRES (OR 12 LARGE JAM JARS)

- 1 small cauliflower, cut into really small florets
- 1 head of broccoli, cut into florets (not too small)
- 2 fennel bulbs, trimmed and cut into 1cm chunks
- 4 fresh red chillies, finely sliced
- 2 fresh green chillies, finely sliced
- 200g fine green beans, trimmed and cut into short pieces
- 225g runner beans, trimmed and cut diagonally into 1cm pieces

- 300g shallots, each peeled and cut into 8 pieces
- 1 red onion, peeled and roughly chopped
- 4 tablespoons sea salt for the flavour base
- 4 tablespoons olive or rapeseed oil
- 2 heaped tablespoons mustard seeds
- 2 level tablespoons ground cumin
- 2 level tablespoons turmeric
- 2 tablespoons dried oregano

- 1 whole nutmeg, for grating
- 3 cloves of garlic, peeled and finely sliced
- 4 fresh bay leaves
- a handful of fresh curry leaves
- 2 level tablespoons Colman's mustard powder
- 2 heaped tablespoons plain flour
- 1 x 200ml bottle of white wine vinegar
- 4 tablespoons caster sugar
- 2 apples, stalks removed
- 2 ripe mangoes

Prep all of your vegetables as I've indicated in the ingredients list, then put them into a large bowl with the sea salt and enough cold water to cover. Leave in a cool place to soak for 1 or 2 hours. Meanwhile, put a large deep saucepan that will be able to hold all the vegetables over a medium heat. Add the oil, mustard seeds, cumin, turmeric and oregano, and stir and cook for a few minutes, until everything starts to smell fantastic. Grate in all the nutmeg, then add the sliced garlic and tear in the bay and curry leaves. Add the mustard powder and the flour, then pour in the entire bottle of vinegar and stir in the sugar. Keep cooking and stirring.

While your sauce bubbles away, grate the apples, core and all, on the coarse side of a box grater. Add them to the pan and stir them in, then halve and stone your mangoes and dice up the flesh. Discard the skin, then slowly stir the mangoes into the mixture.

At this point, drain your bowl of soaked veg really well and add them to the pan. Gently fold them in so they pick up all of the wonderful flavours, but only cook them for around 7 to 10 minutes – no more! That way, the vegetables will still have some nice crunch to them when you eat the piccalilli later. Have a quick taste, and make sure it's well seasoned. Don't be afraid to up the chilli factor if need be; it should have quite a bit of 'oomph'. Once you're happy, divide your piccalilli between your sterilized jars and close the lids tightly. Store in a nice cool place, let it mellow for about 1 month before eating, and that's you sorted for the year!

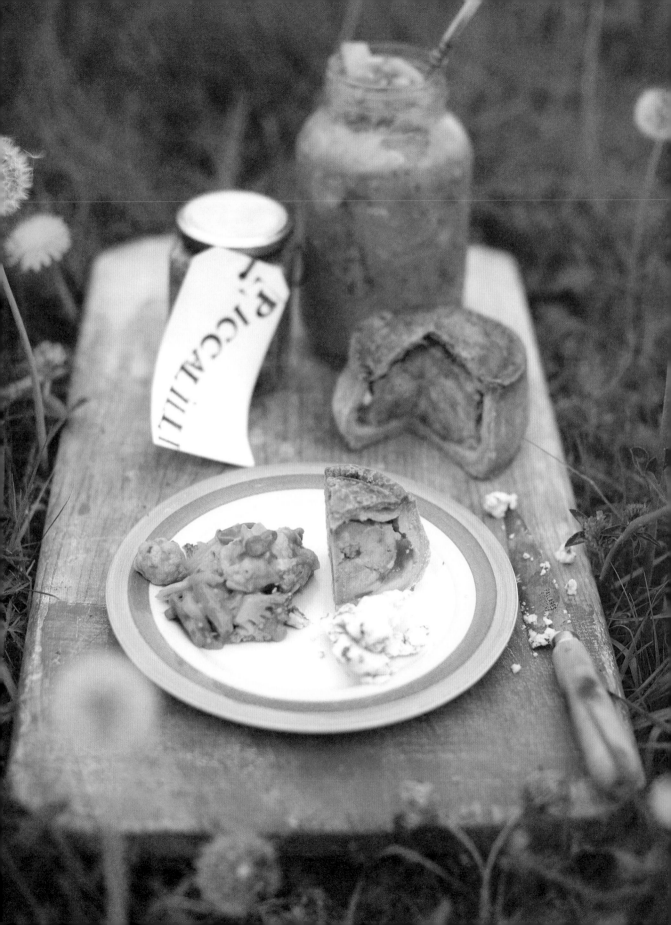

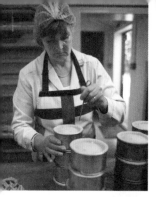

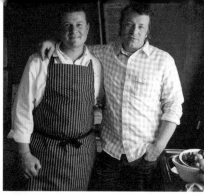

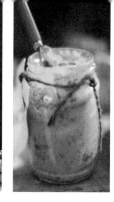

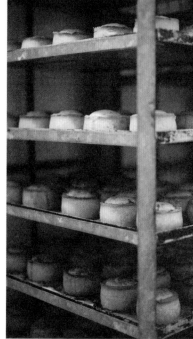

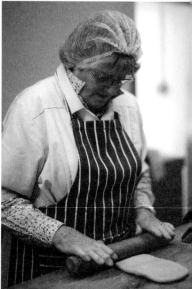

Melton Mowbray Pork Pies

It was an absolute pleasure to meet the guys from F. Bailey & Son butchers in the village of Melton Mowbray in Leicestershire. Their small team make these phenomenal pork pies every day, and have done for a long, long time. It's so nice to see Scott, who is a fourth-generation butcher, still championing local meat. They've got their own abattoir on site and pie-making facilities next door. Now that is old school.

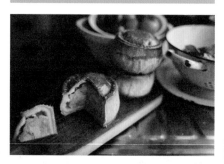

AWARD WINNING PIES

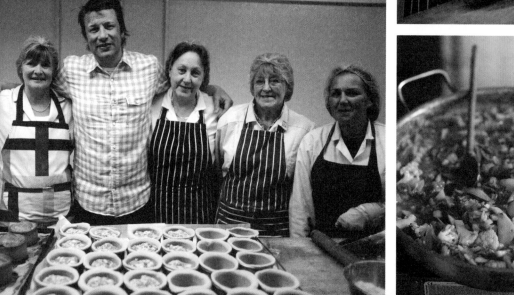

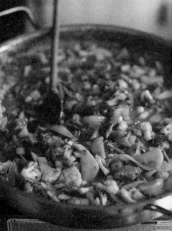

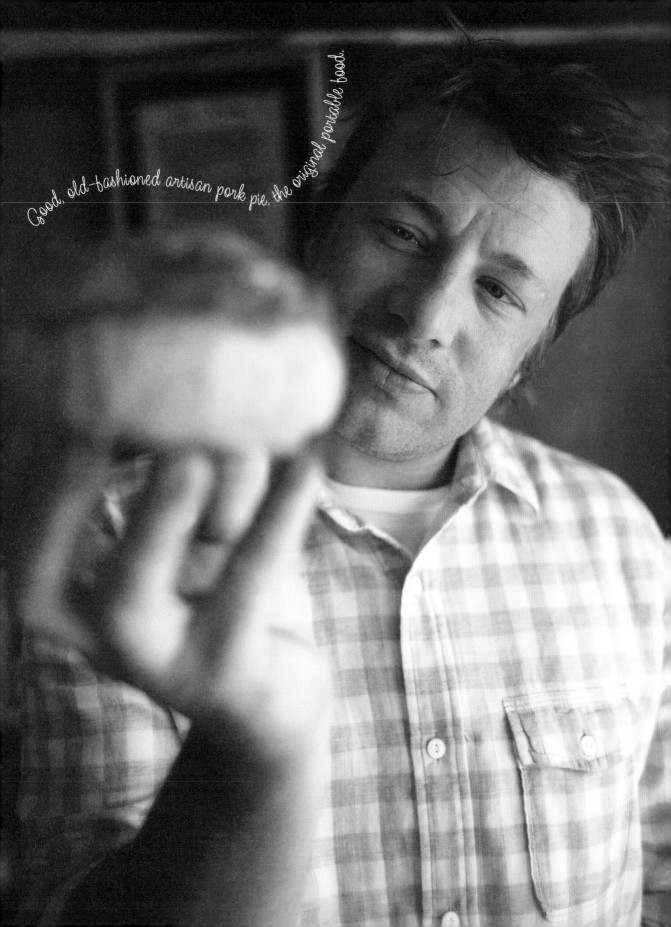

Good, old-fashioned artisan pork pie, the original portable food.

SUNDAY LUNCH SAUCES

No Sunday spread is complete without great condiments and sauces. These four are the great classics of a British table, and I absolutely love them. Of course you can buy them in a supermarket, but honestly they are so easy and quick to make that whipping one or two of these up while your meat roasts in the oven should be no trouble at all. Best of all, you'll be able to get them exactly to your taste. These each make enough for eight people, give them a try.

Orchard Apple Sauce

Wash and quarter 2 **Bramley apples** (roughly 600g). You can also use pears, quinces, or a mixture of all three fruits. Get rid of the cores, then chop the fruit into 1cm dice and put into a pan with 3 heaped tablespoons of **caster sugar**, a few gratings of **nutmeg** and the juice of half a **lemon**. Gently stew the apples until you get the consistency you like, whether that's a purée or a mix of smooth and chunky. Have a taste, and balance with sugar if needed, but keep in mind that you don't want it as sweet as a crumble filling. The acidity from the apples should be able to cut through rich meat like roasted pork. This is also lovely with cold ham or cheese.

Cranberry Sauce

Put 4 heaped tablespoons of **caster sugar** into a pan with the juice of 1 **orange**, 2 **fresh bay leaves**, 2 **cloves** and a couple of pinches of **ground ginger**. Bring to the boil, then turn down to a simmer and add 350g of **frozen cranberries**. Stir well, then cook over a low heat for about 10 minutes, topping up with a little water if you feel it needs it. When the cranberries are soft and tender, remove the cloves and bay leaves with a slotted spoon, have a taste and add a little bit more sugar if need be (though this sauce shouldn't be too sweet - the acid still needs to cut through). Feel free to mash up some of the cranberries for a combination of smooth and chunky, or pop it into a liquidizer and whiz to a purée. Serve with turkey, chicken or cold cuts.

Fresh Mint Sauce

Wash a bunch of **fresh mint**, then gently pat and squeeze it dry in a tea towel. Pick the leaves, roll them into a ball and finely chop them. Once they're nice and fine, put them into a bowl with a couple of good pinches of **sea salt** and a couple of teaspoons of **caster sugar** and just cover with boiling water. Stir in 4 tablespoons of **white wine vinegar** and mix really well. Adjust to taste with a little sugar if needed, and serve with roast lamb, or any other rich meat.

Classic Bread Sauce

Peel and finely slice 1 small **onion**. Put it into a pan with a knob of **butter**, 1 **fresh bay leaf** and 2 **cloves**, and cook slowly for 10 minutes to soften. Add 300ml of **milk** and tear in 2 thick slices of **good-quality white bread**, crusts removed. Simmer for another 10 minutes, then remove the bay leaf and cloves with a slotted spoon. Season to taste with 1 tablespoon of **English mustard** and a pinch of **sea salt** and **ground pepper**. Add a splash of milk to loosen the sauce if needed. Simmer and stir until you get the consistency you like. The more you stir it, the less texture you'll have, and the more you cook it down, the richer and thicker it will be. I love this with roasted chicken, and of course with the turkey on Christmas Day.

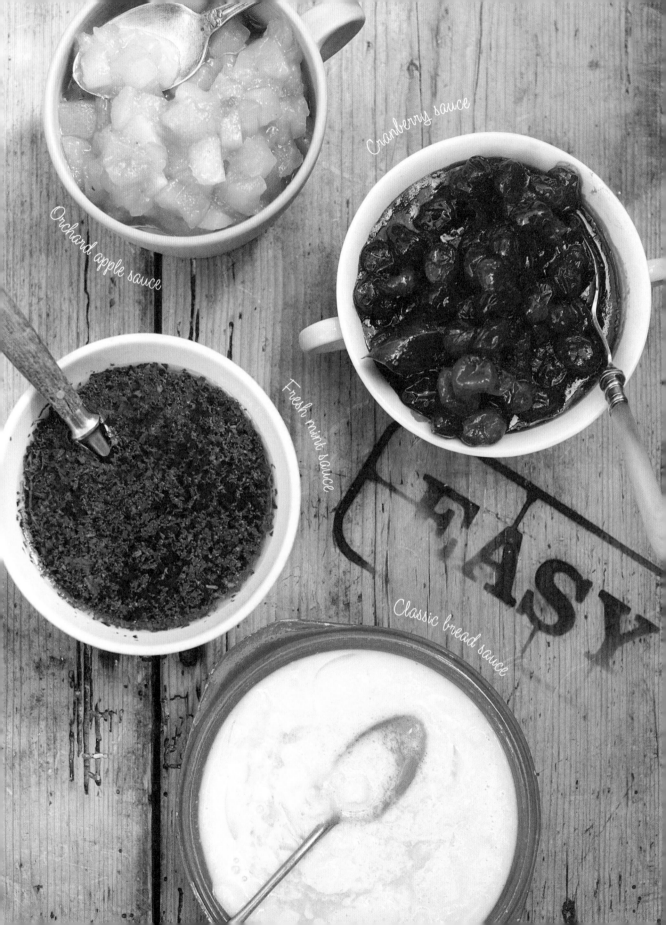

Orchard apple sauce

Cranberry sauce

Fresh mint sauce

Classic bread sauce

SPEEDY PRESERVED CHILLI SLICES

This is a great chilli pickle that will last you about a year and make all sorts of food, from rice dishes, to fish, to salads, sauces, sandwiches and cheeseboards, so much more exciting. Sometimes I'll even nick a splash or two of the salty vinegar from the pickle jar and use it to brighten up stews or curries. Ultimately, when chillies are really good and abundant, your job is to grab a load of them at their best and suspend them for up to a year in salty sweet vinegar so that they're ready and waiting for you whenever you get the urge. This is dead simple. Get yourself 500g of **fresh chillies** – you can mix them or make little batches of different varieties and colours if you like to highlight their unique flavours – you'll be amazed how different they can taste. Remove the green stalks (you can also remove the seeds if you want this to be much milder), then run them through the finest blade on your food processor. Pack an airtight 1 litre Kilner jar as full as you can with the sliced chillies (try not to touch them with your fingers or you could end up with burning body parts later – use a spoon). Add 3 heaped teaspoons each of **caster sugar** and **sea salt**, and a bunch of **fresh mint** if you like, cover with 500ml of your chosen **vinegar** so that all the chillies are covered and sealed, then put the lid on. Give the jar a good shake for a minute to dissolve the salt and sugar then put the jar in a cool dry place. Use as and when you like – after 1 day it will be pickled and suspended at its best, waiting to be used up, so happy days.

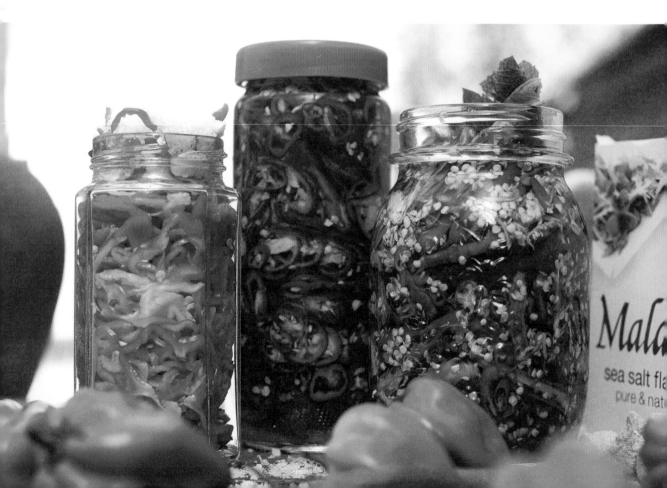

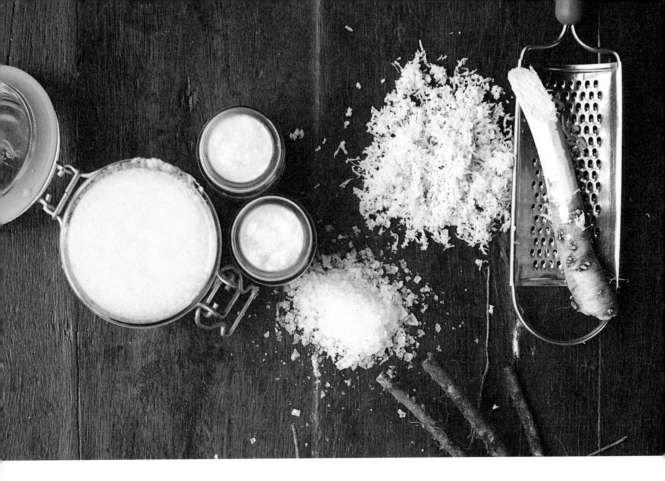

QUICK HORSERADISH SAUCE

I love making my own horseradish, and this recipe only takes about three minutes to make: just peel, buzz, stir and you're done. It makes loads, but divide it between a bunch of little jars and you'll be sorted for the year. I like to add a little to crème fraîche and spread it in sandwiches or burgers, or dollop some next to cold cuts on a platter. Just a spoonful stirred through a dark lamb or beef stew is also heavenly. These quantities will give you 500ml, or enough for 6 good-sized jars. To make the horseradish last a really long time, sterilize the jars before you fill them with the sauce. Check out *www.jamieoliver.com/how-to* to see how it's done. Peel 350g **fresh horseradish** and whack it through the finest grating attachment you have for your food processor. Put it into a bowl with 20g **sea salt**, 250ml **white wine vinegar** and 250ml **water** and mix well. Have a taste – it will be really hot, salty and vinegary too, but that's exactly what you want. Divide evenly between your jars, topping right up with a little more vinegar if you're short on liquid. Now you've got the concentrated stuff. To use this great condiment up you can mix it with yoghurt, mayo or cream to make the most outrageous sauces or dressings for sandwiches, steaks, roast beef dinners, salads or smoked fish.

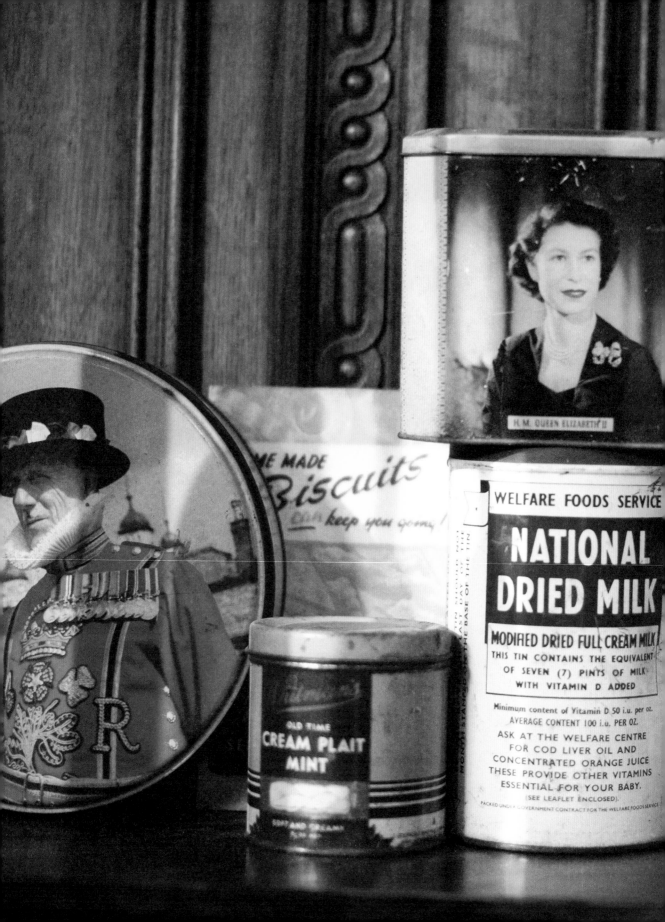

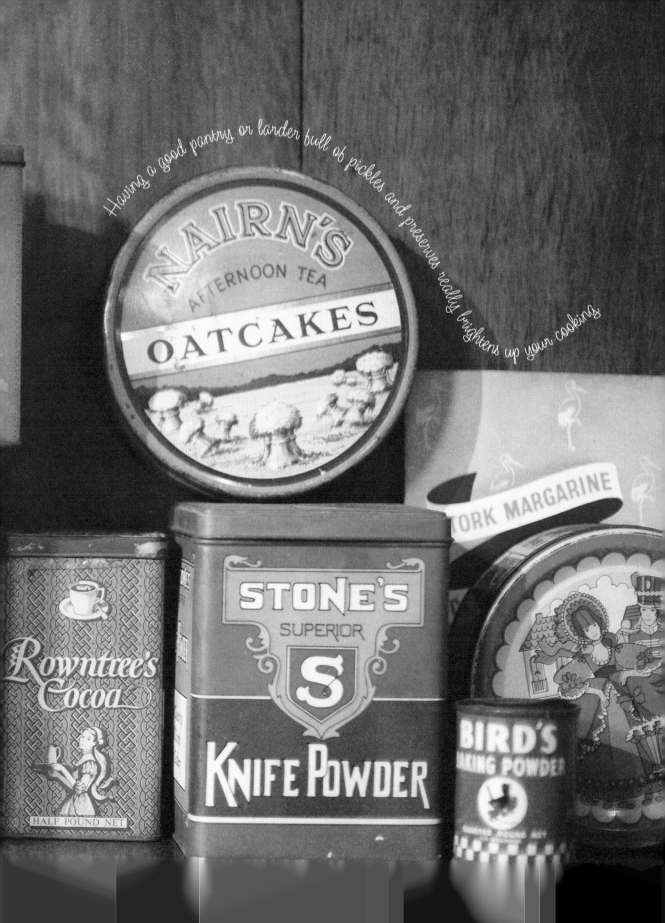

Having a good pantry or larder full of pickles and preserves really brightens up your cooking

MARVELLOUS MUSTARDS

Making mustard will open up a world of possibilities to you. I get excited just thinking about the endless varieties I could try. Some of these mustards will benefit from sitting in the fridge for a couple of days so that the flavours can soften and ripen. Feel free to halve the quantities, but to me, it makes sense to make mustard once a year, to do it well, and then you don't have to think about it. Go to *www.jamieoliver.com/how-to* to see how to sterilize the jars for your mustards.

Beer and Honey Wholegrain Mustard – Makes 3 Standard Jam Jars

You're going to use a standard jam jar to measure everything out here – so stay with me. Put a jarful of **black mustard seeds** and one of **yellow mustard seeds** into a large bowl. Pour in a jar-and-a-half's worth of nice **local smooth ale** and 1 heaped teaspoon each of **dried tarragon** and **dried dill**. Stir it around, cover and leave to sit overnight. The next day, drain the seeds over a bowl, so you can save the beer. Tip the seeds into a liquidizer with 3 tablespoons of **runny honey,** half a tablespoon of **sea salt** and half a jar's worth of **red wine vinegar**. Blitz a couple of times if you like it chunky, a bit more if you prefer it smooth, or go half and half for a bit of contrast. Add some of the reserved beer if needed to help it along, until you get the consistency you're looking for. When you're happy, have a final taste and adjust the saltiness if needed. Divide it between your three jars, pop the lids on and put them into the fridge.

A Quick English Mustard, in Seconds – Makes 1 Standard Jam Jar

It's so easy to make this using **Colman's English mustard powder**, so I say just make a small batch up as and when you need it. Simply put 2 tablespoons of **good-quality red** or **white wine vinegar** and 4 tablespoons of **water** into a bowl, stir in 6 tablespoons of **runny honey** and a good couple of pinches of **sea salt**, then stir in the mustard powder until you get the consistency you like. Season to taste, and serve.

Essex Mustard – Makes 3 Standard Jam Jars

Peel and finely chop 1 **onion**, then peel and finely slice 8 cloves of **garlic**. Put them into a pan with 250ml each of **water** and **cider vinegar**, 12 **peppercorns**, 2 teaspoons of **runny honey,** 4 level teaspoons of **sea salt**, a few **fresh bay leaves** and any **fresh chives**, **tarragon** or **parsley** you've got available. Bring to the boil, then reduce the heat and simmer for 10 minutes. Pour through a sieve into a bowl and whisk in enough **Colman's mustard powder** to thicken it to your liking (roughly 5 x 57g tubs). Have a taste and correct the seasoning with salt, if needed. Place in an airtight jar – this is best enjoyed after it's sat for a day or two in the fridge.

Black Mustard – Makes 3 Standard Jam Jars

Put two 300ml jars' worth of **black mustard seeds** into a liquidizer and blend until you get a nice fine powder (you may need to do this in batches). Rock the liquidizer jug back and forward a bit to make sure all the seeds get to the blade. Simmer 3 handfuls of **raisins** and half a jar's worth of **balsamic vinegar** slowly in a small pan until soft. Tip the raisins and vinegar into the liquidizer and blitz. Add half a jar of **water**, 10 tablespoons of **Worcestershire sauce,** 1 heaped tablespoon of **runny honey** and a couple of level teaspoons of **sea salt**. Liquidize for a minute or so, adding a little more water if needed to help it along. When you've got a good loose mustard consistency, divide it between your jars, pop the lids on and put them into the fridge. VERY IMPORTANT INFO: at this point, the mustard won't taste very nice. But give it a few days and it will develop into an undeniably unique and robust mustard that you will love.

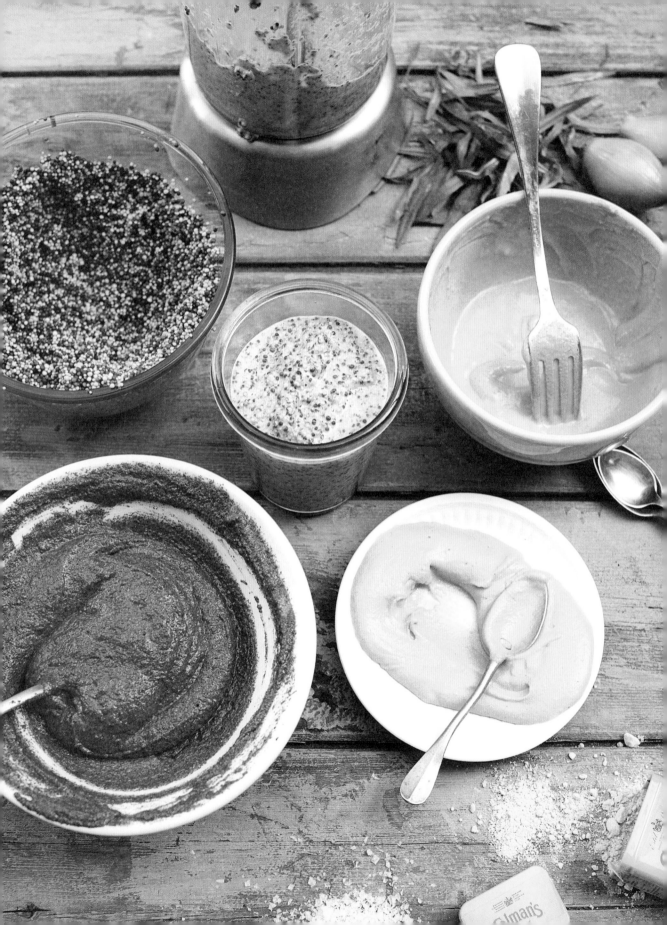

GLORIOUS FLAVOURED VINEGARS

Learning the oh-so-simple (and incredibly cheap!) art of flavouring a vinegar – whatever the variety – is such an important but underrated weapon in your cooking arsenal. So many of the products that we love – pickles, ketchups, sauces, salsas – have either a splash or an abundance of vinegar in them. However, most of them use low-quality, cheap or generic vinegar. If you spend an extra couple of pounds on really nice vinegar and add flavours to it, you'll be doing yourself a massive favour in the long run.

These ideas are quick, fun, they look good and you'll end up with bottles of really diverse acids on your shelf. You'll get to know them all, like characters in a movie, and I promise, before long you'll start to instinctively know which bottles to use for which jobs. Get into this, and you'll be adding a unique edge to your cooking that you just can't buy. For brightness and freshness, it's best to use them up within a year. The flavours will still be delicious at that point, but they will be less vivacious.

GENERAL METHOD: Use any washed bottle or airtight container with a cap, add your choice of flavours (see below) to the vessel, then cover with your chosen vinegar (see above). That's it! I like to buy some of those clear airtight spritzer bottles from Boots and make up a shelf of different flavoured spritzers, then mist those incredible flavours over hot roast chicken and spuds as they come out of the oven.

Meadow Vinegar: Add delicate herbs or flowers like **tarragon**, **dill**, **fennel tops**, **dandelion flowers**, **lavender**, **rose petals**, **pansies**, **violas** and **elderflowers** to your bottle, steep in your chosen vinegar and leave to sit for a month.

Fresh Chilli Vinegar: Use a mixture of **Scotch bonnets** and **habaneros**, steep in your chosen vinegar and leave to infuse for a few weeks.

Dried Chilli Vinegar: Get a nice mixture of all sorts of **dried chillies**, ideally smoked ancho or little bird's-eye chillies for wonderful flavour, steep in the vinegar of your choice.

Bramble Vinegar: Get a few handfuls of any **soft seasonal fruit** such as raspberries, strawberries, blackcurrants or blackberries, place them in a bottle either in a mixture or singly, steep in your chosen vinegar, and leave to infuse for about a month.

Victorian Spiced Vinegar: In a hot pan toast a few pinches of **ground cinnamon**, **five-spice powder**, **ground allspice**, **mustard seeds**, some **black and white peppercorns** and some **orange** and **lemon peel**. Leave to cool, add to the bottle and steep in your chosen vinegar.

Honeycomb Vinegar: When you've used most of the honey from a jar of **honeycomb**, simply top up the jar with vinegar and use after a few weeks.

Apricot Vinegar: Whenever you're eating an **apricot** or **peach**, crack the stone to release the inner nut, place in a bottle with 2 **dried apricots**, cover with vinegar and steep for a month.

Citrus Leaf Vinegar: If you happen to have any **citrus leaves** on your lemons, limes or oranges, twist and roll them up, put them into a bottle, steep in vinegar and leave to infuse.

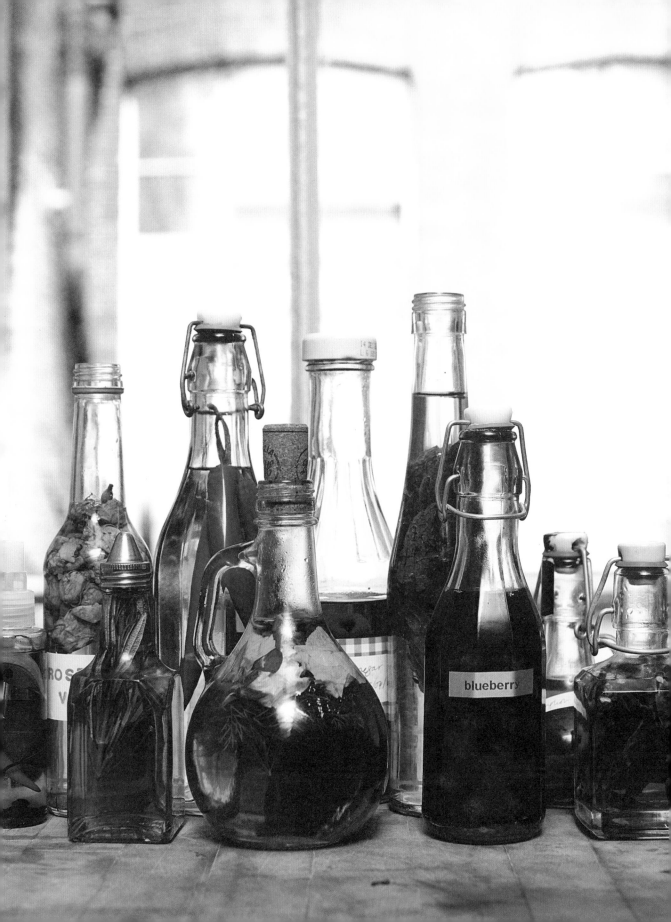

HOMEMADE MAYONNAISE

MAKES 500ml

Plain Mayonnaise

Whisk 2 large free-range **egg yolks** and 1 teaspoon of **Dijon mustard** gently in a large mixing bowl, adding 500ml of **mild olive oil** very, very slowly – almost a drizzle at a time (you don't want the mixture to split). As it starts to thicken, loosen and flavour with roughly 25ml of **white wine vinegar** and a squeeze of the juice of 1 **lemon** (to taste), again a splash at a time throughout the emulsification process. When the oil and vinegar are all whisked in, season to taste with **sea salt**, **freshly ground black pepper**, **lemon** or **vinegar**. Trust your taste buds. Now check out the flavours below to add some excitement.

Marie Rose Sauce

Stir 4 chopped **anchovy fillets**, 2 chopped **cornichons** and 2 heaped tablespoons of **capers** (drained) into 500ml of **mayonnaise**. Add 2 heaped tablespoons of **ketchup**, 1 tablespoon of **brandy**, a few squeezes of **lemon juice** and a pinch of **cayenne pepper**. Season and adjust.

Basil Mayonnaise

Liquidize the leaves from a **bunch of fresh basil** with 4 **anchovies** and half a peeled garlic **clove**. Add a good squeeze of **lemon juice** and a lug of **extra virgin olive oil** until you've got a smooth vivid green liquid. Add this flavoured olive oil to 500ml of **mayonnaise**, season and adjust.

Tartare Sauce

Finely chop 3 **cornichons**, 3 heaped teaspoons of **capers** (drained), 2 **spring onions**, 2 **anchovy fillets** and the leaves from a **small bunch of fresh parsley** (chervil or yellow celery leaves are also great). Add all your chopped ingredients to 500ml of **mayonnaise** then grate in the zest of half a **lemon** and squeeze in the juice. Stir then taste, season and adjust if need be.

Curried Mayonnaise

Finely grate a thumb-sized piece of **fresh ginger** into 500ml of **mayonnaise**, along with 2 heaped teaspoons of **Patak's madras curry paste** and the juice of half a **lemon** (to taste). Season, if necessary, then allow to sit for 15 minutes.

Triple Mustard Mayonnaise

This is simple: Stir in a teaspoon each of **wholegrain**, **English** and **French mustard** into 500ml of **mayonnaise**.

Roasted Garlicky Mayonnaise

Break up a whole bulb of **garlic**, toss it in **olive oil**, then roast it in the oven at 140°C/275°F/gas 1 for 45 minutes. Take it out, and when it's cool enough to handle, squeeze all the garlic flesh out of the skin then mash it up with a fork and stir it through 500ml of **mayonnaise**. Add a good squeeze of **lemon juice**, to taste and season if you think it needs it.

Saffron Mayonnaise

Pop a nice big pinch of **saffron** in a small bowl with a swig of boiling water and squeeze in the juice of half a **lemon**. Leave to sit for a few minutes, then pour every last bit into the **mayonnaise** and add over half a teaspoon of finely grated **fresh red chilli**. Mix well, then have a taste and season if necessary. Leave to sit in the fridge for around 30 minutes before serving.

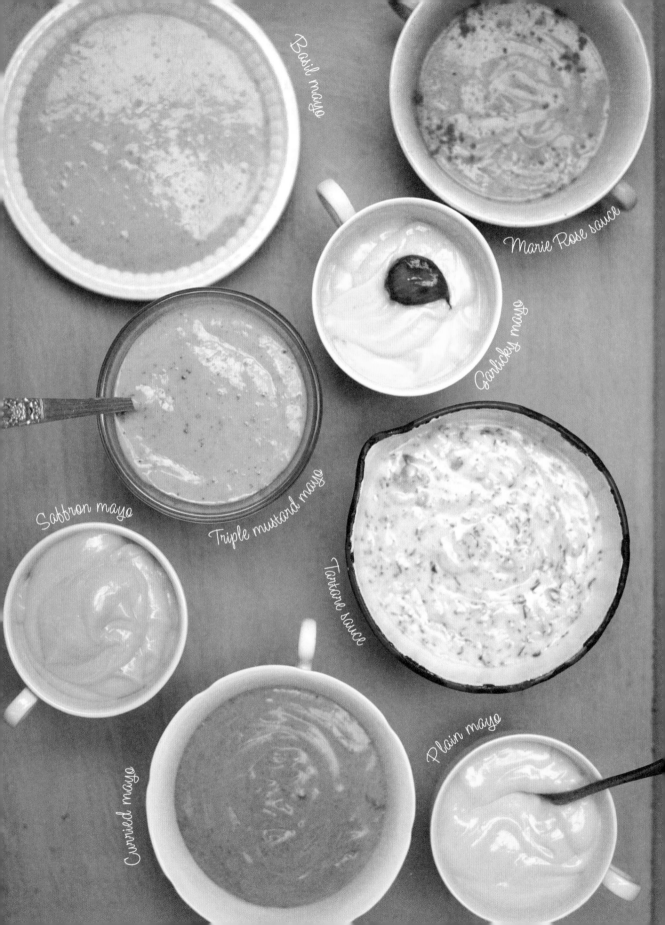

Basil mayo

Marie Rose sauce

Garlicky mayo

Saffron mayo

Triple mustard mayo

Tartare sauce

Curried mayo

Plain mayo

FLAVOURED GIN & VODKA

Adding just a few beautiful things to a humble bottle of alcohol turns it into a sumptuous snapshot of a particular time of year. It's like painting in colour, rather than in black and white. Whatever you drop into the bottle, be it blackberries, blueberries, wild strawberries, sour cherries, wild plums, damsons or sloes, I want you to have the confidence and creativity to complement those delicious juicy fruits with accents of herbs and other flavours. There is an abundance to choose from: fragrant lemon thyme, the crushed-up tutti-frutti flavour of fresh bay leaves, a strip or two of lemon or orange peel, a couple of toasted cloves or a split vanilla pod plopped in the bottom of the bottle … if you think it will taste delicious, it probably will. The sentiment of these drinks is definitely similar to that of the vinegar recipes on page 388. And like vinegar, alcohol is capable of freeze-framing stuff at its ripest, most perfect stage, so that even a year after these lovely fruits have been picked, they're still looking beautiful, and sharing flavour with the alcohol. All you have to do is track down summer or autumn fruit at its best, then pick it, wash it, stuff it into the bottle and pop it into the freezer. This allows the perfumes, colours and flavours of the fruit to burst through the skin. If you don't want to freeze it, you can always cheat by pricking each fruit with a little pin, or the tip of a knife. So if you're lucky enough to pass a bush weighed down with berries you recognize and know are safe, pick the fruit, taste it, and if it's really sour you'll know you need to add a teaspoon or two of sugar when you add it to the alcohol. Place the fruit in a bottle of gin or vodka (you'll need to pour some out first to make room), then pop the cap on and leave to infuse. Give it a swirl round every now and then, and have a little taste every month to see how it's going. Give it a few months, and you'll have a delicious new drink to pull out. **PS:** A splash of flavoured gin or vodka added to a rich meat gravy as it's cooking down, or even drizzled over a steak during the last 30 seconds of cooking with a knob of butter … so delicious.

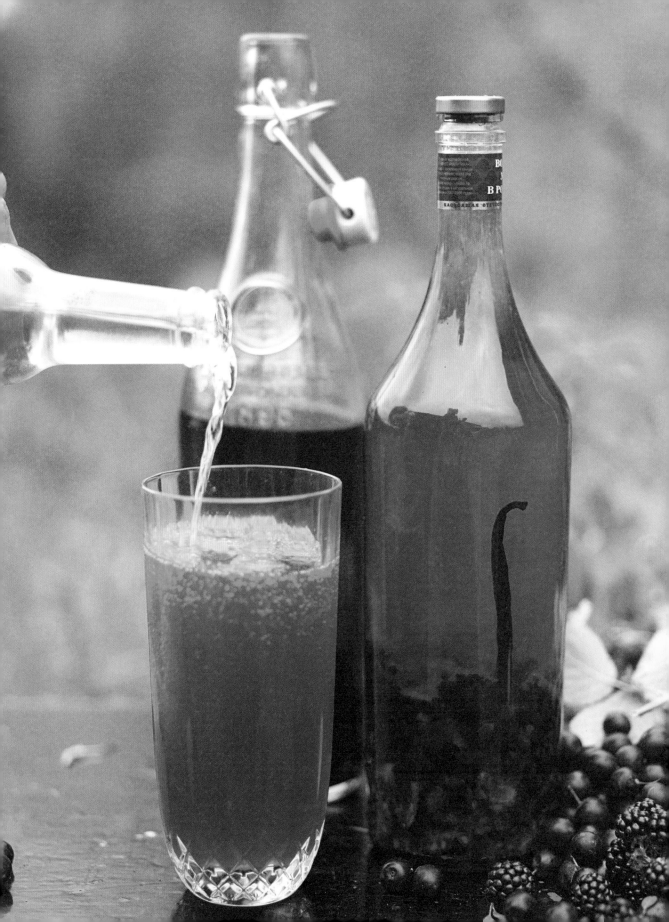

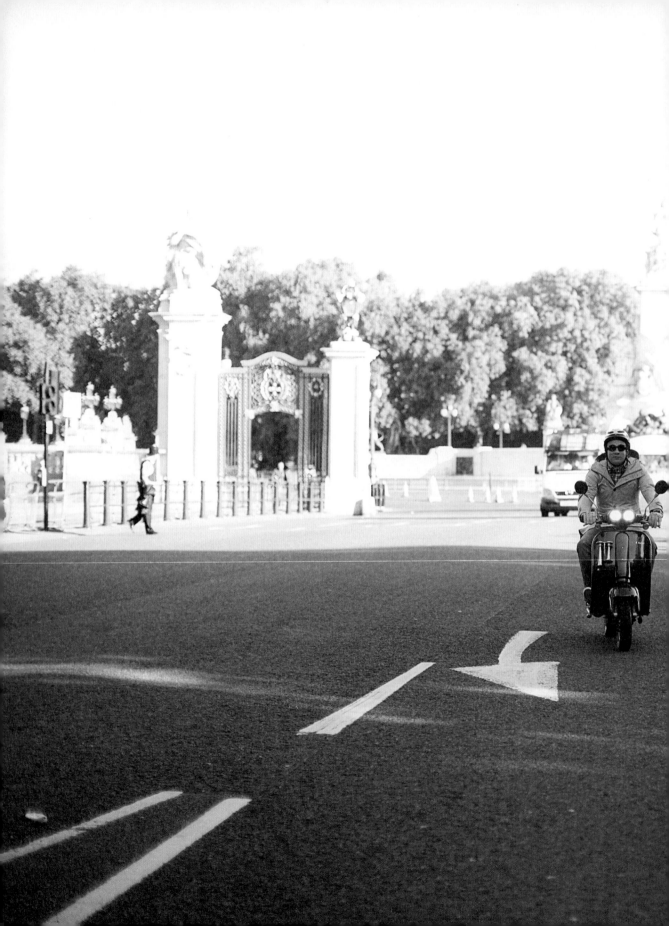

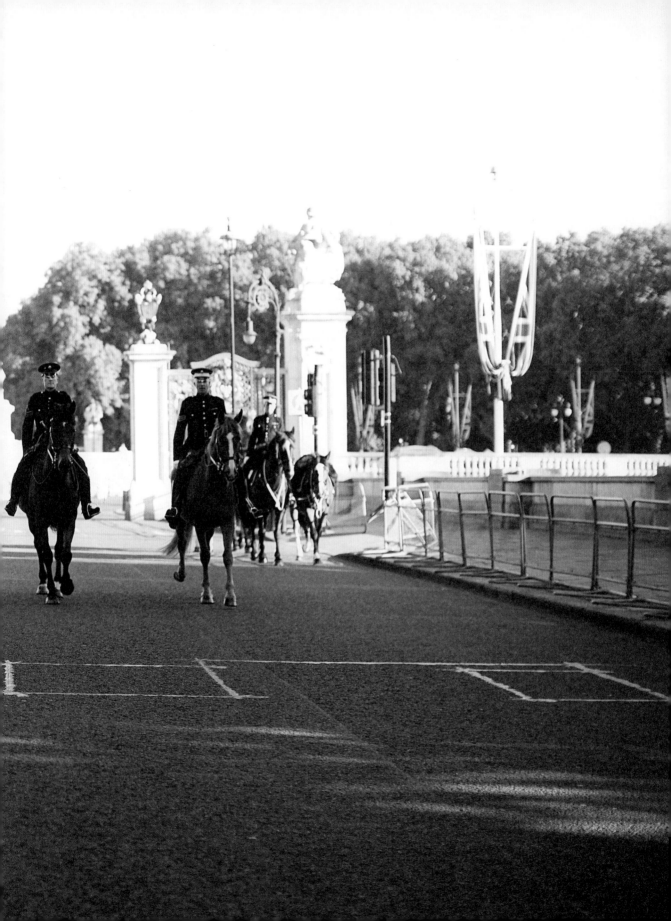

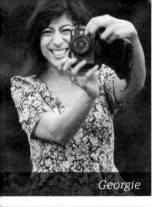
Georgie

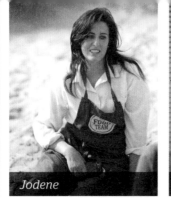
Jodene

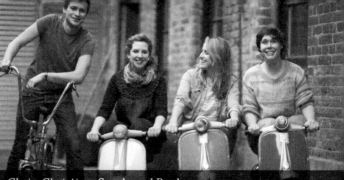
Chris, Christina, Sarah and Becky

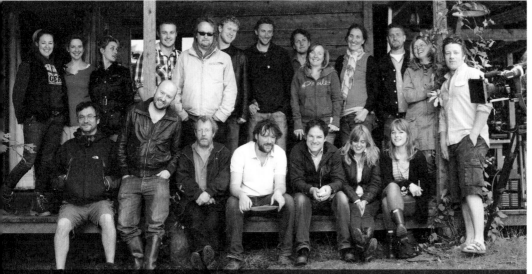
My lovely TV crew

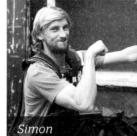
Simon

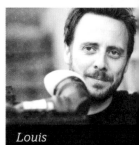
Louis

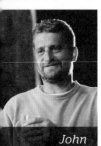
John

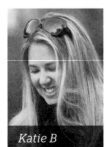
Katie B

Mike M

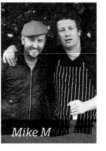
Richard the 1st

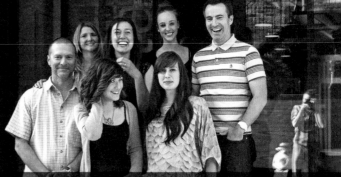
The Interstate team: Brian, Jayne, Lucy, Jessica, James, Christina, Louise and Ben (in the window!)

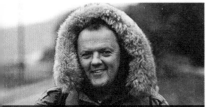
'Lord' Loftus
(Ancestor of Admiral Nelson)

Mike S

Pamela, Ginny, Luke, Dave and Freddie

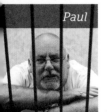
Paul

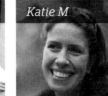
Katie M

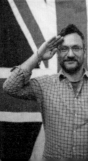

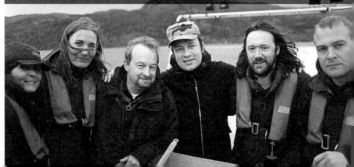

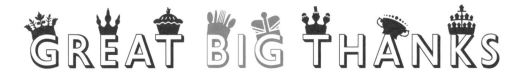

GREAT BIG THANKS

This book is my opportunity to celebrate my own country, and I wouldn't be here without the love and support I get at home. To my beautiful and understanding wife Jools, my gorgeous kids Poppy, Daisy, Petal and, finally, Buddy, my boy! Love and thanks to Mum and Dad for being the first people to teach me what great British food is all about. Thanks and love to 'Lord' David Loftus for being a great friend, great company on the road, and for taking such beautiful pictures. Massive love to my fabulous food and editorial teams. You guys keep me inspired and energized every day. Thank you for all your hard work on these shoots. To the 'divine' Ginny Rolfe, amazing ladies Sarah Tildesley, Georgie Socratous and Christina McCloskey. And of course Chris Gates, Phillippa Spence, Jodene Jordan and Becky Bax. Huge love and thanks to the stellar team at the office, Pete Begg, Claire Postans, Bobby Sebire, Joanne Lord, Helen Martin, Daniel Nowland, and of course the ladies who act as my nutritional conscience, Laura Parr and Mary Lynch. To Becca Hetherston and Abigail 'Scottish' Fawcett - thanks for your part in recipe testing. On words, big thanks to my editor, Katie Bosher, and to Rebecca 'Rubs' Walker and Bethan O'Connor for all their hard work. Shout out to my great friends at Penguin: thanks to my wonderful publisher, Tom Weldon, and art director John Hamilton for your friendship and for always reciprocating my enthusiasm. Thanks to the lovely Louise Moore and Lindsey Evans. Huge thanks to Nick Lowndes, Alistair Richardson, Juliette Butler, Janis Barbi, Laura Herring, Airelle Depreux, Clare Pollock, Claire Purcell, Chantal Noel, Kate Brotherhood, Elizabeth Smith, Anna Rafferty, Nathan Hull, Ashley Wilks, Naomi Fidler, Anna Derkacz and Thomas Chicken. Big thanks as well to my longtime copy-editor - the very lovely Annie Lee. Thanks also to Caroline Pretty, Lizzie Dipple, Pat Rush and Caroline Wilding for all their help. To the talented gang at Interstate Associates for all their hard work on designing another beautiful book with me: thank you - you've done it again. Big love to Jayne Connell and all her team, especially my 'Essex' girls Louise Draper and Lucy Self - before there was TOWIE, there was us! Big thanks as well to the lovely Christina Beani, Jessica Howard, Brian Simpson, James Jeanes and Ben Watts. Massive thanks to my CEO John Jackson, managing director Tara Donovan and manager Louise Holland for all they do (too much to put here!). And to my personal team for looking after me: Richard Herd, Holly Adams, Beth Richardson, Paul Rutherford and Saffron Greening. Thanks as well to my PR manager Mr Peter Berry and the lovely Eloise Bedwell on marketing. And to everyone at my office for their hard work and energy - lots of love. Love to my Fresh One TV gang - to Zoe Collins, Jo Ralling and Roy Ackerman and everyone who came on these trips with me: the brilliant Claire Wingate, Mike Matthews, Pamela Gordon, Claire Whalley - the very lovely Katie Millard, Sally Wingate, Amy Ruffell, Nicolanne Cox, Viki Kolar, Francesca Bassett, Alex Buxton, Rose Walton and Charlotte Sinden. To the cracking crew: Luke Cardiff, Mike Sarah (and his lovely son Joe), Dave Miller, Simon Weekes, Godfrey Kirby, Freddie Claire, Pete Bateson, James Vivian, Louis Caulfield, Mihalis Margaritis, Crispin Larratt, Steve Hudson, Jake Scott and Lee Meredith. You guys kept me laughing and worked really hard - so thank you. Shout out as well to Mark Manning at Directors Cut Films and all the energetic runners who've supported us on these trips: Ashley Day, Siggy Stone, Basil Khalil, Leona Ekembe and Katie Eaton. Special thanks as well to Kate Colquhoun, who helped us out loads with the historical details for TV and book. Again, big thanks to Paul, for looking after the pub, and to Zoot (aka Paul Flak) for his help. Massive respect and appreciation to Daryll Group and Mark Hedgecock from the Fullbridge Restoration Company (*www.fullbridgerestoration.co.uk*), and the rest of their team. Honestly, these guys are the business. What they can do with just about any vehicle is truly incredible. Finally, the biggest thanks of all goes to all the wonderful British people I met on my travels. You welcomed me, and my motley crew, into your homes, gardens, businesses and community centres to share your food and your stories. You've each reinforced my belief that we have so much to be proud of in this incredible country of ours. Big love, and thanks for everything you do and have done.

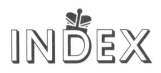

INDEX

- Page references for illustrations are in **bold**
- Recipes marked v are suitable for vegetarians

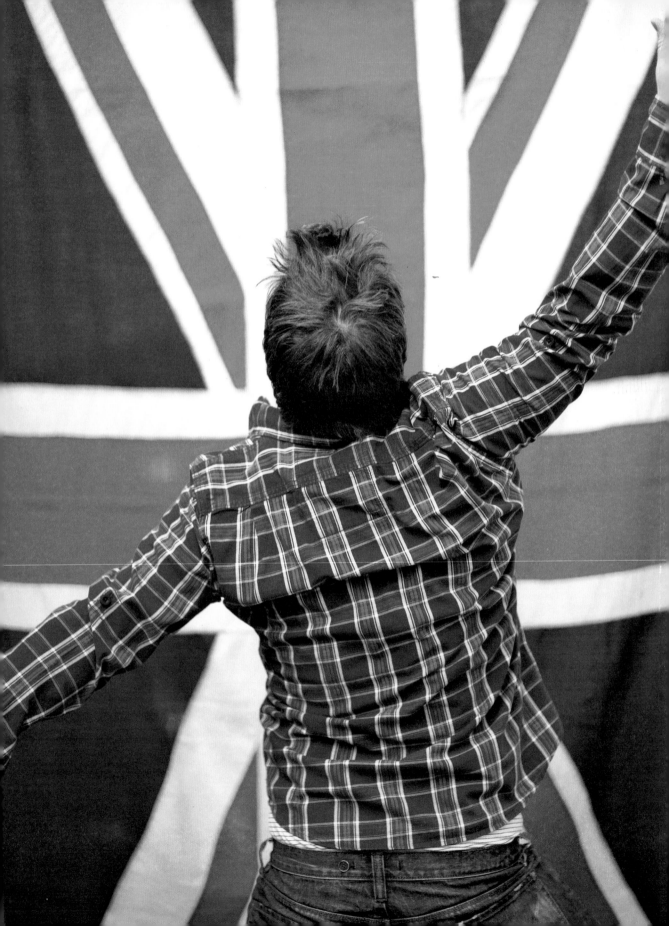

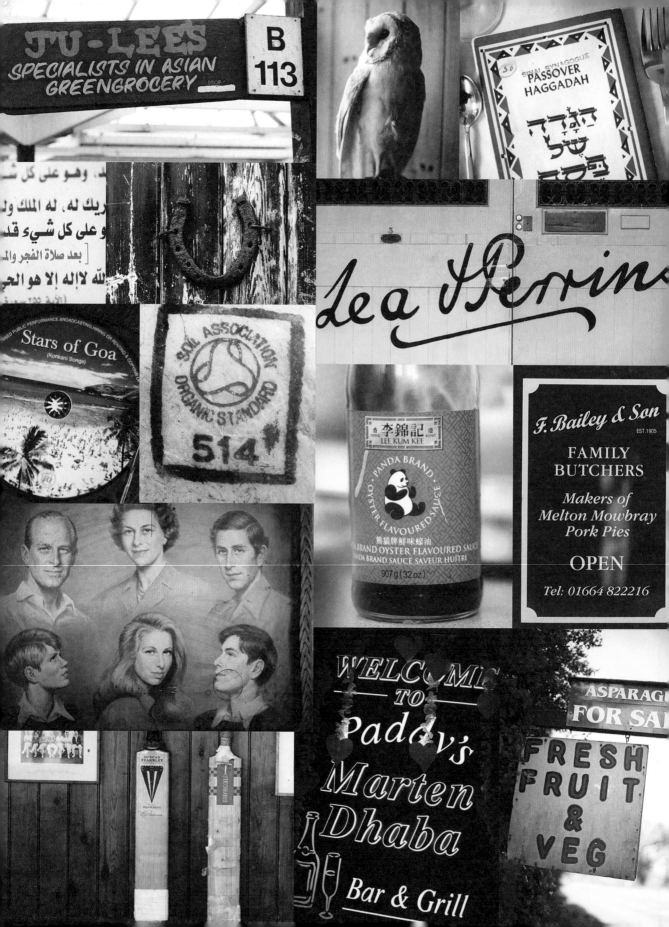